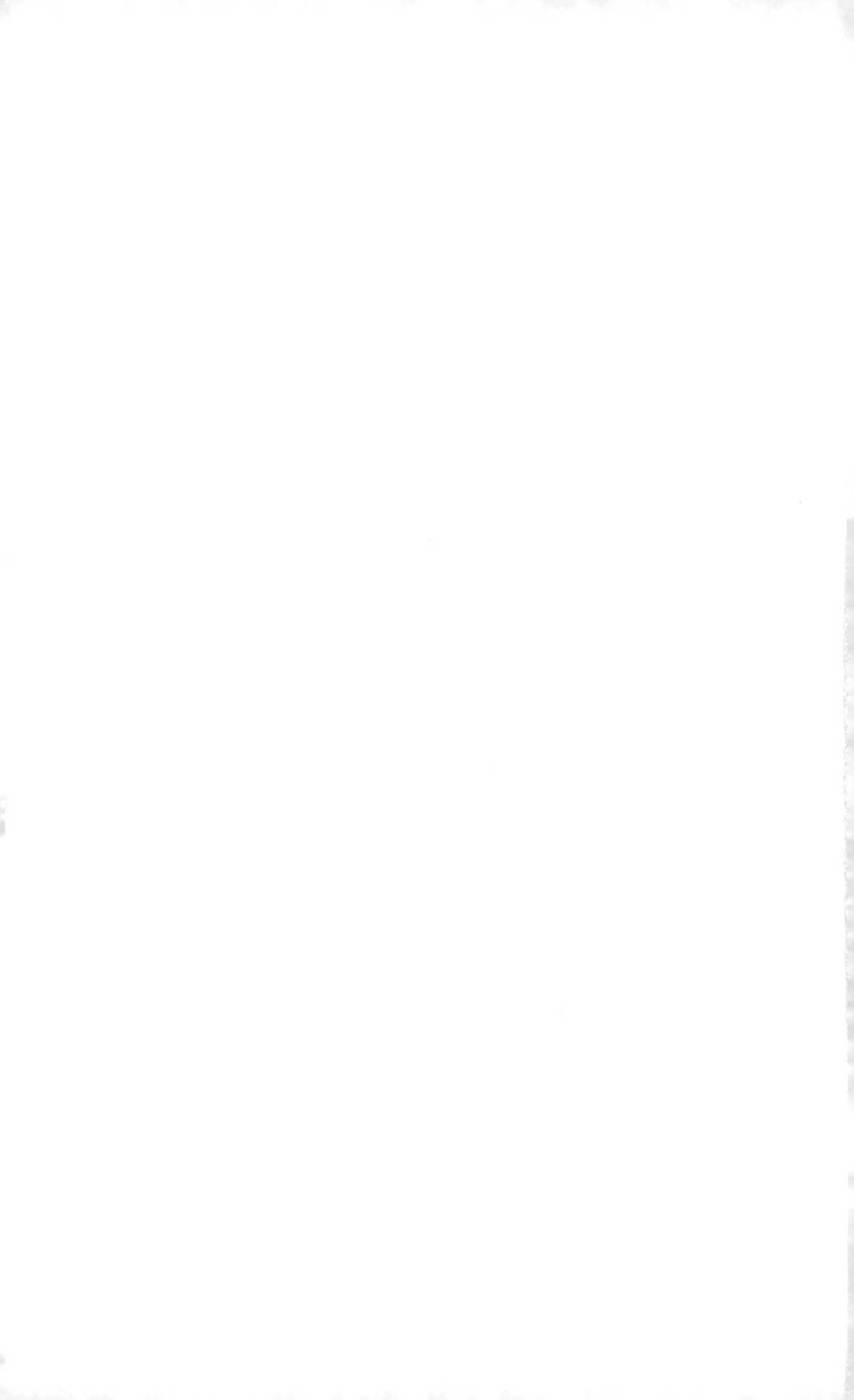

IBS

IBS

Finding and Treating the Root Cause of Irritable Bowel Syndrome

Izabella Wentz, PharmD

AVERY
an imprint of Penguin Random House
New York

AVERY

an imprint of Penguin Random House LLC
1745 Broadway, New York, NY 10019
penguinrandomhouse.com

Copyright © 2026 by Wentz LLC
Illustrations by Dave Kinzel
Illustration on page 456 by Tina Chan

Penguin Random House values and supports copyright. Copyright fuels creativity, encourages diverse voices, promotes free speech, and creates a vibrant culture. Thank you for buying an authorized edition of this book and for complying with copyright laws by not reproducing, scanning, or distributing any part of it in any form without permission. You are supporting writers and allowing Penguin Random House to continue to publish books for every reader. Please note that no part of this book may be used or reproduced in any manner for the purpose of training artificial intelligence technologies or systems.

Avery with colophon is a registered trademark of Penguin Random House LLC.

Most Avery books are available at a discount when purchased in quantity for sales promotions or corporate use. Special editions, which include personalized covers, excerpts, and corporate imprints, can be created when purchased in large quantities. For more information, please e-mail specialmarkets@penguinrandomhouse.com. Your local bookstore can also assist with discounted bulk purchases using the Penguin Random House corporate Business-to-Business program. For assistance in locating a participating retailer, e-mail B2B@penguinrandomhouse.com.

Book design by Ashley Tucker

ISBN 9780593420805
Ebook ISBN 9780593420812

Printed in the United States of America
1st Printing

The authorized representative in the EU for product safety and compliance is
Penguin Random House Ireland, Morrison Chambers, 32 Nassau Street, Dublin D02 YH68, Ireland, https://eu-contact.penguin.ie.

To my beloved Michael—your love makes the impossible possible, and I cherish every step of this life we walk together

CONTENTS

Introduction: My IBS Success Story and How to Create Your Own 1

PART I
Understanding IBS and the Root Cause Approach 19

Chapter 1
What Is Normal Digestive Function and What Is IBS? 21

Chapter 2
The Conventional Medical Approach to IBS 39

Chapter 3
What's Really Going On and How the Root Cause Approach Can Help 57

PART II
The Root Causes 81

Chapter 4
Dietary Triggers 83

Chapter 5
Digestion and Digestive Enzymes 139

Chapter 6
Depletions 173

Chapter 7
Deficiency of Beneficial Bacteria, Excess Pathogenic Bacteria 199

Chapter 8
Intestinal Permeability 231

Chapter 9
Intestinal Overgrowth 255

Chapter 10
Gut Infections 295

Chapter 11
Alterations in Stress Hormones 339

Chapter 12
Thyroid Hormones and Autoimmunity 359

Chapter 13
Inflammation and Inflammatory Bowel Disease (IBD) 387

Chapter 14
Toxins and Chemical Triggers 423

PART III
Creating Your Healing Plan 451

Chapter 15
Where to Start 453

Chapter 16
Symptom Solutions While You Heal 465

Author's Note 483
Acknowledgments 485
Index 489

INTRODUCTION

My IBS Success Story and How to Create Your Own

Why write a book focused on irritable bowel syndrome (IBS)? I have a lot of reasons, some of them simple, some a little more complex! Let's start with the simple . . .

The simple reason is because I was diagnosed with IBS in my early twenties, during my first year in pharmacy school. The year was 2002, and, unfortunately, I didn't get much help from modern medicine, despite being a student of it myself! I struggled with recurring bouts of painful cramping and explosive diarrhea until I eventually figured out how to resolve it, and I have spent the last decade helping others solve their digestive issues, too. I want to share what I learned with you so you don't have to suffer needlessly.

At the time of my own struggles with IBS, I thought (and was told) that my digestion was just overly sensitive and that my digestive symptoms were my "normal." I thought everyone's stomach hurt after eating and bloating was just a part of life. Many of my clients think the same, accepting painful bloating, bowel urgency, excessive flatulence, and

Introduction

inconsistent bowel patterns (i.e., frequent diarrhea or "going" every two weeks and/or a mix of both) as "just the way their bodies work."

Some may seek medical advice and only get Band-Aid approaches like over-the-counter or prescription medications that barely mask symptoms and even present with unpleasant side effects instead of solving the problem. Many people just learn to live with uncomfortable gastrointestinal symptoms without realizing there are real solutions. Does any of this sound familiar to you?

I remember like it was yesterday when my symptoms started. It was actually a school night, and I was in my first year of my doctor of pharmacy program (PharmD) and I decided to stay after class to study with classmates for a big pharmaceutics exam happening the next day. I usually studied at home by myself because some friends mostly goofed off instead of studying, but this day was different. I remember my professor seeing us as he left for the evening and nodding approvingly at his students studying so diligently.

Later, that evening, after the Chicago traffic died down, I drove home and delightfully made myself a microwaved feast of my favorite go-to dish—ramen noodles covered in soy sauce, à la graduate student—to refuel after my late-night studying session. I went to bed at around two a.m., feeling very confident about my ability to ace the exam, as I had studied long and hard.

But alas, my plans were foiled. I was awakened at around four a.m. with the worst kind of stomach cramping. I crawled out of bed and nearly doubled over in pain before I made my way to the bathroom and experienced a bout of explosive diarrhea. (I apologize for the TMI, but you *did* pick up a book about IBS.)

It was the first of many that night, and I was still running back and forth between the bathroom and my bed when it came time to leave for my exam.

I felt awful.

I was also in a panic, because I didn't know how I could possibly take my exam when I felt so weak, exhausted, and sick! My family doctor suggested I had food poisoning. He told me to stay hydrated and wrote me a note. I initially thought my digestive distress would be a onetime thing, but unfortunately, the symptoms kept coming back. And worst of all, they came back at the most random and inconvenient times.

- At my morning pharmaceutical calculations lecture, while I was avidly taking notes.
- During work at the pharmacy. Sometimes, I'd have to sprint to the bathroom while in the middle of a patient conversation.
- On a date.
- While out with friends enjoying a fun evening.
- In the middle of the night. I'd wake up with horrific cramps, and strangely, on days when I had to wake up very early, I would be overtaken by cramps and diarrhea soon after getting up.

As my symptoms persisted, I returned to my doctor. He wisely suggested stress; understandable, since I was in grad school. But while stress can be a relevant cause, I didn't receive a relevant solution to the stress or symptoms it was causing.

I got a diagnosis of IBS and a prescription for Levsin (hyoscyamine), a medication that works by blocking the effects of the neurotransmitter acetylcholine to slow down digestive secretions and gut motility.

At first, I was excited as it seemed to work . . . But unfortunately, I soon realized this old-school drug had many side effects. My diarrhea stopped, but rather than "normal" bowel function, I ended up with constipation. That would have been fine and perhaps even welcome, but it also slowed down *all* the other secretions in my body, including my saliva, leading to dry mouth, and my tears, leading to blurry vision. As pharmacy students, we used the acronym SLUD to remember the side effects of anticholinergic drugs: side effects related to S (salivation), L (lacrimation, tear production), U (urination), and D (defecation). Some of my more linguistically creative colleagues used the slogan: *"No sh*t, no spit, no see, no pee."*

Furthermore, it slowed down my brain function, making me dizzy, a bit clumsier, and a touch disoriented. Once, I used it right before a dinner out with friends, and it made the waiters at my favorite restaurant do a double take when I stumbled in and almost fell over. Acetylcholine supports learning, memory, and movement, so blocking it isn't ideal if you want a sharp mind and agile body. Long-term anticholinergic use has even been linked to cognitive decline.

Since I couldn't drive or focus in class with blurry vision and a disoriented brain, the medication was a no-go for me. Instead, I resolved to carry a sh*t kit around: Imodium AD tablets, Pepto-Bismol (the pink stuff), and baby wipes for unexpected bouts that were often painful and unresponsive to regular toilet paper. Also, an extra pair of underwear and pants, just in case.

I also wondered whether what I was eating had a potential impact on my symptoms. A part of me suspected the ramen and soy concoction may have had something to do with my digestive issues. After all, it was the last thing I ate before I got sick. Nutrition was not the focus of my studies, but I was taking microbiology and knew that dried goods were an unlikely source of food poisoning. So what could it be?

Cooking and eating real food was also not something that I was doing much of in graduate school. Most of the food I ate was fast food and/or came in a package. Some staple items I received at my school's "health fair" for free, including my go-to breakfast—a meal replacement shake. I eventually realized that my bouts of diarrhea often occurred during my first morning class, so I asked the pharmacist at my weekend job whether the shakes could be the culprit.

She noticed that the shakes were made with soy lecithin, a potential cause of food intolerance.

Because my IBS started right after my "college gourmet" meal of soy and ramen, this made a lot of sense to me. I decided to exclude soy from my diet and the diarrhea improved, but I still had occasional stomach pains and stomach cramps, especially if I didn't get enough sleep, which was happening five out of seven days each week. I was not out of the woods yet but didn't really know where to turn for help.

Before bloggers, social media gurus, and virtual consults, we were limited to getting help from people within our own circles and communities. In my culture (I grew up in Poland), getting advice from psychics was commonplace, so I was delighted when my friends and I came across a psychic, curiously at the mall, while on a trip to Las Vegas the following year. The psychic told me two very useful pieces of advice:

1. Break up with my boyfriend.
2. If I stopped eating red meat, my stomach problems would improve.

I had already been thinking about breaking up with said boyfriend but hadn't mentioned it to anyone, so I was intrigued. "This man knows things about me," I thought to myself, so in addition to breaking up with that boyfriend, I also decided to give up red meat to see if the Vegas psychic was as good of a medical intuitive as he was a life coach.

It turns out he was right about both things. I met my future husband within six months of the breakup. And I saw further improvement in my digestion by eliminating red meat. I only wish the psychic had given me lottery numbers as well . . . but I digress.

Getting off soy and red meat kept me from having explosive diarrhea (I was grateful for that), but my digestion was still off. I often had

Introduction

stomachaches, was constantly bloated, and would have daily loose stools. As time went on, I began to feel more and more unwell. I was fatigued most days, and then I began to experience memory loss, anxiety, and panic attacks . . .

After that, I started getting a strange chronic cough that would wake me up at night. I was diagnosed with acid reflux and was taking multiple medications to keep it at bay. If that wasn't enough, I started dealing with environmental allergies, seemingly becoming more sensitive to everything in my life.

Working, living, and enjoying life as a normal twentysomething was a struggle. I had such a hard time waking up in the mornings and struggled with anxiety and fatigue during my workdays. I would have coughing fits during work presentations and often had to excuse myself from meetings to make a beeline for my second office, the bathroom.

Vacations were not much better. On a trip to visit family in Europe with my new husband, I struggled with hives and nonstop diarrhea for almost two weeks straight! The worst was when I went to visit my great-aunt in rural Poland who only had an outhouse and not an in-home bathroom. I ran out of her house but didn't make it all the way to the outhouse across the property and had to squat ASAP. My husband recalls that I was in my pretty dress talking to my great-aunt, when I suddenly ran out of the home crying. He found me squatting in a random patch of grass next to the barn.

Upon my return, I started to have even more symptoms and felt like my life and body were falling apart. I felt like an old woman because my joint pain and carpal tunnel syndrome prevented me from my two favorite hobbies: yoga and writing. And to top it all off, I began to lose my hair. As a Leo, losing my beautiful lion's mane was too much and was the impetus to taking charge of my health.

By this time, I was already a practicing pharmacist and realized that not all practitioners were created equal. I decided to seek out more opinions. After seeing an urgent care doctor, a primary care doctor, a gastroenterologist, an allergist, a cardiologist, a dermatologist, and an endocrinologist, I was eventually diagnosed with Hashimoto's thyroiditis, an autoimmune thyroid condition.

....

My life changed with that diagnosis. It became my path to healing, as well as the path to my life's work helping others heal.

If you are familiar with my work, you'll know I have written three books on thyroid health and founded an informational website called thyroidpharmacist.com in 2013. As the name suggests, I am both a pharmacist and a thyroid expert. This expertise didn't come from school, rather, it came from being a human guinea pig, and later a health adviser to others with the condition.

My IBS symptoms were an important clue to the root cause of my Hashimoto's disease, and since recovering my own health, I have been determined to help others as well.

After getting the autoimmune diagnosis, I wanted to know what caused my immune system to attack itself and what I could do about it. In my quest for answers, I came across the work of Dr. Alessio Fasano, a gastroenterologist who proposed a theory that intestinal permeability is a key factor that allows for autoimmune conditions to occur. Intestinal permeability or leaky gut, in which the junctions between the epithelial cells (cells that line the small intestine) become damaged and loosen, allows toxic substances such as partially digested food, pollen, feces, dead cells, and bacteria to escape from the digestive system and pass into the bloodstream, triggering an immune response. The immune system will attack these invaders but may also attack the body itself (including the thyroid gland).

While some individuals may be asymptomatic, the symptoms typically attributed to intestinal permeability include digestive distress such as bloating, gas, cramping, food sensitivities, diarrhea, constipation and you guessed it—IBS symptoms! Additionally, fatigue, pain, mood and skin issues as well as an autoimmune diagnosis may also signal intestinal permeability.

After reading this theory, I realized something. The IBS, acid reflux, chronic fatigue, anxiety attacks, carpal tunnel syndrome, and hair loss were all connected, and in addition to correcting my thyroid levels with hormones, I focused on digging at the root cause of my Hashimoto's.

After a lot of trial and error, I was able to get my Hashimoto's into remission through addressing the many imbalances impacting my immune system, including food sensitivities, infections, stress, nutrient deficiencies, toxic overload, and of course intestinal permeability.

Addressing these issues helped me feel vibrant, calm, healthy, and strong. After so many years of struggling, all of my symptoms (including the IBS symptoms) were now a thing of the past!

But I stumbled a bit before I got better. After initially coming across a study documenting improvement in thyroid function after gluten elimination in people who had both celiac and Hashimoto's, I took a food sensitivity test that revealed I was sensitive to gluten and dairy. Within three days of getting off gluten and dairy, my digestive symptoms virtually vanished. The bloating was gone and I was no longer in pain after eating! I had no idea stomachs were not supposed to hurt after eating. My acid reflux was gone, and I gladly threw my Tums, Prilosec, and Pepcid in the trash. My previously loose stools were well formed for the first time since I could remember. While some thyroid markets and symptoms began to improve, sadly my healing came to a halt, and I continued to struggle with brain fog, fatigue, anxiety, skin breakouts, and hair loss . . . and after a few months the bloating started to come back.

Determined that food was the answer, I cut out more foods. I felt better temporarily. So I cut out even more foods, until I was left with a very limited diet. I looked and felt malnourished, despite eating a "very clean diet." Unfortunately, this is all too common; many patients and even integrative professionals just focus on cutting out more foods, without realizing there could be an underlying cause. Eventually I invested in functional medicine testing, and a stool test revealed I had *Blastocystis hominis,* a common yet controversial parasitic protozoan infection. Studies have shown that treatment of this pathogen can induce a remission of IBS, hives, food sensitivities, and even Hashimoto's, yet most conventional medical doctors don't test for it and don't believe it could be problematic. But by treating this infection, I was able to get myself into remission and reintroduce most foods! It was at this point that I wrote my first book, *Hashimoto's Thyroiditis: Lifestyle Interventions for Finding and Treating the Root Cause*, in 2013, and started working with people with Hashimoto's to help them achieve remission, too. My hope now is to enlighten people about possible root causes to IBS (including *B. hominis*) so people with IBS can find relief from their symptoms. While I didn't intend to specialize in IBS (or even thyroid conditions initially), many of my clients with Hashimoto's also had IBS, and a big part of helping them with Hashimoto's has focused on their gut!

Conventional medicine often works in silos, looking at each organ system as operating individually. But my experience made me realize that the body works as a whole and everything is connected. As I began to unravel some of my own symptoms, I discovered functional medicine, a patient-centered approach to healing focused on addressing the root causes of disease, not just the symptoms.

After attending an Institute for Functional Medicine training, I learned that IBS often precedes an autoimmune diagnosis by five to ten years. I wondered whether my Hashimoto's might have been prevented if I had found the cause of my IBS sooner? What if we treated IBS symptoms as a sign from the body that we need to dig deeper, instead of it being an annoying symptom that needs to be suppressed with symptom-relief drugs? I often wonder if addressing the root cause of IBS could have also helped twenty-four million people in the United States with an autoimmune condition and the millions more who are as yet undiagnosed?

While it's hard to know exactly how many people with IBS also have an autoimmune condition, and vice versa, there does appear to be significant overlap between the two conditions, and a number of people with autoimmune disease will present with symptoms that are very similar to IBS, which can sometimes make disentangling the two conditions challenging. For example, a 2019 population-based study found that having an autoimmune disease is a risk factor for developing IBS and about 20 percent of people with rheumatoid arthritis had IBS, while a small study of 80 people with IBS found that 18.5 percent of them also had thyroid dysfunction.

Since my initial IBS diagnosis, I've grown both as a researcher and as a functional medicine practitioner, and more research has emerged regarding IBS.

I have been wanting to write this book for over ten years, but a bit of impostor syndrome kept me from writing it. After all, my expertise is in thyroid health, not in gastroenterology. But during that time, I had to learn all I could about gut health to help clients who sought out my help. When I was starting off, I thought going gluten-free and dairy-free was the answer for everyone. Spoiler alert: It isn't for everyone, and it wasn't even the complete answer for me.

What I learned helped me recognize that there are numerous treatable conditions that can cause digestive issues and are often misdiagnosed as IBS. Each of these conditions requires a different treatment approach.

A final reason why I felt I had to write this book was because of an unexpected illness that nearly devastated my happy little family at the most vulnerable time. My dear husband was diagnosed with inflammatory bowel disease (IBD) two weeks after the birth of our precious son. He went from an energetic ultra-marathon-running superhero to someone with horrific digestive symptoms who was barely waking up at eleven a.m. I am fortunate that we had an amazing doctor who recognized his symptoms and recommended a diagnostic workup right away instead of brushing the symptoms off as just "IBS and stress." The correct diagnosis allowed us to know what we had to work with and helped us create an effective plan for healing.

Fortunately, through the knowledge I've gained on my healing journey and from functional medicine trainings and the generous advice of colleagues, we were able to get his IBD into remission within a month. I have seen firsthand the devastating effects that inflammatory bowel disease can have on people, many of whom go misdiagnosed for several years and struggle to find the right treatment. If you have IBD, I hope to share how you can heal once and for all, too.

But this experience further highlighted that my individual triggers and biochemistry were different from the triggers and biochemistry of my clients and my husband. Not only do different conditions require different treatment, but also the treatment approaches for different people need to be specialized. I've realized that IBS is considered a "throwaway diagnosis" or a "wastebasket diagnosis" and is given to people who have a particular set of unexplained gastrointestinal symptoms. Being able to apply an IBS label is convenient, but it doesn't explain why a person has digestive symptoms, and consequently the treatment approaches often fall short. Most of the conventional information about IBS is too general to work for everyone with an IBS label.

Additionally, not all doctors do the proper workup before giving this diagnosis.

Your symptoms may be labeled as IBS while they actually may be caused by a different medically identifiable, treatable, and often testable condition, such as celiac disease, SIBO (small intestinal bacterial overgrowth), or IBD. In other cases, your symptoms may be caused by conditions that have not yet been recognized by conventional medicine but are largely known in functional medicine and natural medicine circles, such as enzyme deficiencies, protozoal infections, and bacterial imbalance in the gut.

To help you address your unique triggers, I decided to organize this book by the causes of digestive issues with their corresponding protocols. I hope that with this book, I can shed light on triggers I have identified so you can find the most helpful approach to healing and say goodbye to your digestive symptoms. I hope to even help potentially prevent or reverse an autoimmune diagnosis. And perhaps this book will teach you, or a practitioner you are working with, a new methodology for finding triggers and patterns.

....

Even if you don't have a doctor guiding you at the moment, or if you have a doctor who doesn't know what to do about your symptoms, the good news is there are plenty of things you will learn to do on your own by reading this book. And these things will help you get your symptoms under control and get your life back.

Conventional treatment for IBS typically focuses on eating more fiber and taking laxatives and/or a variety of prescription meds (meant in some cases for other conditions) that may help manage symptoms . . . or not. As I experienced, some of these methods may even contribute to unpleasant side effects. According to research, less than 25 percent of people with IBS gain complete relief from any particular symptom with conventional methods. By reading this book and following the recommendations, it is my hope that at least 80 percent of IBS patients will find a full resolution of their symptoms.

In addition to limited symptom relief, the conventional approach to IBS carries significant long-term risks. Without proper symptom resolution, people are at risk for malabsorption of nutrients and an overall diminished vitality and quality of life.

They may also experience "symptom shifting" or an "evolution" of symptoms, indicating the development of another condition in addition to IBS. New research is emerging every year on how the causes of IBS and fibromyalgia, chronic headaches, chronic fatigue syndrome, back pain, and chronic pelvic pain, among others, are often the same. In 2023, for example, researchers determined that IBS and fibromyalgia are both driven by microbiome alterations and the gut-brain axis.

IBS is also associated with depression, suicidal behavior, and an increased frequency of invasive surgical procedures, such as hysterectomies, appendectomies, and cholecystectomies (gallbladder removal surgery). In the elderly, and I believe especially in those with undiagnosed IBD, IBS may be associated with higher rates of colorectal cancer.

In my experience and that of other functional medicine providers, people often receive an autoimmune diagnosis five to ten years after an IBS diagnosis.

You Can Feel Better by Cutting Branches and Digging at the Root

If you've picked up this book, you're probably dealing with some or all of the most common digestive symptoms labeled as IBS, such as abdominal pain and cramping, gas and bloating, or changes in bowel habits, including constipation and diarrhea. Perhaps you're also feeling some of the other commonly co-occurring symptoms such as acid reflux, heartburn, fullness after eating, belching, nausea, depression, or anxiety.

While most conventional doctors will label these symptoms as IBS and consider the case closed with no clear action plan to resolve them, functional medical practitioners like me view these symptoms as signs that your body, and especially your gut, need some attention.

In order to feel better and heal, we need to put on our detective hats. Rather than accepting the label of IBS, I want to encourage you to take charge of your health and shed your IBS symptoms and diagnosis by identifying and treating the root causes of your symptoms.

There are so many innovators in the world of IBS, yet most doctors, even gastroenterologists, are not aware of every cause.

In my personal experience I have seen many drivers for IBS, including celiac disease, food sensitivities, digestive enzyme deficiencies, dysbiosis, medication side effects, bacterial infections, viral infections, nutrient deficiencies, hormonal imbalances, mitochondrial dysfunction, toxicity, and protozoal infections including *Blastocystis hominis* to be potential triggers.

If you have been given the label of IBS by a primary care doctor or have self-diagnosed, I would highly recommend that you have a comprehensive workup from a qualified gastroenterologist who is well-versed in screening for celiac disease, inflammatory bowel disease, SIBO, and bile acid diarrhea. Knowing the right diagnosis can help you create a plan for remission.

If you've already gone the gastroenterologist route and have not come out with helpful strategies or have perhaps received a diagnosis that wasn't fully resolved with the recommended treatment, I also want to offer more hope that there are additional causes (and protocols) that could be the answer for you.

Research-backed causes that will be covered in this book include:

- Dietary triggers, such as celiac disease, non-celiac gluten sensitivity, non-celiac wheat sensitivity, dairy, high-nickel foods, high FODMAP foods, fructose intolerance, sucrose intolerance, alcohol, caffeine, carbonated beverages, and food additives

- Digestive enzyme deficiencies
- Bile acid malabsorption
- Nutrient depletions, especially zinc and glutamine
- A deficiency of probiotics, or good bacteria, in the gut microbiome
- Intestinal permeability, also known as leaky gut
- Intestinal overgrowths, including bacterial and fungal in the small intestine (SIBO and SIFO) and intestinal candidiasis
- Gastrointestinal hypomotility, or slowed transit time through the digestive tract, also known as slowed gut motility
- Infections, including residual parasitic, bacterial, and viral infections
- Alterations in stress hormones
- Thyroid imbalances and autoimmunity
- Inflammation
- Inflammatory bowel disease
- Toxins and chemical triggers, including certain medications
- Western lifestyle factors such as stress, alcohol use, dehydration, poor bowel habits, low-fiber diet, lack of exercise, poor sleep habits, and smoking

While you may have never heard of these conditions, rest assured that they are treatable, and proper treatment can result in a remission of your symptoms. To me, the diagnosis of IBS is a very convenient term to describe a cluster of symptoms, but it does a disservice to people and practitioners because the many causes are clustered under one umbrella, and thus it's difficult, if not impossible, to create an effective treatment protocol with only an IBS diagnosis.

For example, if your diarrhea is caused strictly by SIBO, a temporary low FODMAP diet may help with symptoms and a SIBO targeted antimicrobial will be helpful to achieve remission. But if it's due to celiac disease, a lifelong gluten-free diet may be more appropriate.

Furthermore, if your diarrhea is caused by a parasite, using an antiparasitic drug or herb will be a better choice. Of course, it's important to note that one person may have more than one cause, and one cause may have numerous consequences. For example, a person with celiac disease is at greater risk for parasitic infections and may require a gluten-free diet and an antiparasitic protocol for full symptom resolution. Protozoan parasites like *Giardia* may lead to fat malabsorption, so a person with *Giardia* may need to take enzymes as well as antiparasitics to have full symptom resolution.

Based on my years of research, patient study, and work with thousands of clients, this book is designed to help you take charge of your own health by breaking down the symptoms, relevant tests, and protocols of each potential root cause so you can easily figure out if it could apply to you and what to do next. You may need a combination of conventional medicine, integrative medicine, and good old-fashioned self-management strategies to have a full remission of symptoms.

While some of these tests and protocols are considered experimental by conventional medicine, they can offer a path to healing when conventional test results show "all of your labs are normal." Unfortunately, the testing methods utilized by most conventional medicine practitioners often fail to find the treatable causes of IBS symptoms. Based on the latest findings, *IBS: Finding and Treating the Root Cause of Irritable Bowel Syndrome* offers a comprehensive root cause workup of what's really going on with you and clear, actionable steps to get rid of your IBS symptoms and prevent a host of chronic illnesses.

How My Approach Is Different

While the conventional approach to IBS routinely doesn't dig deep enough into specific underlying root causes, I have also seen various integrative, functional, and holistic medicine experts focus too narrowly on a sole root cause of IBS symptoms, such as an imbalance in gut flora, SIBO, or food sensitivities.

Some individuals new to integrative medicine may limit their recommendation to taking probiotics or doing an elimination diet for every individual with IBS, without considering that an impaired gut flora, a small bowel bacterial overgrowth, and food sensitivities can be symptoms of a deeper root cause, like an underlying infection or toxin. If the infection is not addressed, symptom relief will only be partial or temporary. Not only is this discouraging, it leaves the person open to more health challenges and a future diagnosis of autoimmune disease.

I know digging for root causes can seem overwhelming. But healing from any chronic condition and moving toward better health is a journey. It took me several years and a few stumbles before I found what made me feel better—and it was 100 percent worth it! I believe it will be worth it for you, too.

How to Use This Book

Part I lays the groundwork for uncovering the root causes of your IBS. You'll learn about the symptoms, types, and co-occurring conditions of IBS and gain insight into why conventional medical approaches often fall short.

Part II guides you on your healing journey, helping you identify the root causes behind your specific symptoms. It covers testing where necessary and provides treatment options, including diets, medications, and supplements.

Part III brings it all together, offering guidance for creating a plan for resolving your IBS symptoms and strategies for relieving your symptoms while you dig for root causes.

I encourage you to take your time with each of the chapters—they'll give you the foundation you need to create a personalized health plan that truly fits your needs.

PART I

Understanding IBS and the Root Cause Approach

CHAPTER 1

What Is Normal Digestive Function and What Is IBS?

Digestive distress is so common that many of us have started to believe that it's normal. I often meet people who only poop once every two weeks or rely on laxatives for years. This, of course, is not normal digestive function. I also see those who plan their lives around bathroom accessibility and carry around their own sh*t kits and extra underwear everywhere they go! That isn't normal, either. In 2022, people in the United States spent more than $1.7 billion on over-the-counter (OTC) laxatives to ease constipation and almost $350 million on OTC antidiarrheal medications.

Now, as someone who has worked with thousands of clients to take back their health, I know it doesn't have to be that way! IBS symptoms are associated with many other identifiable and treatable conditions, and in order to heal, we have to look beyond laxatives or antidiarrheal meds to the underlying source of symptoms.

Before we get into treating the causes of IBS, I would love to share what healthy digestion actually looks like. I know many of my family members, friends, clients, and even colleagues often disregard symptoms of digestive distress just as I did. I personally thought having a stomachache after eating was part of the normal digestive process, and I didn't realize how truly compromised my digestion had been prior to getting off dairy and taking digestive enzymes!

What Does Healthy Digestive Function Look Like?

Many of us have learned to live with our digestive troubles for so long we may not even know what healthy digestion looks and feels like. Here are a few signs of healthy digestion:

- Most foods can be digested without causing bloating, cramps, fatigue, or pain. (Shocking, I know!)

- Regular and frequent bowel movements pass approximately one minute after sitting on the toilet, without pain or strain, and without needing to use your fingers to press on your anus to poop.

- Regularity is defined as bowel movements that come at a predictable time, often in the morning, twenty to forty minutes after eating, or twenty to forty minutes after other daytime meals.

- Frequency varies from person to person, ranging from one to three times daily to every other day. However, going fewer than three or four times a week may indicate constipation.

- Soft, well-formed, brown stool ranging between type 3 ("a sausage shape with cracks in the surface") and type 4 ("like a smooth, soft sausage or snake") on the Bristol Stool Chart, or as I like to call it, "The Official Poop Chart." (Types 1 and 2 indicate various stages of constipation, while types 5 through 7 are considered loose stools or diarrhea.)

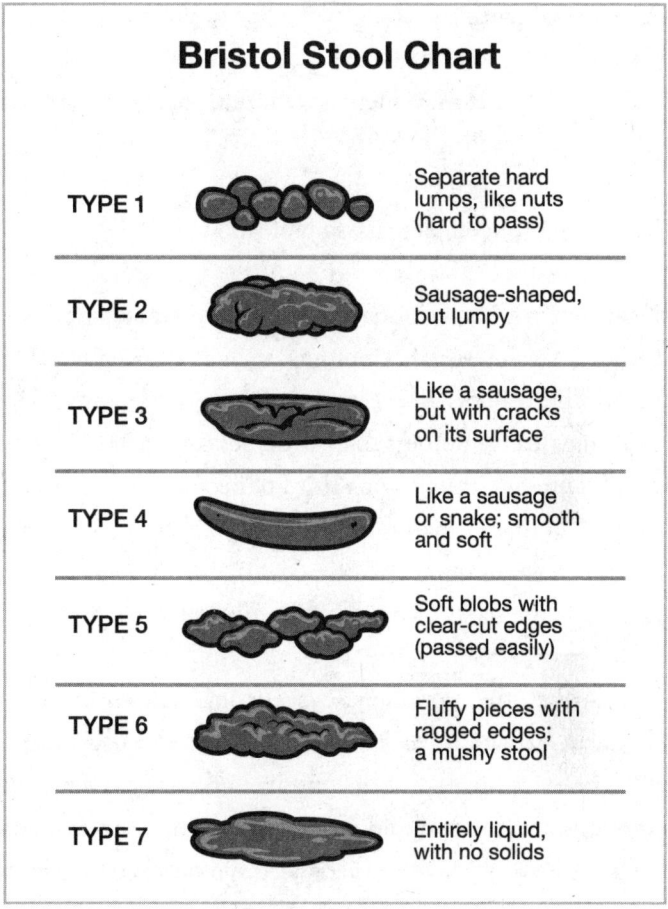

This diagnostic tool was developed by researchers in England to help clinicians determine how long it takes for food to pass through the body and leave as waste.

The Symptoms That Lead to the Diagnosis of IBS

If you're reading this book and have a personal history of digestive distress, it's likely that you're well aware of the many symptoms of IBS, but for the sake of completeness, let's start by taking a closer look at the most common symptoms that may lead to a diagnosis of IBS.

People with IBS can have a variety of symptoms, including:

- Abdominal pain, cramping
- Changes in bowel frequency
- Change in bowel movement appearance (pellet shaped, watery)
- Bloating or swelling
- Relief of pain with bowel movement
- Sensation of incomplete passing of stools
- Mucus in stool
- Difficulty with bowel movements, such as straining
- Other gastrointestinal symptoms, such as excess gas, acid reflux, heartburn, fullness after eating, belching, and nausea
- Psychological symptoms such as depression and anxiety (which may be present in up to one third of people, with some studies indicating that as many as 60 percent of people with IBS patients have anxiety)
- Symptomatic flares or periods of remission

There can be other common co-occurring symptoms, such as fatigue, frequent urination, back pain, headache, and bad breath or an unpleasant taste in the mouth. In contrast to occasional bowel distress, IBS symptoms are frequent and chronic. One large survey found that 57 percent of people with IBS experienced symptoms daily and 50 percent had symptoms for more than ten years! Another study found that people with IBS experienced symptoms an average of 8.1 days per month, and two-thirds of people having IBS stated they had reduced activity levels due to their symptoms.

IBS and Mucus

The presence of noticeable amounts of mucus, a clear or whitish jellylike substance that helps lubricate the colon, has been reported in 50 percent of people with IBS. This may be due to de-

> hydration or constipation but also has been observed as a characteristic in the diarrhea-predominant type of IBS. In IBS-D, seeing increased mucus in the stool is likely the result of an increase of mucin-degrading bacteria, which influences mucus shedding.

Types of IBS

With such a range of associated symptoms, it's not surprising that IBS can present slightly differently in various people. While one person with IBS may be regularly running to the bathroom with urgent diarrhea, another person may struggle to pass a painfully hard stool. To reflect these differences, four distinct diagnostic types of IBS have been created:

- **IBS with constipation (IBS-C):** More than 25 percent of abnormal bowel movements consist of lumpy and hard poop. Constipation happens when food moves too slowly through the digestive tract and the colon or large intestine absorbs too much water from the partially digested food, making it dry and difficult to pass. Studies suggest women are significantly more likely to develop IBS-C than men.

- **IBS with diarrhea (IBS-D):** More than 25 percent of abnormal bowel movements consist of watery and loose poop. In this case, waste is passing through the digestive system too quickly for the colon to absorb enough water, so the stool is very runny. This is the most common type of IBS, reported by about 40 percent of people.

- **IBS with mixed bowel habits (IBS-M):** As the name implies, a person with this type of IBS will have a mixture of constipation and diarrhea, which can alternate as quickly as within a few hours or on a daily, weekly, or monthly basis.

- **IBS unclassified (IBS-U):** Most poop is normal, but the person has recurring stomach pain and other IBS symptoms.

Individuals can experience different combinations of symptoms, and symptoms and even IBS types can change over time.

How Is IBS Diagnosed?

Up until recently, there has not been a definitive test to rule out or confirm IBS, so diagnosis is based on medical history (including family history), self-reported clinical symptoms (relating primarily to bowel habits), and evaluation of current medications. One report found it takes about four years on average for people to be given a diagnosis of IBS.

In the past, doctors have referred to irritable bowel syndrome as nervous colon, spastic bowel, colitis, and mucous colitis. It wasn't until 1948 that (aptly named) P. W. Brown finally coined the term "irritable bowel syndrome" to describe the trifecta of constipation, diarrhea, and abdominal pain when no infection was to blame.

Until the 1970s, IBS was a diagnosis of exclusion, meaning it was given after extensive lab testing and procedures—even surgery—were done to rule out other potential diagnosable diseases. If everything came back "normal," doctors would label the condition IBS.

Because the diagnostic methods and tests utilized at the time were not showing any abnormalities, guidelines were created to reduce unnecessary testing and standardize a definition of IBS. As a result, doctors came up with a set of symptom-based criteria to positively diagnose IBS. I'll share why that's a problem later in this chapter!

The Manning Criteria

The Manning criteria was the first diagnostic algorithm, based on asking people fifteen symptom-related questions, such as whether they experienced looser or more frequent stools with the onset of pain or felt pain relief after a bowel movement. This algorithm was found to be too broad and unable to adequately distinguish people with IBS from those with other gastrointestinal conditions.

The Rome IV Criteria

In 1989, an international expert consensus in Rome developed a more refined set of criteria, updated three times since. The Rome IV criteria, now the most widely used, requires recurrent abdominal pain for at least three months (averaging at least once a week) with symptom onset six months prior. For a diagnosis of IBS, patients must also meet two or more of the following:

1. Pain specifically related to defecation. Pain is the most common symptom of IBS and could involve the presence of abdominal pain (often described as severe muscle tension and cramping) associated with straining and constipation and/or the urgency to pass loose stool and diarrhea. Pain typically decreases after a bowel movement.

2. Changes in frequency of stool (how often, urgency). People can have a combination of normal bowel habits (regular and easy to pass) that alternate with frequent loose stools, including a heightened sense of urgency to defecate, and/or constipation that can last for days or longer. Defecating may include a feeling of incomplete relief after defecation.

3. Changes in form (appearance) of stool (diarrhea and/or constipation and the presence of mucus in the stool). Stool may be hard, lumpy, and difficult to pass, characteristic of constipation, or watery, mushy, and shapeless, characteristic of diarrhea.

There are also two tools practitioners may use to measure the degree of pain and symptoms a patient is self-reporting.

The Functional Bowel Disorder Severity Index (FBDSI): This scale rates severity based on the level of pain at the current visit, number of physician visits in the previous six months, and an assessment focused on functional abdominal pain from mild (<36) to severe (>111).

The IBS Symptom Severity Scale (IBS-SSS): This scale measures the intensity of IBS symptoms during a ten-day period, including abdominal pain, bloating, stool frequency and consistency, and interference with life in general. The sum of these five items is each scored on a scale from 0 to 100.

Emerging Diagnostic Testing

New blood tests are emerging that may help doctors make an IBS diagnosis, based on findings that IBS-D can be triggered by food poisoning and has autoimmune components. Blood tests measure two antibodies: anti-CdtB, which forms in response to bacteria from food poisoning, and anti-vinculin, an autoimmune response against a gut protein.

Those with elevated levels of either anti-CdtB or anti-vinculin antibodies can be diagnosed with IBS with 96 percent certainty, while elevated levels of both antibodies indicate IBS-D or IBS-M, with up to 100 percent certainty. The antibody tests are not effective for diagnosing IBS-C, as these antibodies aren't elevated in most IBS-C cases. Please note that current medical guidelines do not recommend testing for people who meet diagnostic criteria, so patients often need to self-advocate.

- IBSchek: The IBSchek was developed by Commonwealth Diagnostics International and was the first test introduced to measure anti-CdtB and anti-vinculin antibodies for IBS diagnosis. It was launched around 2015 but has been discontinued.

- IBS-Smart: The IBS-Smart test, developed by Dr. Mark Pimentel, is the currently available and patented version of the antibody test. Only a licensed physician can order IBS-Smart. You can work with either your primary care doctor or an online doctor through the IBS-Smart website (https://www.ibssmart.com).

While the test won't likely give you the *cause* behind IBS, it may be a helpful tool on your journey.

Is Testing Ever Recommended by Conventional Guidelines?

Current medical guidelines do not recommend testing for patients who meet Rome IV diagnostic criteria for IBS and do not have red flag or "alarm" symptoms.

However, additional tests are recommended for people with red flag symptoms that may indicate a differential diagnosis—i.e., a diagnosis other than IBS—such as IBD (inflammatory bowel disease), celiac disease, a polyp, or even cancer.

Red flag symptoms include:

- IBS symptom onset after age fifty
- Rectal bleeding
- Unexplained weight loss
- Nighttime symptoms such as diarrhea (IBS symptoms are usually better at night when an individual is asleep)
- Abdominal mass
- Iron deficiency anemia
- Persistent pain not relieved by flatulence or bowel movement
- Fever
- Elevated white blood count
- Unexplained vomiting
- Difficulty swallowing

Other red flag concerns physicians should screen for include:

- Food allergies, as a genetic predisposition toward developing allergic diseases, known as atopy, may be a source of symptoms.
- Family history of gastrointestinal diseases such as colon cancer, inflammatory bowel disease, or celiac disease, as research suggests an increased risk.
- Recent travel, contributing to an increased risk for bacterial infection or parasite.

If you were to see a gastroenterologist who was well versed in gastrointestinal disorders presenting with any of the above-mentioned symptoms, you would likely get a more comprehensive diagnostic workup, such as a complete blood cell count (CBC), a comprehensive metabolic panel, a C-reactive protein test (to screen for inflammation), a test for celiac disease, a stool test, and sigmoidoscopy or colonoscopy to rule out other conditions such as colon cancer, rather than just getting an IBS label based on symptoms. Yet sadly, some general practitioners who may not be as up-to-date on their diagnostics may miss these red flag symptoms and still give people an IBS label without further investigation.

Differential Diagnosis in IBS: Conditions That Can Be Misdiagnosed as IBS

Your gastrointestinal symptoms may be labeled as IBS, but digging at the root can help identify what's really going on.

Common conditions that may be mistaken for IBS with constipation include:

- Diet and lifestyle: inadequate fiber intake, immobility, stress
- Endocrine: hypothyroidism, diabetes, hypercalcemia

- Neurologic: Parkinson's disease, multiple sclerosis, spinal cord injuries, pelvic floor dysfunction

- Drug side effects: antidepressants, opiate analgesics, calcium-channel blockers, clonidine, anticholinergics, antihistamines

- Other: endometriosis, colorectal cancer, ovarian cancer, diverticular disease, bowel obstruction, hemorrhoids, intestinal cancer, tumors, gallstones, biliary colic

Common conditions that may be mistaken for IBS with diarrhea include:

- IBD: Crohn's disease, ulcerative colitis, microscopic colitis

- Dietary: lactose intolerance, fructose intolerance, sorbitol intolerance, alcohol intake, excess caffeine intake, intolerance to fatty foods, poor breakdown of gas-producing foods, other food sensitivities or allergies

- Gastrointestinal infections: bacterial or viral gastroenteritis, parasitic infections such as *Giardia*, bacterial overgrowth (including small intestinal bacterial overgrowth or SIBO), HIV

- Malabsorption: celiac disease, bile acid diarrhea

- Drug side effects: proton pump inhibitors (PPIs), antibiotics, nonsteroidal anti-inflammatory drugs (NSAIDs), beta-blockers, ACE inhibitors, chemotherapy

- Enzyme deficiency: exocrine pancreatic insufficiency (EPI)

- Other: endometriosis, ovarian cancer, colorectal cancer, carcinoid, vasoactive intestinal peptide-secreting tumors (VIPoma), ischemic colitis, hyperthyroidism, stress, anxiety disorders, abdominal angina, cholecystitis, pancreatitis

Whether a practitioner does further evaluation or testing to exclude any of these other differential diagnoses depends on how well a patient reports their symptoms and health history, as well as the knowledge and determination of the practitioner to peel back the onion and figure out what's really going on. As a young and bushy-tailed pharmacy student, I really thought all doctors had a certain level of competence, but after a few months of working at a pharmacy in East Los Angeles, I realized that was sadly not the case in the real world.

I'm an advocate for anyone presenting with IBS symptoms to get more comprehensive testing. Infections, inflammatory bowel disease, and even cancer (especially in the early stages) may not always present with red flag symptoms.

I know too many people who have been told they had irritable bowel syndrome, when indeed they had another condition, such as inflammatory bowel disease, cancer, or celiac disease. Statistics say a whopping 10 percent of people with IBD may be misdiagnosed with IBS, and in one study, 25 percent had celiac disease!

My Manifesto for More Testing!

In the past thirty years, we've identified numerous treatable causes and diagnostic tools for IBS, yet most doctors still rely on symptoms alone to diagnose it.

Once a doctor labels someone's symptoms as IBS, there's rarely any further investigation into the real underlying issues. And since conventional treatment for IBS is about managing symptoms, not curing the condition, that label can feel like a life sentence. I believe everyone experiencing IBS symptoms deserves a thorough investigation to uncover the root causes.

Why don't conventional doctors explore more testing—even with red flag symptoms for IBS? The reasons for this are varied. One reason is that more than 94 percent of patients with IBS symptoms are seeing family doctors or general internists, instead of specialists. Generalists may skip tests that may have been offered by gastroenterologists. One study found that 0 percent of patients with IBS were diagnosed with all the recommended tests! Only 13 percent of IBS patients see a gastroenterologist before or after diagnosis. The inclination to avoid "unnecessary" and "expensive" testing is also likely at play, too. Remember, the conventional IBS diagnostic criteria were established to avoid too much testing, as most of the tests that were done were not revealing any apparent causes. This is certainly a worthy goal within reason—no one wants to spend too much money on tests—but it seems the pendulum may have swung too far in the opposite direction to the detriment of patient care, especially considering that the Rome IV guidelines were based on an incomplete set of tests!

Unfortunately, there is also a lag between when mainstream medicine identifies best practices and those best practices are fully embraced as a conventional standard of care. One now-famous 2001 study found it takes about seventeen years for evidence-based research findings to be integrated into daily patient care practices. Seventeen years! Not to mention the light-years of lag time behind emerging research as well.

I, along with many of my functional medicine colleagues, consider IBS to be a wastebasket diagnosis, a label so vague and broad that it's almost meaningless as to what the best approaches to treatment should be.

As a patient advocate and functional medicine practitioner, I often shake my head in disbelief when I hear someone say their tests came back normal, only to realize they didn't have the right tests done in the first place.

In addition to the red flag tests I shared above, I would love for every patient and practitioner to be aware of more comprehensive tests that can be utilized to discover the cause behind the symptoms.

Recommended Tests for IBS-Related Symptoms with Red Flag Symptoms

- Complete blood cell count (CBC) (screens for anemia, inflammation, and infection)
- Comprehensive metabolic panel (to evaluate for metabolic disorders and to rule out dehydration or electrolyte imbalances)
- C-reactive protein (CRP) test (signifies inflammation)
- Calprotectin stool test (suggestive of IBD)
- Anti-*Saccharomyces cerevisiae* antibodies (ASCA) (to help identify Crohn's disease)
- Celiac disease (tTG, DGP, and EMA antibody blood tests)
- IBS-Smart test (tests for anti-CdtB and anti-vinculin antibodies that are present in IBS-D and IBS-M)
- Comprehensive stool analysis (such as the GI-MAP, which will show calprotectin levels)
- Imaging procedures (such as X-ray, CT scan, or MRI to evaluate intestinal tissues)
- Endoscopic procedures (such as an upper endoscopy, capsule endoscopy, sigmoidoscopy, or colonoscopy to rule out IBD and other conditions such as colon cancer)

Is IBS Real?

You may have heard some integrative medicine practitioners say that IBS is fake (or have seen some clickbait with the same headline), and I want to assure you that despite the attention-grabbing headlines, your symptoms are 100 percent real.

Pain, bloating, constipation, diarrhea, and the long list of other frustrating symptoms of digestive distress you may be experiencing are not "all in your head" or the result of poor stress management or just the way your body works. They are not inconsequential or something you need to live with. They are signs that your body, and especially your gut, are out of balance. And they can be resolved.

Because IBS is such a vague diagnosis and many people diagnosed with IBS are ultimately found to have another treatable condition with similar symptoms, even conventional medical practitioners are debating the usefulness and validity of an IBS diagnosis.

The good news is the functional medicine approach looks beyond the IBS label to figure out what's really going on in the body. By digging into the root cause of your symptoms and addressing the underlying cause, you can take back your health and your life.

Common Co-Occurring Conditions

IBS often goes hand in hand with other conditions, likely due to shared root causes!

Some of the most notable co-occurring conditions include:

- Chronic fatigue syndrome: CFS patients frequently complain of gut dysfunction and are more likely to report having a previous diagnosis of IBS. One study found that 92 percent of people with chronic fatigue syndrome had IBS! Conventional medicine offers very little for CFS besides perhaps stimulant medications, while *Giardia* is a treatable cause of both!

- GERD (gastroesophageal reflux disease): Up to 79 percent of IBS patients report GERD symptoms and about 71 percent of GERD patients report IBS symptoms. I used to have terrible GERD symptoms and used every acid reflux med I could find, to no avail. Nothing helped until I found and treated my root causes, which were dairy intolerance, a *Helicobacter pylori* infection, and low stomach acid.

- Psychiatric disorders: Depression, anxiety, and somatization disorder (converting a mental state such as depression into physical symptoms such as bowel pain) occur frequently in IBS. One study found that 20 percent of people with IBS have depression, 60 percent have anxiety, and 20 percent have other psychological disorders. The gut and brain are in constant contact, and the gut is often called the "second brain" because many of the neurotransmitters associated with emotional state, such as the "happy" hormone serotonin, are produced in the gut. An imbalanced gut can influence the brain, resulting in mood issues.

- Fibromyalgia: Found in 60 percent of IBS patients, with 70 percent of fibromyalgia patients having IBS. One study found that 100 percent of people with fibromyalgia had SIBO, a potential root cause for both.

- Temporomandibular joint syndrome (TMJ): Some 64 percent of people with TMJ (jaw pain) were found to have IBS, and people with IBS had more than three times the risk of a disorder of the jaw, jaw joint, and facial muscles than controls.

- Certain female health conditions and surgeries: Between 48 to 79 percent of people with chronic pelvic pain, dysmenorrhea (pain with menstrual cramps), dyspareunia (painful intercourse), or a history of numerous abdominal surgeries also have IBS. Women who have had a hysterectomy for chronic pelvic pain are twice as likely to have IBS.

- Metabolic disorders: Diabetes, obesity, and thyroid dysfunction are all linked to higher rates of IBS.

The good news? Treating the root causes can address several conditions at once. The key is to address the root causes, not just manage symptoms. More research supports this approach, focusing on true healing rather than medication alone.

The Takeaway

If you've only seen a primary care doctor or perhaps self-diagnosed your IBS, I encourage you to see a gastroenterologist to get a comprehensive workup, especially if you have red flag symptoms. Gastroenterologists are more aware of how to diagnose the various differential diagnoses, such as IBD, celiac disease, and colorectal cancer.

If you have gone that route and still found "nothing wrong," there's still hope you will have a full remission of symptoms, but you may need to do a little more digging and self-advocacy.

It is important for you to become self-educated and self-empowered to get the results you deserve. Your gastrointestinal symptoms may be labeled as IBS when actually they are caused by different medically identifiable, treatable, and sometimes testable conditions. In other cases, it is likely caused by conditions that have not yet been recognized by conventional medicine but are largely known in functional medicine and natural medicine circles. Despite research texts and guidelines that have identified various causes of symptoms associated with IBS bowel distress, the average person who presents to his/her primary provider with symptoms of diarrhea or constipation is likely to be given an

IBS diagnosis without any further investigation as to what is really going on.

The shortcomings of the conventional approach to diagnosing IBS leads to boilerplate treatments that don't deliver for most people, as we'll see in the next chapter.

Chapter Summary

- Signs of healthy digestive function include easy digestion of most foods—no bloating, cramps, fatigue, or pain—and regular and frequent bowel movements, which are soft, well-formed, and sausage-shaped.

- People with IBS may experience a variety of symptoms, including abdominal pain, changes in bowel frequency and shape, bloating, excess gas, acid reflux, depression, and anxiety, among others.

- Emerging diagnostic tests and functional medicine testing can help identify the medically identifiable and treatable condition often underlying the "wastebasket" diagnosis of IBS.

Visit https://ibsrootcause.com/bonus for notes on this chapter.

CHAPTER 2

The Conventional Medical Approach to IBS

IBS has been a poorly understood condition since symptoms of abdominal pain and mucus discharge with stool were first recorded by Western physicians in the late nineteenth century. Early theories proposed it was caused by a mental disorder and associated with hysteria and hypochondria. Lovely, right?

While the conventional medical view has come a long way since then, I think many would agree it hasn't come far enough. As we've discussed, IBS continues to be frequently misdiagnosed and ineffectively treated. So why can't we just invent a drug that treats digestive issues and also gives us all baby-smooth, glowing skin?

One reason for this frustrating situation is that conventional medicine is focused on trying to answer the question "What *condition* does a person have?" rather than "What is the *cause* behind a person's symptoms?" Without access to comprehensive root cause testing for digestive issues, even the most well-intentioned and up-to-date conventional doctor is left to cluster a variety of symptoms with an unknown cause under a convenient, yet sadly non-actionable "umbrella" label that offers imprecise treatments options.

And without tailoring treatments to a cause, treating IBS can be difficult. Symptom relief following conventional treatment for IBS is incredibly poor, as mentioned, with one study finding fewer than 25 percent of people gaining complete relief from any given symptom. Current conventional management therapies for patients with IBS result in up to 50 percent of patients remaining significantly symptomatic as long as six years after diagnosis.

Another reason for poor outcomes in the real world is the research-to-practice gap. During my time in pharmacy school, the understanding was that current guidelines were around twenty years behind emerging research, and during my public health training, I learned about a theory known as the diffusion of innovation, which explains how innovative research and current guidelines make it into real-world medical practices.

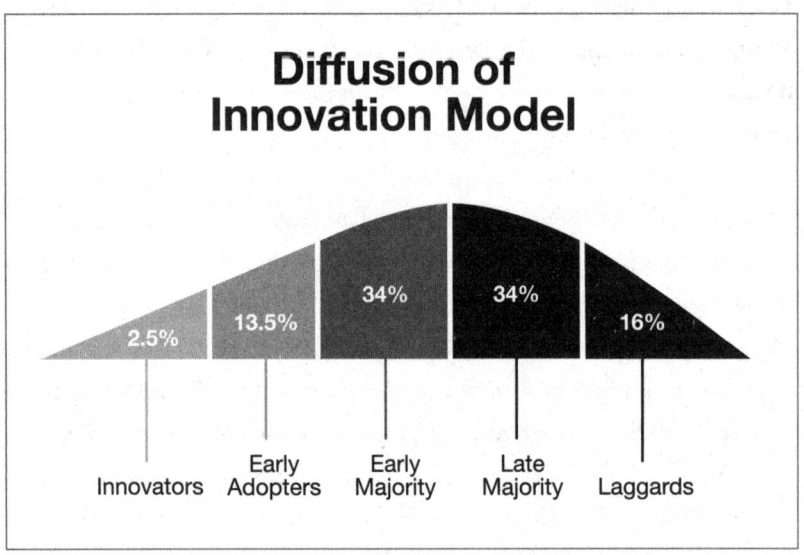

Everett Rogers identified different stages that individuals and organizations go through when adopting innovation. He identified five categories of adopters, based on how much time it took them to incorporate the innovation into their current practice or organization. Innovators are the first to adopt, followed by early adopters. The early majority adopt ahead of the average person, and the late majority adopt innovations afterward. Lastly, there are the laggards, who are of course the last to adopt. As you can see by the chart, innovators are a rare breed.

The health care professionals currently in practice may be innovators and well versed in the latest research and how to implement it, or they may be on the other end of the spectrum, sometimes the "last to know" that a new solution is available to them! You may get different recommendations and results depending on where your practitioner falls. The truth is: Some people don't know what they don't know. This is why it's so imperative for you to be self-educated.

Despite the shortcomings of the conventional approach to IBS, many of the conventional medical treatments for IBS may be helpful in some cases, such as when the right treatment is matched to the right cause, or when someone is looking for help with symptom management until the cause of IBS is identified.

As a pharmacist certified in medication therapy management, I am passionate about advocating for safe and appropriate medication use when warranted, as well as avoiding potentially harmful medications. If you're a person diagnosed with IBS, I hope this chapter helps you advocate for the most helpful treatments for yourself and know which treatments may not be a good fit. If you're a practitioner, I hope it helps you get better patient outcomes while minimizing side effects. Additionally, my hope is to speed up the diffusion of innovation by getting this book in front of innovators so they can spread the word and teach others.

Conventional Targets for IBS Therapy

Despite thousands of studies pointing to root causes of IBS, the conventional standard of care model is based on a one-size-fits-all approach that aims to relieve individual symptoms but does not address the root causes of the condition.

Most conventional practitioners view IBS as a chronic condition (like diabetes, high blood pressure, and hypothyroidism) requiring ongoing *management* (with no attempt to resolve it). People are often given Band-Aid treatments such as antidiarrheal medications, fiber, laxatives, and other medications (even antidepressants!) focused on symptom management.

Conventional medicine has identified several key areas as targets for therapy in IBS, focused on symptom management. While conventional medicine guidelines may call these "causes," a more appropriate term in my humble opinion for most of them is "symptoms." Here are the main targets that guide conventional treatment approaches:

- Altered gut motility: Medications can help regulate the contractions of the intestinal muscles. For diarrhea-predominant IBS, treatments aim to slow motility, while those with constipation benefit from medications that speed it up.

- Lower pain tolerance (visceral hypersensitivity): Visceral hypersensitivity in IBS refers to an increased sensitivity in the nerves of the digestive system, making individuals more prone to experiencing pain and discomfort from normal gut activities like digestion. This heightened pain response is a key factor in IBS symptoms, such as bloating, cramping, and abdominal pain, even when no structural abnormalities are present. It plays a significant role in the chronic discomfort many people with IBS experience. Conventional therapy often targets nerve sensitivity with medications like antispasmodics, antidepressants, or pain modulators, which aim to reduce the gut's hypersensitivity to normal digestive processes.

- Intestinal inflammation: Anti-inflammatory medications, while more common in conditions like IBD, can be used in cases where immune cell activity is heightened in IBS, providing some symptom relief.

- Psychosocial distress: Since stress and mental health are major contributors to IBS, conventional treatments may include stress management strategies, antidepressants, or therapy to improve the brain-gut connection and reduce symptom severity.

- Altered brain-gut communication: Medications that address neurotransmitter signaling, such as antidepressants or gut-targeted drugs, are often used to regulate the communication between the brain and gut, aiming to ease symptoms such as pain and motility issues.

- Bacterial overgrowth (SIBO): Antibiotics are frequently used to treat SIBO, along with dietary changes to reduce the overgrowth of bacteria in the small intestine and improve IBS symptoms. This can be helpful, but only if the other reasons SIBO developed in the first place are addressed. A reduction in SIBO has been found to correlate with improvement of IBS symptoms in some clinical trials (but not others).

Conventional Approach to Treating IBS

I'm excited to see that some of the currently available research has been making its way into medical guidelines, and current treatment options are much more sophisticated compared to the treatment options offered to me twenty years ago! I'm also excited that current American College of Gastroenterology (ACG) treatment guidelines recommend non-drug measures, as well as newer-generation medications for treating IBS, instead of just those old-school medications that made me blurry eyed!

It's important to note that not every doctor will recommend the "emerging therapies," and I do think knowing the cause will be most helpful, but these treatments can be a great place to start if you're looking for symptom improvement while you look for the cause of the IBS. If you've been helped or partially helped by some of these interventions, perhaps understanding their mechanism of action could provide clues to the causes of your digestive symptoms.

Please also note that under the conventional medicine model, all of these would be lifelong therapies to manage but not resolve symptoms. In contrast, the aim of the root cause approach is to implement temporary healing methods that would produce a full symptom resolution with a less aggressive maintenance plan (with the exception of perhaps a few conditions such as celiac disease, which does require lifelong abstinence from gluten, the triggering protein).

Diet and Lifestyle
Exercise
Exercise can support bowel motility, especially in those with constipation, low muscle tone, or a sedentary lifestyle. Movement may stimulate intestinal contractions by increasing circulation, breathing, and core strength. However, excessive exercise, potentially due to causing nutrient deficiencies like L-glutamine, can worsen IBS-D. I cover L-glutamine and supportive nutrients in chapter 6.

Low FODMAP Diet
Studies have shown the low FODMAP diet, which limits nondigestible fermentable carbohydrates, can improve IBS symptoms. This diet can be very helpful for symptom management if your IBS is caused by SIBO, but in my experience, you will likely need additional intervention to actually get rid of the SIBO (see chapter 9).

Avoiding Gas-Producing Foods

Avoiding foods such as celery, carrots, bananas, raisins, onions, beans, prunes, apricots, pretzels, caffeine, and alcohol may be especially helpful for people with food sensitivities, dysbiosis, digestive enzyme deficiency, SIBO, and gut infections.

Lactose-Free Diet

Avoiding lactose will help tremendously if you have lactose intolerance, but you may not get a full resolution if you have other causes, even other dietary triggers. I'll be diving deeper into lactose intolerance in chapter 5.

Psychological Therapies

Relaxation therapy, psychological therapy, cognitive behavioral therapy (CBT), mindfulness therapy, and gut-directed hypnotherapy may improve IBS symptoms, but multiple treatments are needed.

Pharmacological Treatments

If you were to go to a pharmacy to seek some over-the-counter recommendations for IBS, you would probably get some of the following suggestions.

If you were constipated . . .

1. The pharmacist would hopefully ask if you were taking any medications or supplements that cause constipation, such as antihistamines, calcium, iron, or opioids, and suggest less constipating alternatives. For more on the role of medications, see chapter 14.

2. You would potentially get recommendations for getting plenty of liquids, fiber, and physical activity in your daily routine.

3. The pharmacist may recommend some over-the-counter osmotic laxatives such as Miralax (polyethylene glycol), bulk laxatives such as psyllium, or stimulant laxatives such as bisacodyl or senna if the others aren't effective.

OTC Recommendations for Constipation
- Soluble fiber supplements like psyllium husk (Metamucil, Citrucel, FiberCon) act as bulk-forming laxatives by absorbing water, softening stool, and stimulating intestinal contractions. They may also support gut health by feeding beneficial bacteria. However, in cases of SIBO or dysbiosis, fiber can worsen symptoms. It's best to increase fiber slowly to a target of 21 to 38 grams per day with water. Insoluble fiber (like bran) may trigger bloating and pain.

- Laxatives: While laxatives can be helpful in extreme circumstances, they are not a long-term solution, as they can become habit-forming and people can become dependent upon them to have regular bowel movements. Long-term use of laxatives can cause the intestines to lose their normal tone and nerve response, resulting in the inability to have a natural bowel movement. Guidelines suggest taking them for only seven days without supervision, and side effects can include IBS symptoms such as cramping, abdominal pain, and diarrhea.
    - Stimulant laxatives increase intestinal muscle contractions and fluid secretion into the bowel to aid in bowel movement. Examples are sennosides (Ex-Lax) and bisacodyl (Dulcolax).
    - Osmotic laxatives draw water from surrounding tissues into the bowel to increase the water content of stool, softening it and making it easier to pass. Polyethylene glycol (Miralax) is one example.

- Lubricants: These agents, as the name suggests, provide lubrication to the intestines to help stool pass through more easily. Laxative lubricants such as mineral oil are typically consumed orally. Please note that mineral oil is not usually recommended due to increased risk of aspiration pneumonia.

- Stool softeners: Stool softeners work by drawing water into the stool and softening it, helping it move through the colon. Docusate sodium (Colace) is a popular brand.

- Suppositories: These medications are inserted into the rectum to do their duty at the site where we do our doody. Some suppositories work by softening the stool, whereas others provide lubrication and/or stimulation to promote peristalsis Bisacodyl (Dulcolax) is an example.

OTC Recommendations for Diarrhea
- Loperamide: Loperamide works on mu opioid receptors in the gut wall to slow intestinal contractions and gut transit time, allowing more water to be absorbed back into the body through the intestinal wall and making stool less watery and frequent. A common brand name is Imodium. This medication was a mainstay in my personal sh*t kit! It is very helpful in the short term but should not be used for infectious diarrhea.

- Bismuth subsalicylate: The active ingredient in "the pink stuff," aka Pepto-Bismol, has anti-inflammatory and antacid properties that can help treat a range of digestive problems, including heartburn and upset stomach. It's also a powerful antibacterial and antimicrobial found to be very effective at relieving diarrhea triggered by an infection, particularly those caused by bacteria including *Escherichia coli*, *Clostridium difficile,* and *Salmonella,* among other pathogens, with one study finding that bismuth subsalicylate had a prevention rate of traveler's diarrhea greater than 60 percent. Bismuth subsalicylate is also often used with other medications as part of a treatment regimen to eradicate *H. pylori*, the most common cause of ulcers. It should not be used alone to self-treat active, bleeding ulcers as salicylates can cause intestinal or stomach bleeding when used in this way, and it should be avoided if you are allergic to salicylates, which include aspirin and NSAIDs (ibuprofen, naproxen).

- Soluble fiber supplements, such as psyllium husk (Metamucil): A multitasking recommendation for both constipation and diarrhea is often to get more fiber. By soaking up water in the digestive tract, soluble fiber firms up loose stool and slows its passage through the colon. It can also feed the "good" bacteria and help with rebalancing the microbiome. Some individuals with IBS caused by SIBO and dysbiosis may have a worsening of symptoms with the use of fiber supplements. Guidelines suggest gradually increasing dietary fiber to 21 to 38 grams per day (depending on age and gender) plus water. Insoluble fiber (bran) may exacerbate bloating and pain.

OTC Gas and Bloating Medicine
- Simethicone: Simethicone helps break up gastrointestinal gas bubbles, helping it exit the body more easily and relieving fullness and bloating. The marketing geniuses behind one common brand name of this medication have come up with the name GasX, which I feel fairly summarizes its action.

> ### Emerging OTC Recommendations Supported by the American College of Gastroenterology
>
> I'm so excited probiotics are recommended by many pharmacists and by the American College of Gastroenterology for IBS. Certain strains can support the microbiome, enhance gut motility, and reduce symptoms like bloating, constipation, and diarrhea. They may also help fight off pathogens. However, not all probiotics are helpful, some may worsen SIBO or histamine-driven IBS. As they say, the devil's in the details! I'll cover the best strains in chapter 7.

Prescription Medications

When people don't get relief with the over-the-counter interventions, conventional practitioners may choose to utilize prescription medications.

The main prescription players when I was in pharmacy school were the three A's: antibiotics, antispasmodics, and antidepressants.

Antibiotics and antispasmodics are used to resolve diarrhea by changing the gut microbiome and slowing down gut contractility, respectively. Tricyclic antidepressants are thought to work by blocking pain receptors and are used for diarrhea, while SSRI (selective serotonin reuptake inhibitor) antidepressants are thought to keep more serotonin in the gut, helping with constipation.

In recent years, scientists have come up with new variations of medications that impact serotonin receptors and may be useful for diarrhea and constipation. New drugs focused on partially blocking opiate receptors have emerged as an option for opiate-induced constipation. Additionally, a new class of drugs for constipation, known as secretagogues, has also become available.

While the options have definitely improved over the years, practitioners are advised not to expect miracles, even with the newer drugs, as many people continue to struggle with IBS symptoms, despite taking medications. Please also make note that some of the less innovative and up-to-date practitioners may only have the three A's in their toolbox.

Antibiotics for Diarrhea
Rifaximin (Xifaxan)
This nonabsorbable antibiotic with a broad antimicrobial spectrum has activity against a variety of pathogenic bacteria that can cause diarrhea, inflammation, and bloating, as well as some notable antiparasitic properties. It is an antibiotic that primarily stays in the intestines and does not cause systemic side effects. It can be especially helpful if the IBS-D is caused by SIBO. It may also be helpful for postinfectious IBS, if it's caused by bacteria/parasites within its killing spectrum. The challenge with this medication is that it can cost more than $2,000 for fourteen days and is often not covered by insurance. About 50 percent of people who use it need to repeat another course in six months. I personally believe it works best when combined with other methods for addressing SIBO to produce a complete resolution of symptoms.

Antidepressants
Tricyclic antidepressants (amitriptyline, desipramine)
Tricyclic antidepressants can help to relieve diarrhea due to their anticholinergic effects, as well as modulate visceral hypersensitivity, through their effects on neurotransmitters.

SSRIs
Although not FDA-approved for constipation, some selective serotonin reuptake inhibitors (SSRIs) (sertraline, fluoxetine, citalopram) are sometimes used for this purpose. They work by blocking the reabsorption of serotonin, leaving more serotonin available for cells to use. More serotonin can improve gastrointestinal (GI) motility as well as help reduce

visceral pain and address depression (SSRIs are the most common type of antidepressant).

Newer Serotonin Modulators

Depending on what you do with the serotonin receptors, you can either slow down or speed up the movement of stools.

Alosetron Hydrocholride (Lotronex)

A selective serotonin type-3 antagonist, it is FDA-approved for adult females with severe IBS-D who have failed other therapies. It is contraindicated for people with constipation and other GI conditions such as Crohn's disease and ulcerative colitis. Side effects include pain, nausea, and constipation. Due to concerns of causing ischemic colitis, alosetron was withdrawn as a generally available medication. It is now only available to women with special approval.

Ondansetron (Zofran)

This medication is traditionally used for nausea and vomiting, and while not FDA-approved for IBS, it has a similar mechanism of action to alosetron but with a safer side effect profile, so physicians have started using it off-label for IBS. Ondasetron blocks the action of serotonin, reducing urgency and stool frequency in severe diarrhea. Studies have shown it can shorten diarrhea from viral gastroenteritis as well, so it can be a very helpful tool.

Antispasmodics

Antispasmodics are typically prescribed for all IBS types relating to abdominal pain and cramping, but they are predominantly used for diarrhea, as they can cause constipation as a side effect. The antispasmodics that are available in the United States include hyoscyamine (Levbid, Levsin, Anaspaz, NuLev), and dicyclomine (Bentyl). These act as smooth muscle relaxants and work to increase colon transit time, reduce stool frequency, and improve stool consistency. They are useful for abdominal pain, as they mediate smooth muscle contraction. Unfortunately, they have anticholinergic activity, which can cause dry mouth, dry eyes/blurry vision, urinary retention, and constipation. Hyoscyamine was the drug I was prescribed many years ago (and the one I stopped due to all of the side effects!).

Drotaverine: Antispasmodic Without Anticholinergic Effects

Drotaverine is an antispasmodic drug approved to treat symptoms of IBS in the European Union. Like other antispasmodics, it helps reduce smooth muscle spasms in the GI tract. It has been shown to significantly reduce pain frequency and severity in patients with IBS. In a prospective double-blind, randomized placebo-controlled study, eighty patients with IBS were given either drotaverine or a placebo for four weeks. At the end of the study, pain frequency and severity were reduced by 71.4 percent.

Even more impressive, drotaverine does not have anticholinergic activity, and therefore it produces none of the side effects associated with anticholinergic drugs. In fact, no significant adverse effects have been reported in studies, and side effects of drotaverine are classified as rare. Of the antispasmodic drugs, drotaverine would be my first choice and a good reason to visit Europe.

Intestinal Secretagogues

Intestinal secretagogues are a newer class of drugs prescribed for IBS-C that work by increasing the amount of water in the intestines, allowing stool to soften so it becomes easier to pass as well as increasing the transit time of food through the digestive tract. They include linaclotide (Linzess), plecanatide (Trulance), and lubiprostone (Amitiza).

These medications may also relieve intestinal pain and cramping by reducing abdominal muscle contractions. On average, most of them lead to one to two more bowel movements per week. An editorial published in *Gastroenterology* in 2018 suggests linaclotide at 290 mcg per day may be the most effective option, but results may vary among patients.

Tenapanor, the newest secretagogue approved by the Food and Drug Administration in 2019, claims a triple mechanism of action. In addition to increasing water in the gut to support faster transit times and softer stool, like the others, animal studies suggest that tenapanor can also decrease intestinal permeability by improving the function of the tight junctions of the small intestine and reduce visceral hypersensitivity, leading to less pain.

Side effects of the intestinal secretagogues include diarrhea, abdominal pain and distension, gas, diarrhea, nausea, and dehydration.

Opiate Receptor Modulation
Opiate medications such as the painkiller morphine are notorious for inducing constipation and slowing down GI transit, so drug manufacturers have focused on this mechanism of action to modulate gut motility.

Loperamide, an over-the-counter opioid receptor agonist that binds to opiate receptors in the gut, is the go-to for most people with noninfectious diarrhea, but eluxadoline (Vibrezi), a prescription medication that acts on numerous opioid receptors, has recently come to market.

Additionally, *opiate-blocking* medications are available to manage constipation that occurs as a side effect from chronic opiate use.

- *For diarrhea:* Eluxadoline (Vibrezi) acts on opioid receptors to slow down gut motility and can help with abdominal pain and loose stools. It is FDA approved for IBS-D but is considered a controlled substance due to abuse potential and has numerous contraindications and drug interactions.

- *For opiate-induced constipation:* A few medications have been specifically designed for opioid-induced constipation because they are opioid antagonists, meaning they block opiate receptors. The medications include methylnaltrexone bromide (Relistor), naldemedine (Symproic), and naloxegol (Movantik) and are used in patients who take opioid medications for chronic, non-cancer-related pain. The drugs have been created to preferentially block opiate receptors in the gut, but some of the medications can lead to opioid withdrawal symptoms and can cause the opioid medications to be less effective if the opioid blockade goes beyond the gut.

Prescription Medication Options for IBS Available in the United States

NAME	CLASS	INDICATION (May Include "Off-Label" Use)
Alosetron hydrochloride (Lotronex)	Serotonin modulator, selective serotonin type-3 antagonist	IBS-D
Dicyclomine (Bentyl)	Antispasmodic	IBS-D
Eluxadoline (Vibrezi)	Mu- and kappa-opioid receptor agonist and delta-opioid receptor antagonist	IBS-D
Hyoscyamine (Levbid, Levsin, Anaspaz, Nuley)	Antispasmodic	IBS-D
Linaclotide (Linzess)	Intestinal secretagogues	IBS-C
Lubiprostone (Amitiza)	Intestinal secretagogues	IBS-C
Methylnaltrexone bromide (Relistor)	Opioid receptor antagonists	Opioid-induced constipation

NAME	CLASS	INDICATION (May Include "Off-Label" Use)
Naldemedine (Symproic)	Opioid receptor antagonists	Opioid-induced constipation
Naloxegol (Movantik)	Opioid receptor antagonists	Opioid-induced constipation
Ondansetron (Zofran)	Serotonin modulator, selective serotonin type-3 antagonist	IBS-D
Plecanatide (Trulance)	Intestinal secretagogues	IBS-C
Rifaximin (Xifaxan)	Antibiotic	IBS-D
Scopolamine (Buscopan)	Antispasmodic	IBS-D
SSRIs (sertraline, fluoxetine, citalopram)	Antidepressants	IBS-C
Tenapanor (Ibsrela)	Intestinal secretagogues	IBS-C
Tricyclic antidepressants (amitriptyline, desipramine)	Antidepressants	IBS-D

The Takeaway

The diet, lifestyle, and medication suggestions for IBS have come a long way since I was in pharmacy school and I do think some of them may be helpful and effective, but this, of course, depends on the cause of your IBS.

If your IBS is caused by SIBO, you may feel better with rifaximin and a low FODMAP diet. But if your IBS is caused by a pancreatic enzyme deficiency, these tools may be of little use to you, and reducing fatty foods and supplementing with pancreatic enzymes just might do the trick!

Thus, one of the downfalls of the conventional approach is that it doesn't consider individual causes of IBS. We'll dig deeper into the tailored, functional medicine root cause approach in the next chapter!

Chapter Summary

- The conventional medical approach focuses on managing symptoms rather than resolving the underlying root cause.

- Typical IBS treatments can be a good starting place for symptom relief while you search for the root cause, but know there are more answers if these treatments have failed you.

Visit https://ibsrootcause.com/bonus for notes on this chapter.

CHAPTER 3

What's Really Going On and How the Root Cause Approach Can Help

Conventional medicine has made headway since I was initially diagnosed with IBS, but it is still light-years behind the insight of medical researchers and root cause practitioners. For over ten years I have been aware of most of the causes of IBS I am sharing in these pages, and the body of evidence keeps growing in the medical journals, yet the average patient isn't going to get most of this information from their pharmacist or doctor.

Emerging research and clinical experiences of functional medicine practitioners are showing that irritable bowel syndrome is not a condition you are stuck with forever and ever, and it's not a chronic condition that needs long-term treatment with prescription medications. Rather, it is a set of symptoms with various underlying root causes that can be addressed and resolved.

I first became fascinated with getting to the root cause when I was working in public health as part of a government-sponsored project to improve health outcomes for people with chronic health conditions, by focusing on health care systems. I was trained in root cause analysis, a method that helps to differentiate symptoms from causes. We know that focusing on symptoms can help temporarily but feel a bit like a game of Whac-A-Mole, while focusing on root causes can solve the problem and prevent it from recurring.

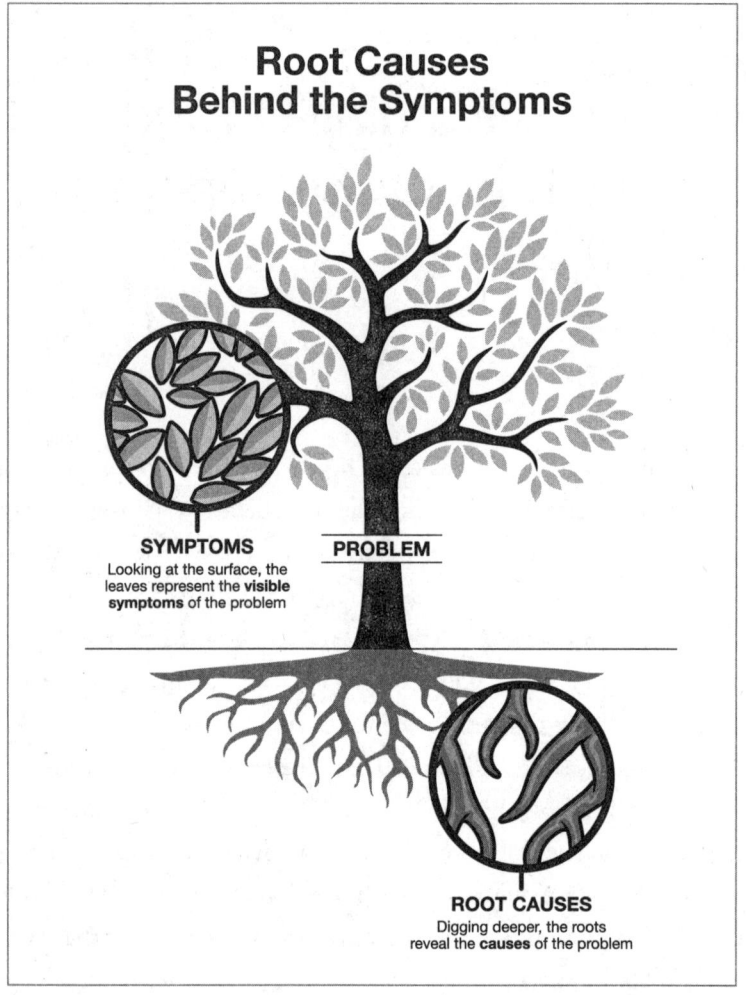

Image inspired by art in Lari Numminen, "What Is Root Cause Analysis?," Workfellow, https://www.workfellow.ai/learn/what-is-root-cause-analysis

While I was initially trained in root cause methods to improve health care systems, I found the methods are just as effective at promoting long-lasting improvements in human bodies. The root cause approach helped me get my own Hashimoto's and IBS into remission and I was excited to find a newly emerging branch of medicine called functional medicine that also focused on root causes.

Functional medicine practitioners focus on why a person developed a particular condition, what they can do to reverse the condition, and/or how to prevent its progression.

Investigating to figure out what's really going on to cause symptoms can take a lot more time (certainly more than a typical ten-to-fifteen-minute doctor's office visit) and requires a more rigorous review of medical histories, additional lab testing, and more ongoing support. However, it does get results. In my clinical experience, about 80 percent of people diagnosed with IBS will find a resolution to their symptoms by following the root cause approach.

In this chapter, you'll discover why the root cause approach is necessary to treat IBS, the potential root causes for your symptoms, and how to become a root cause detective and find the source of your individual IBS.

Discovering Root Causes

There are various root causes to IBS, and some people may present with more than one root cause. Complicated cases are often described as peeling back multiple layers of an onion. Many researchers and innovators have advanced our understanding of potential root causes. These are just a few I would love to highlight:

Dr. Mark Pimentel is one of the leading researchers in the field of IBS and SIBO (small intestinal bacterial overgrowth). He was the first to demonstrate a strong link between SIBO and IBS, particularly IBS with diarrhea (IBS-D), shifting the understanding of IBS from a purely functional disorder to one with a microbial and motility-related root cause. Dr. Pimentel developed breath-testing protocols for diagnosing SIBO, pioneered the use of rifaximin as a targeted antibiotic treatment, and helped identify methane-producing archaea (now called IMO) as a cause of constipation-predominant IBS. His research has transformed how we diagnose and treat chronic bloating, diarrhea, and constipation by focusing on underlying bacterial imbalances in the small intestine.

CONVENTIONAL APPROACH	ROOT CAUSE APPROACH
Focused on trying to answer the question "*What* condition does a person have?"	Focused on trying to answer the question "*Why* did this person develop a particular condition, and how can we intervene?"
IBS diagnosis is based on medical history and self-reported symptoms according to the Rome IV diagnostic criteria.	IBS is an umbrella term for a cluster of symptoms with various root causes that can be identified and treated.
Lab testing is not required for a diagnosis and generally not deemed necessary. Potential for misdiagnosis is high.	Targeted testing and sometimes protocol trials in addition to a person's symptoms can identify potential root causes.
Treatment involves chronic symptom management with medications and sometimes diet.	Seeks to resolve symptoms by treating the body as a whole integrated system, providing protocols targeted to address each unique root cause and support complete digestive system health.
Band-Aid approaches mean IBS symptoms can persist and progress, allowing for immune system imbalances and potential progression to autoimmune conditions.	Treatments address the underlying root cause of IBS symptoms, helping to restore gut and immune system balance.

Dr. Saad Habba identified that 98 percent of 303 patients with IBS-D actually had treatable causes behind the diarrhea, such as celiac disease, non-celiac gluten intolerance (sensitivity to gluten but not having celiac disease), carbohydrate intolerance, and bile-acid-induced diarrhea. He discovered a syndrome he coined as Habba syndrome (now called bile acid malabsorption), which connects some cases of chronic diarrhea to too much bile in the intestines due to gallbladder dysfunction. Using low-cost, generic prescription drugs that reabsorb bile, he is able to see symptom resolution for most of his patients.

These two innovative gastroenterologists have helped to raise awareness about two very important causes of IBS. However, there are so many other potential causes. I get excited about finding the causes, because when we find the right cause, the treatment becomes more obvious.

A large review published in 2022 by *Scientific Reports* found that the prevalence of five conditions causing IBS-like symptoms went undiagnosed (misdiagnosed as IBS). Those conditions included pancreatic exocrine insufficiency, SIBO, microscopic colitis, carbohydrate malabsorption, and bile acid diarrhea.

Dr. Benjamin I. Brown published an article in the journal *Gastrointestinal Disorders* focused on even more causes to consider, including stress, circadian rhythm disruption, physical inactivity, lactose intolerance, food sensitivities, non-celiac gluten sensitivity, nickel sensitivity, vitamin D deficiency, low-grade inflammation, intestinal permeability, dysbiosis, and parasitic infections.

Let's take a closer look at some of the most common root causes for IBS symptoms.

While these are causes I see most frequently in my clients, it's important to remember that these aren't the *only* potential root causes. I have done my best to summarize all of the causes I am aware of (either the ones I have personally seen driving IBS and ones I have mostly learned about from research), but there could be other causes as well. Furthermore, while I have done my best in this book to summarize the most helpful healing protocols that I am aware of, there may be others.

Over time, as I've evolved as a functional medical practitioner and additional research has emerged, medical professionals have discovered more root causes, but most people will find that one (or more) of the following root causes is driving their symptoms. Addressing them will significantly reduce and may even completely resolve IBS symptoms.

Genetic Predisposition for Any Number of Physiological Processes Related to Gastrointestinal Function

These include gut motility, pain tolerance, bile acid synthesis, serotonin synthesis and reuptake, emotional and psychological status, neuropeptide signaling (associated with pain), gut microflora makeup, and food allergies, among others. Researchers are still hunting for a genetic connection, but a rare mutation of the SCN5A gene, found in 2 percent of people with IBS, is associated with disruptions in bowel function and abdominal pain. The FUT2 gene has also been associated with lowered amounts of *Bifidobacteria,* which contributes to IBS, and linked to IBD, with studies finding an increased risk of developing Crohn's disease in people with the non-secretor phenotype (about 20 percent of Caucasians). I think genetic information can occasionally be helpful in offering us some actionable insights, but I often say genes are not our destiny, because in most cases of IBS, it's the *gene expression* from environmental factors that leads to illness, not the genes themselves.

Dietary Triggers

My work with Hashimoto's thyroiditis really opened my eyes to the world of dietary triggers on overall health and disease development, as well as the profound effect these can have on digestive symptoms. Studies have found that between 50 and 80 percent of people with IBS identify a particular food as a possible trigger for their symptoms.

Up to 25 percent of people with an IBS diagnosis may actually have celiac disease, but others may react to gluten due to other mechanisms of food reaction. There are different types of food reactions managed by different branches of the immune system. *Food allergies* are often the food reactions that get the most attention due to their life-threatening nature, but most physicians don't test for other types of food reactions that can cause the digestive symptoms associated with IBS, such as food sensitivities and intolerances. Symptoms of food sensitivity/intolerance can mirror those of IBS: diarrhea, constipation, bloating, cramping, acid reflux, stomach pain, burping, nausea, gas, and anxiety. This means food sensitivity alone could be misdiagnosed as the chronic condition of IBS!

Many of my clients have found that removing or limiting reactive foods for a period of time (except in the case of celiac disease, which requires a lifelong removal) resolved many if not most of their IBS symptoms.

Digestive Enzyme Deficiencies

IBS-like symptoms can occur due to a person's inability to digest different food types including protein, fat, and/or starches. This can often be corrected by taking the right digestive enzyme in the correct dose. Some enzyme deficiencies can be uncovered by comprehensive testing, while others are best trialed if symptoms suggest deficiency. Some people may benefit from broad-spectrum enzymes while others from very targeted enzymes.

A retrospective analysis over a ten-year period examined the effect of broad-spectrum enzyme therapy on 104 patients who experienced IBS-like symptoms. Patients were given a broad-spectrum enzyme supplement to take before meals, which contained protease, lipase, amylase, amyloglucosidase, cellulase, hemicellulase, and lactase. Of the 86 patients with follow-up data, 71 of them reported an improvement or elimination of their symptoms. In terms of specific enzymes, researchers have shown 6.1 percent of people diagnosed with IBS-D actually have a deficiency in pancreatic enzymes (this can be measured by a simple fecal test), and pancreatic enzyme therapy may reduce diarrhea and abdominal pain.

Bile Acid Malabsorption

Bile helps to break down fat in the small intestine. If it's inadequately reabsorbed after doing its work, bile can make its way into the colon and trigger diarrhea. Treating bile acid malabsorption may help clear up diarrhea in 30 percent of cases of IBS-D.

Nutrient Depletions

Deficiencies in a few key nutrients related to gut health, such as glutamine, vitamin D, thiamine, carnitine, vitamin A, zinc, and others, may contribute to IBS symptoms. For example, glutamine, zinc, and vitamin A are essential to the integrity of the gut lining, and deficiencies may lead to intestinal permeability, which we know can contribute to the development of IBS. Meanwhile, thiamine deficiency can alter gut microbial composition and can lead to low stomach acid, resulting in SIBO and slowed motility. Carnitine and choline deficiency have also been linked to slowed motility.

A Deficiency of Probiotics, or Good Bacteria, in the Gut Microbiome

A 2020 meta-analysis utilizing the findings from twenty-three studies and some 1,340 participants found people with the IBS diagnosis often have a microbiome pattern characterized by not enough good bacteria and too many bad bacteria and/or yeast in the gut microbiome. The report also concluded that commensal bacteria (such as *Lactobacillus* and *Bifidobacterium*) were found to be deficient and potentially pathogenic bacteria populations (*E. coli* and *Enterobacteriaceae*) increased in people with IBS compared to healthy controls. An imbalance in beneficial bacteria can affect signaling between the gut and brain, which is associated with IBS, and result in altered levels of serotonin, an important neurotransmitter for mood and digestive function that plays a role in gut motility, pain sensitivity, and the amount of fluid in stool, poor digestion of fibrous foods, and intestinal permeability.

Intestinal Permeability

Studies have found that people with IBS are likely to have increased intestinal permeability, though not everyone with IBS will have it. Certain types of IBS are more prone to it, with one study finding that barrier function was most likely compromised in people with IBS-D (37 to 62 percent), followed by post-infectious IBS (17 to 50 percent), and IBS-C (4 to 25 percent).

Intestinal permeability may also be the cause of visceral hypersensitivity.

Intestinal Overgrowth of Bacteria or Yeast, Often in the Small Intestine (Where They Don't Belong)

One 2018 meta-analysis of over fifty studies found one third of IBS patients tested positive for small intestinal bacterial overgrowth, or SIBO. An overgrowth of *Candida,* an opportunistic yeast and member of the fungal family, in the small intestine has been found in about 25 percent of people with previously unexplained GI symptoms, like those associated with IBS.

Gastrointestinal Hypomotility (Also Known as Slowed Gut Motility)

The walls of the intestines are lined with layers of muscle that contract as they move food through your digestive tract (referred to as gut motility). Slow or weaker contractions are associated with low muscle tone in the gut, vagus nerve issues, mitochondrial dysfunction, hypothyroidism, certain medications, and other metabolic conditions such as diabetes and obesity.

Slower gut motility typically leads to constipation, but it can also cause diarrhea along with a host of other IBS-like symptoms, such as abdominal discomfort, bloating, flatulence, and nausea. A slower transit time has been shown to result in lower numbers of bacteria that produce the beneficial fatty acid butyrate, thereby reducing gut barrier integrity and increasing the risk for pathogen infections.

Hypomotility has been shown to resolve with mitochondrial and vagus nerve support and prokinetics to increase transit time.

Infections

Chronic infections are an overlooked source of intestinal permeability and IBS-like symptoms, and identifying and treating them correctly can have a tremendous impact on how you feel. While conventional medicine practitioners believe these infections are self-limiting and refer to this phenomenon as post-infectious IBS or PI-IBS, I have seen many persistent cases, sometimes lasting many months or even years after an initial infection. These include viral, bacterial, and protozoal infections, which have been found to be a strong risk factor for developing IBS, with exposed individuals 4.2 times more likely to develop PI-IBS within twelve months after infection. *Borrelia burgdorferi,* the bacteria that causes Lyme disease, is one potential trigger for IBS, while one long-term population-based study found people with a *Helicobacter pylori* bacterial infection were nearly three times more likely to develop IBS than those who had not been infected.

Additionally, several studies have found a higher rate of parasitic infection in people with IBS. In one study, 30 percent of participants with IBS had at least one intestinal parasite. The most common include:

- *Blastocystis hominis,* a protozoa found in 13 to 73 percent of people with IBS (studies vary), in particular diarrhea-predominant IBS.
- *Giardia,* found in 5 to 10 percent of those with IBS. Individuals infected with *Giardia* are more likely to have a subsequent IBS diagnosis.
- *Dientoamoeba fragilis,* which a 2010 study found in up to

4 percent of people with IBS and suggested those infected with *D. fragilis* may be "misdiagnosed" with IBS.

As parasite detection methods are not 100 percent reliable (and can give many false negatives), these rates could be even higher. Proper treatment of these unwanted guests resolves IBS symptoms in most cases!

Alterations in Stress Hormones

While most people with common sense can connect stress to IBS, researchers have explained how this happens. A 2008 study by Lutgendorff and colleagues highlighted that stress reduces beneficial bacteria in the gut and allows pathogenic bacteria to proliferate. Intestinal bacteria have an ability to sense a stressed host and upregulate their virulence.

Thyroid Imbalances and Autoimmunity

A dysregulation of thyroid hormones can lead to digestive distress and is a very common finding in IBS, with one study determining 18.5 percent of people with IBS have some degree of thyroid dysfunction, with subclinical hypothyroidism accounting for 15 percent. Hypothyroidism causes a slowing down in the digestive process, often resulting in constipation. On the other hand, hyperthyroidism (having an overactive thyroid gland) can lead to diarrhea. That being said, autoimmune hypothyroidism is associated with an autoimmune attack against the thyroid, resulting in fluctuating thyroid hormone levels. Some people may initially experience a surge in thyroid hormone levels during the early stages of the autoimmune attack, followed by low levels of thyroid hormone, resulting in fluctuating GI symptoms. Thyroid disorders are considered a differential diagnosis of IBS, yet despite their common co-occurrence and potential to cause IBS symptoms, they are rarely tested for by conventional doctors.

When Was the Last Time You Felt Well?

This is a common question I ask my clients, and if the answer is that they felt well until they developed a bout of "food poisoning," I often expect to find a lingering infection as the cause. One gentleman I worked with who was in his fifties recalled that his symptoms started after a bout of diarrhea while traveling the world in his twenties. A comprehensive test for parasites showed that the likely culprit, a protozoan parasitic infection, was still lingering thirty years later.

Post-infectious IBS (PI-IBS) has been described as a variant of IBS that develops after a severe bout of gastroenteritis, caused by bacteria, parasites, or a virus. Conventional practitioners typically attribute this to long-lasting changes in the gut microbiome after the infection clears. However, functional medicine testing often reveals that many infections persist, continuing to fuel IBS symptoms. Research shows a fourfold increase in IBS risk after infectious enteritis, especially from bacteria and parasites. While conventional medicine tends to *assume* that these infections clear on their own or with a short course of antimicrobials, lingering infections are a common culprit in my experience and, unfortunately, standard tests often miss them. And we all know that "assume" is spelled "A-S-S-U-M-E!"

Inflammation

Although the extent of the inflammation is not as severe as in cases of IBD, people with IBS have been found to have markers indicating higher levels of chronic, low-grade inflammation compared to healthy controls.

Inflammatory Bowel Disease

IBS and IBD share several of the same symptoms, and there are many instances when IBD is missed. According to some studies, as many as

10 percent of people with IBD may be misdiagnosed with IBS, and IBD patients were three times more likely to have had a previous diagnosis or treatment for IBS. Getting a proper diagnosis and addressing IBD with a treatment plan may be the path to healing.

Toxins and Chemical Triggers
We are exposed to countless toxic substances on a daily basis through the foods we eat, the air we breathe, and the products we apply to our skin. They can disrupt the microbiome and cause widespread inflammation, including in the gut.

While it is impossible to remove all toxins from our lives, we can significantly reduce our exposure and eliminate a few key ones that could be at the root of IBS symptoms, such as mold and glyphosate, a widely used herbicide.

Medications
Digestive distress is a common symptom of many medications, including NSAIDs, antibiotics, proton pump inhibitors, iron supplements, allergy meds, metformin, opiates, diuretics, oral contraceptives, and many others. More gut-friendly alternatives can be considered.

Western Lifestyle Factors
Stress, alcohol use, dehydration, poor bowel habits, low-fiber diet, lack of exercise, poor sleep habits, and smoking, elements of the so-called Western diet and lifestyle, are associated with a higher prevalence of IBS found in North America.

While it may take some time and experimentation to get to the root of your digestive issues, it is possible. I have seen the root cause approach help so many people take back their health and transform their lives. I wholeheartedly believe it can do the same for you!

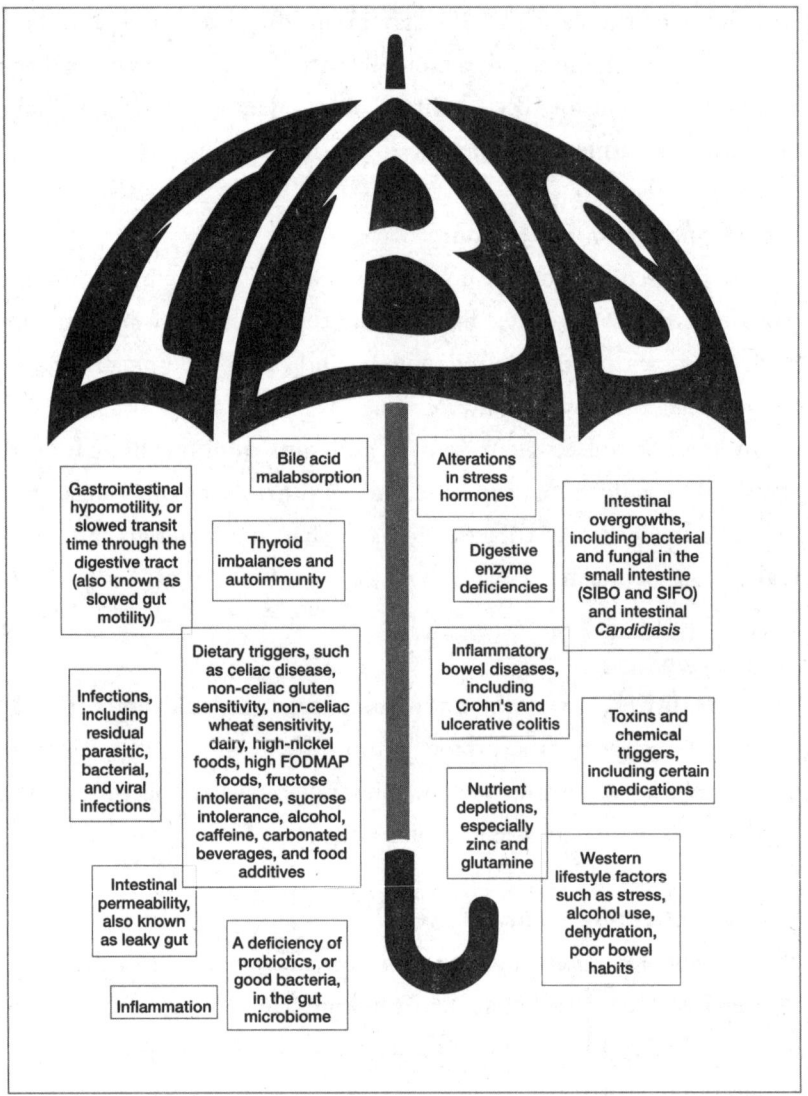

Do Women Have More IBS?

If you've got IBS, there's a good chance you might just be one of the "hot girls" TikTok is talking about! In 2022, women on the platform started opening up about living with IBS, sparking a movement that raised awareness and created a space for women to bond over their digestive struggles. It also helped shatter the age-old taboo: Yes, women poop, too. By May 2022, the TikTok hashtag #IBStiktok had over 62.7 million views, and #hotgirlswithIBS surpassed 11.8 million views. That's a lot of hot girls with IBS!

It's no coincidence that the trend to share about IBS is coming from young women. After all, the prevalence of IBS is twice as common in women as in men, and symptoms most often start in young ladies (teens and early twenties) and are less likely to occur in hot women (sometimes called women over fifty).

Estrogen and progesterone, which have receptors throughout the digestive tract, affect gut function in various ways, influencing symptoms such as bloating, diarrhea, and constipation. Hormonal fluctuations during the menstrual cycle, pregnancy, and perimenopause can also play a significant role in altering gut motility and sensitivity.

- Menstrual cycle and period diarrhea: Many women experience a spike in digestive symptoms like diarrhea during their periods due to a surge in prostaglandins, hormonelike chemicals that cause the uterus (as well as the intestines!) to contract. "Period diarrhea" can occur in both women with and without IBS, though women with IBS may be more sensitive to it. Scientists have noted that women with IBS have an increased perception of pain linked to the decrease in levels of progesterone during their period.

- Pregnancy and constipation: During pregnancy, women are often constipated. This can be due to the rise of progesterone and estrogen levels, which can slow down gut motility. Pressure from a growing uterus on the intestines may also play a role as the baby grows. In contrast, if you feel a relief from your digestive symptoms during pregnancy, please be sure to look into IBD.

- Perimenopause and constipation: As women enter perimenopause, estrogen dominance often emerges, where estrogen levels remain high relative to progesterone. This imbalance can slow down digestion and increase constipation, a common issue starting in a woman's thirties. Estrogen dominance is often exacerbated by factors like gut dysbiosis and poor detoxification, further contributing to IBS symptoms. See page 199 for more info.

Are Salads the Reason Women Have More IBS?

Hear me out on this . . . In Western culture, salads are often seen as a "feminine" choice, and women tend to choose them more frequently, viewing them as a healthy, low-calorie option.

For people with IBS, salads can be tricky. Raw vegetables are harder to digest, and their high insoluble fiber content can irritate the gut, leading to bloating, gas, and diarrhea.

Many salad staples, like onions and cruciferous veggies, are also high in FODMAPs. Additionally, cold foods like salads can slow digestion, causing discomfort, while certain dressings containing gluten, dairy, soy, and food additives may further trigger IBS.

Last but not least, raw vegetables can carry harmful bacteria, making them a potential source of foodborne illness. Prewashed greens and ready-to-eat kits are often linked to outbreaks of *E. coli*, *Salmonella*, and *Listeria*. To minimize symptoms, try incorporating more cooked vegetables and avoiding high FODMAP ingredients in your salads, as well as washing produce thoroughly to prevent infections.

Changeable Factors: Diet, Exercise, and Birth Control

While conventional medicine has focused on the influence of female hormones on digestive function, rest assured, you're not destined to have IBS just because of your hormones.

Certain lifestyle choices can worsen IBS in women. For instance, many women opt for salads, which are culturally considered a "female food" in many Western societies. Salads can be a major digestive trigger, not to mention they carry a higher risk of picking up gut infections. For ways to address digestive triggers and gut infections, see chapters 4 and 10, respectively.

Women are generally more likely to have their ears pierced, increasing the risk of nickel sensitivity, also addressed in chapter 4.

Young women are often more likely to focus on cardio exercises that can deplete glutamine, an amino acid crucial for maintaining gut health. For ways to replenish glutamine, see chapter 6.

Furthermore, women also tend to have a higher exposure to potential toxins. For example, women on average use thirteen personal care products, compared to eleven by men, many of which are endocrine-disrupting substances. Women are also the primary recipients of breast implants, which can lead to breast implant illness. For ways to reduce your toxic exposure, see chapter 14.

External hormones can play a role, too. Most notably, hormonal contraceptives, particularly those containing drospirenone (like Yaz), have been recognized as an IBS trigger. Postmenopausal women who use hormone replacement therapy (HRT) seem to be more likely to develop IBS than women who are not using HRT. For more, see chapter 14.

Root Cause Testing for IBS Symptoms

Depending on what your symptoms might be, you can test for many of the IBS root causes:

- Elevated antibodies associated with gastrointestinal infections, such as food poisoning, which may indicate IBS-D and IBS-M (IBS-Smart) *(optional)*

- Food sensitivities (Alletess Lab 96 IgG Food Sensitivity Panel and Alletess Lab 184 IgG Food Sensitivity Panel)

- Dysbiosis, pathogenic bacteria, and parasites (comprehensive stool analysis tests such as Diagnostic Solutions GI-MAP, Vibrant Wellness Gut Zoomer 3.0, Genova Diagnostics GI Effects, Mosaic Diagnostics Comprehensive Stool Analysis, and Doctor's Data GI360, and targeted microbiome analysis stool tests such as Enbiosis and Viome Gut Intelligence Test)

- Yeast, mold, *Candida* and *Clostridia* metabolites, elevated ammonia, neurotransmitter metabolites, and many other root causes (Mosaic Diagnostics Organic Acids Test [OAT])

- Estrogen metabolism, stress hormones, and other markers of hormone imbalance (Precision Analytical DUTCH Complete)

- Parasites (comprehensive stool analysis tests such as Diagnostic Solutions GI-MAP, Vibrant Wellness Gut Zoomer 3.0, Genova Diagnostics GI Effects, Mosaic Diagnostics Comprehensive Stool Analysis, and Doctor's Data GI360, ParaWellness Research Comprehensive Parasite Stool Test, and Ova and Parasite x3 Test)

- SIBO (Genova Diagnostics 3-Hour Lactulose Kit, Gemelli Biotech Trio-Smart SIBO breath test, Commonwealth Diagnostics SIBO and IMO test)

- Mycotoxins (Mosaic Diagnostics Organic Acids Test [OAT], Mosaic Diagnostics MycoTOX Profile, RealTime Laboratories Mycotoxin Panel, Vibrant Wellness Mycotoxins Test, and comprehensive stool analysis) *(optional)*

- Glyphosate (Mosaic Diagnostics Glyphosate Test) *(optional)*

- Thyroid hormones (Full thyroid panel, which includes not only TSH and T4, but also T3, and the two most common Hashimoto's antibodies, TPO and TG antibodies)

How to Get Started as a Root Cause Detective

To find the root of your IBS-like symptoms and the types of changes that will help you feel better, you must DIG AT IT. The acronym stands for the common root causes plus additional strategies for easing top symptoms:

D: Dietary triggers, Digestion and Digestive Enzymes, Depletions, Deficiency of beneficial bacteria
I: Intestinal permeability, Intestinal overgrowth
G: Gut infections

A: Alterations in stress hormones
T: Thyroid hormones and autoimmunity

I: Inflammation and IBD
T: Toxins and chemical triggers

The chapters in Part II of *IBS: Finding and Treating the Root Cause* will explain all of the above root causes in detail, providing a research-backed explanation of how they contribute to IBS-like symptoms and how we know those symptoms can be reduced or resolved by addressing them. For each root cause, I'll share information to help you determine if it could be a factor in your situation and what to do about it if you think it is. You'll discover:

- how to determine if the root cause could apply to you based on your symptoms
- testing options to consider (many of which can be self-ordered)
- a plan for treatment including conventional and natural treatment options (nutrition, supplements, and lifestyle changes)
- details for how to manage in the long term

As you read the following chapters, pay attention to the root causes that resonate with you based on the clues from your symptoms and personal health history. Keep track of the interventions you try and how they impact your well-being alongside your symptoms. Create a health journal or use any physical notebook or digital journal that works for you. You will see improvement with each root cause you address!

I know root cause detective work can feel overwhelming, given that many people may have more than one root cause for their IBS symptoms as well as potentially multiple layers to peel away and consider. The best thing you can do is to just start.

Tackle one thing at a time.

My recommendation is to start by addressing dietary triggers with an elimination diet focused on commonly reactive foods. You may find that this one simple step quickly resolves one or more symptoms. (Yes, I know not eating a favorite food may not be *easy*, but if it relieves your symptoms, won't it be worth it?)

If eliminating common reactive foods doesn't help, take another step. The best thing you can do is keep moving forward. Addressing one root cause may even help with another. For example, you may treat an underlying *H. pylori* infection and find it also helps to resolve your SIBO. Or you may restore a healthy gut microbiome and find you no longer have as many food sensitivities. So while there are many potential root causes, I do want to point out that we may not always need to find every single one to feel better. Sometimes just taking one small step can make a world of a difference.

It can take some time and experimenting to dig at it, but this approach will help reverse the IBS symptoms you've been hoping to get rid of for so long. That said, please don't abandon your conventional medical therapy, prescriptions, or doctor without consulting with a new health care provider first and ensuring you have continued care and guidance. If you have Hashimoto's and choose to begin any lifestyle changes to address IBS symptoms, especially supplementation, I encourage you to work with your doctor to monitor your thyroid symptoms, thyroid hormones, and thyroid antibodies.

I am excited for you to turn the page and discover a diet or lifestyle change that helps you start feeling like yourself again!

Choosing Supplements

As part of the treatment options for each root cause, I often include supplement suggestions. Supplements can be a powerful tool for healing.

But it is important to keep in mind that not all supplements are created equal. As a pharmacist, I can share that many supplements are ineffective and some are downright unsafe. Most supplements do not undergo the same scrutiny and testing that pharmaceutical products do, as many of the quality tests required of pharmaceutical companies are "voluntary" for supplement companies. For this reason, most supplement companies do not take the extra steps to test their products to ensure safety and purity.

Evaluating the safety, efficacy, and cost of various treatments was a large part of my training as a pharmacist. I have put my training to good use, evaluating the best supplement brands and developing my own supplement line, Rootcology. The name "Rootcology" is derived from a blend of my two passions and areas of expertise, root causes and pharmacology: root—going after the root cause of disease—and cology (as in "pharmacology"), understanding how tiny amounts of substances affect the human body.

Rootcology is dedicated to creating innovative, bioavailable products made with the greatest care and with the highest-quality ingredients available. All of the supplement ingredients have been carefully chosen by yours truly, and all Rootcology supplements are gluten free, dairy free, pesticide free, toxin free, pharmaceutical grade, and free from potentially harmful fillers.

Furthermore, all Rootcology supplements undergo third-party testing to ensure that the ingredients on the label are safe, are effective, and match what's actually inside the bottle. I created Rootcology to give you a trusted source of supplements that are safe and effective for people with multiple sensitivities and chronic health conditions.

In addition to Rootcology, high-quality supplement brands include Pure Encapsulations, NutriDyn, Integrative Therapeutics, Klaire Labs, Allergy Research Group, Metagenics, Designs for Health, Thorne, Jarrow Formulas, NOW Foods, Biotics Research, and Xymogen.

Throughout this book, you'll find the supplements I recommend as well as the specific brands, my own and others', to use. I hope this information is helpful on your journey!

The Takeaway

IBS is not a chronic condition that needs long-term treatment with prescription medications, rather it is a set of symptoms with underlying root causes that can be addressed and resolved. To find those underlying root causes, we need to DIG AT IT, one step at a time.

Chapter Summary

- The root cause approach and the testing and treatment recommendations in this book can help you identify and address the causes driving your symptoms.

- Common root causes include dietary triggers, digestive enzyme depletions, nutrient depletions, a deficiency of probiotics, and gut infections and overgrowths.

- Going through the list of root cause factors, testing for confirmation, and incorporating the solutions mentioned can improve and eliminate IBS-related symptoms. The root cause approach can help you heal and take your life back!

Visit https://ibsrootcause.com/bonus for notes on this chapter.

PART II

The Root Causes

CHAPTER 4

Dietary Triggers

If you've dealt with IBS for some time, you may have noticed that food has an impact, but when trying to track down what might be causing your digestive symptoms, you might find conflicting information. Is it gluten, dairy, or soy? Spicy food or sugar? Red meat? Alcohol or caffeine? High-histamine foods, high-fat foods, or certain carbohydrates known as FODMAPs? Carbonated beverages, fructose, or yeasty beers? Processed foods or raw foods? High-fiber fruits and vegetables? Artificial sweeteners like erythritol and mannitol?

As many as 84 percent of people with IBS report that food triggers do indeed play a role in their digestive symptoms. When I began to look into food triggers as a potential root cause, I found getting off gluten and dairy were big game changers for my IBS and acid reflux, so when I first started working to advise people on their health, I thought everyone's digestive symptoms were caused by those two foods... And of course, I was surprised that some people continued to be symptomatic despite removing gluten and dairy.

In recent years, the low FODMAP diet has become a popular recommendation for treating the symptoms of IBS, with studies reporting improvement. But for all of the people who feel better with this approach, there are many others who don't! Meanwhile, more fiber is often a mainstream recommendation for IBS, yet some people find that it triggers IBS symptoms. So, then, what is the right IBS diet?

Spoiler alert: There isn't just one!

Remember, IBS is an umbrella term for digestive symptoms that may have various origins. We might see some improvement with general digestive health-promoting strategies, but if we want a full resolution of symptoms, we need to determine the cause so we can tailor the approach.

Digestive symptoms could be caused by infections, celiac disease, gut dysbiosis, food intolerance, nutrient deficiencies, and digestive enzyme deficiencies, among other things! Some people may have more than one cause, and oftentimes the underlying cause may lead to issues with specific foods.

There are various types of reactions one can have to foods. Some of them can be immune-mediated and others are not, but all of them can cause the minor to severe chronic gastrointestinal distress associated with IBS.

In other instances, foods such as caffeine, alcohol, carbonated beverages, spicy foods, and fatty foods can trigger symptoms by irritating the digestive tract, and fiber may be an issue if the gut microbiome is out of balance.

Regardless of the cause of IBS, most people will find that eliminating reactive foods will lessen or even resolve their IBS symptoms. In my experience, I've found the elimination of triggering foods to be one of the fastest-acting interventions for people with digestive issues. For many, foods can be reintroduced after a period of elimination once the gut is more balanced and has a chance to heal. However, some individuals, including those with celiac disease, will require lifelong removal of the offending food.

In this chapter, we will review the reasons why foods cause reactions, dive into some of the common reactive foods, and cover how to tell if a food is reactive for you. I will also share my helpful protocols for each type of food reaction.

The Main Types of Food Reactions

Studies have found that between 50 and 80 percent of people with IBS identify a particular food as a possible trigger for their IBS symptoms! I think this can actually be higher in real life, as not everyone is aware that a food may be triggering for them.

Reactions to food can be the result of several different mechanisms that occur in the body. We might use terms like "allergies," "sensitivities," "hypersensitivities," or "intolerances" to describe food reactions interchangeably, but they are all unique types of food reactions, and the devil is in the details.

I remember casually telling Craig, a colleague of mine, that doing a blood test with my doctor and removing my reactive foods helped me get rid of the acid reflux and IBS I struggled with for many years, in just three days! Unbeknownst to me, he excitedly made an appointment with an allergist and went through extensive and expensive testing, yet the tests were inconclusive and did not help his symptoms at all. I wish I had been more specific with him as to which exact tests to get, so I want to make sure I make it very clear in this book for you so you don't waste your time and money on irrelevant testing.

While all food reactions can cause similar symptoms, each type is driven by a different mechanism. The mechanism is relevant because it determines which tests and treatment approaches to utilize. So let's get into the details.

Food reactions can be immune-mediated or non-immune-mediated. Food allergies and food sensitivities both result in immune system responses, but they are moderated by different branches of the immune system and cause reactions of different types and intensities.

Type I hypersensitivity reactions, mediated by the IgE branch of the immune system, are known as allergies and are the ones most people think of when first learning about whether foods could trigger symptoms. Peanuts and shellfish that cause people to stop breathing within minutes of ingestion are the most common and life-threatening examples. They are relevant for some but not all people with IBS and have their unique protocols—this is what my colleague Craig tested for without relevance—but there are two additional types of immune-mediated reactions to food that can occur.

Type III hypersensitivity reactions are delayed reactions, known as food sensitivities, and in my experience, they are far more likely to be causative of IBS symptoms than Type I hypersensitivity. They are mediated by the IgG branch of the immune system, and testing for Type III hypersensitivity reactions is what helped me.

Type IV hypersensitivity reactions to foods are also very relevant to IBS and include celiac disease and systemic nickel sensitivity. These are important causes of digestive issues, but they're often missed, and people receive an IBS diagnosis instead of a plan for healing.

(I will spare you the college immunology lesson, but in case you're wondering, Type II hypersensitivity reactions are not related to ingested foods; rather they're related to immune-system mediated cell destruction, blood transfusions, and autoimmune disease.)

In contrast to immune-mediated reactions, food intolerances are non-immune-system-mediated reactions that occur due to poor digestion or absorption of a particular food, often due to digestive enzyme deficiencies. They are often reversible once the correct enzymes are supplemented.

In my experience, other intolerances occur due to a metabolic buildup of a particular metabolite (component) of a food, usually due to a microbial imbalance that can lead to excess production of the metabolite and a depletion of the cofactors needed to break it down. These include histamine intolerance, salicylate intolerance, sulfur intolerance, and oxalate intolerance.

"Mechanical triggers" is a term I coined to describe food reactions that don't seem to be immune mediated or due to any enzyme deficiency or metabolic buildup to my knowledge (perhaps further studies will reveal otherwise), but they do seem to be irritating to the average IBS gut, potentially by causing intestinal permeability. Food additives, alcohol, caffeine, carbonated beverages, citrus, spicy foods, and caffeine fall into this category.

How to Determine Which Foods Are Triggering Your IBS

If you already know the foods that are reactive for you, that's great! Hopefully the strategies in this book will help you become less reactive when possible. If not, here are some ideas on how to determine your food reactions.

If we were living in a perfect world, where everyone had access to the best testing, private chefs, and limitless resources, I would recommend comprehensive testing, as well as a comprehensive elimination diet.

Following an Elimination Diet

An elimination diet focuses on eliminating one or more potentially reactive foods (such as gluten, dairy, and soy) at a time, and observing whether your symptoms have improved. It's recommended to follow the diet for at least three weeks, and benefits can often be seen in just a few days. Elimination diets that are helpful for uncovering dietary triggers of IBS symptoms include the gluten-free diet, the dairy-free diet, the soy-free diet, the low FODMAP diet, the additive-free diet, grain-free diets (Paleo, Autoimmune Paleo), the low-nickel diet, the low-histamine diet, the low-oxalate diet, and the low-salicylate diet.

One of the most popular recommendations for IBS at the time of writing this book is to eliminate high FODMAP foods, and indeed this approach can be very helpful for people with SIBO-induced IBS, helping 50 to 86 percent of people with abdominal pain, bloating, and flatulence, depending on the study. Please note that a low FODMAP diet should not be a stand-alone SIBO treatment (see chapter 9) and should not be used long term.

According to Dr. Liz Lipski, author of *Digestive Wellness*, a one-year elimination diet of seven foods—wheat, corn, dairy, coffee, tea, citrus, and chocolate—resulted in an 88 percent reduction of bloating/distension, 90 percent reduction of colic, 85 percent reduction of diarrhea, and 54 percent reduction of constipation.

In my experience, I have found that a simple elimination diet is a great place to start for many people, and I tend to focus on common reactive foods including gluten, dairy, soy, corn, sugar, spicy foods, alcohol, and caffeine. Over the course of three to four weeks this diet helps 70 to 80 percent of people with digestive symptoms.

If you suspect that food additives are an issue for you, focus on a nutrient-dense diet of whole foods, be more mindful of the ingredients in foods, and practice moderation when it comes to your favorite sweet treats and packaged foods. The negative effects of many food additives kick in at higher doses.

Some people who start with the elimination of just one or two foods (gluten, dairy, and soy being the most likely suspects) find all of their digestive symptoms resolve and they decide not to reintroduce these foods into their diet. If this is you, know that you don't have to reintroduce foods if you don't want to. Your body, your choice!

Are There Tests to Help Us Figure Out Whether a Food Is Reactive?

Tests can uncover various reactions to foods and, in some cases, may provide more guidance than the elimination diet.

For example, a celiac disease test can reveal whether a person should avoid gluten lifelong or just temporarily, and a test for nickel sensitivity may reveal that the person may need to minimize nickel exposure not just in food but also in their daily routine.

IgE tests can offer additional protocols and alternatives to food elimination in the case of atopy, while an Organic Acids Test (OAT) may point to metabolic buildups. Additionally, some people may have a difficult time doing an elimination diet, or they may find that the elimination diet misses some foods that may not be "the usual suspects." Randomly, pineapple turned out to be a trigger food for me on a food sensitivity test, and I would have never thought to eliminate it from my diet! For me personally, IgG food sensitivity testing helped me take action. While I had heard that gluten and dairy could be a cause of my symptoms, I needed to see it on paper!

> ### What Causes Reactions to Foods?
>
> Something I learned the hard way when I first discovered reactive foods is that if we're not mindful of the big picture as to why we are reacting to certain foods, we can really get hung up on diet culture. I used to think a food was either good or bad depending on how my body responded. While that may be true on an individual basis for a moment in time (right now, blueberries might be bad *for you* because they trigger your IBS), but that does not mean that food is inherently bad for everyone. It doesn't even mean it will always be bad for you. Restoring proper digestive function and microbiome balance can make blueberries good for you again in no time!
>
> Food reactions can develop for a variety of reasons, but I have come to believe that a common cause is often a lack of the necessary digestive enzymes to properly break down and digest the foods we frequently consume. Improperly broken-down food particles can lead to intestinal inflammation and even trigger an immune system response.

> Gut infections, deficiencies in nutrients that support proper gastrointestinal function and the breakdown of food metabolites (such as B_6 and glycine), intestinal permeability, intestinal overgrowths, and microbial imbalances in the gut can increase the risk of food reactions.

Will I Have to Avoid Problematic Foods Forever?

I consider the elimination diet or other highly restrictive diet as short-term Band-Aid-like tools to give the digestive system a break from inflammatory reactions rather than a long-term solution. The goal with dietary changes is to heal the gut so we can tolerate as many foods as possible!

As you rebalance your gut flora, clear out gut infections, and resolve other root causes driving your symptoms, you will be able to reintroduce most foods. Depending on how many foods you are sensitive to and how damaged your gut is when you begin eliminating foods, the amount of time you'll need to wait before reintroducing those foods will vary. Everyone starts from a different place, and your own timeline may be different from the next person's.

Food elimination is such an important part of healing IBS symptoms and I hope you will take this important step after identifying your reactive food. My hope for you is also to be able to reintroduce most foods so that you can live a healthy and balanced life!

Common Food Triggers

Now that we've covered the pathways to reactivity, let's dive into the common reactive foods. It's important to note that one food may have multiple pathways by which it can cause a reaction. For example, people may react to gluten found in wheat due to celiac disease or due to non-celiac gluten sensitivity. It's also important to note that while there are some patterns, food reactions may vary depending on a person's health status and even their geographical location.

In an observational study of 197 U.S. adults with self-reported food intolerances, 59 identified a lactose intolerance, 61 reported intolerances to a non-lactose food, and 77 had both a lactose and a food intolerance. Lactose was the most common food trigger, followed by wheat and eggs. The most commonly reported digestive symptoms were gas, abdominal pain, and diarrhea. For most, symptoms occur within minutes of ingesting the food, and the symptoms lasted for hours.

In my work with people with Hashimoto's, primarily based in the United States and Europe, I've identified gluten, dairy, soy, and eggs as some of the most common food sensitivities based on food sensitivity testing. Oftentimes, this is because they're more difficult to digest, but I believe also because they're a mainstay of the Western diet.

In my experience with people with IBS and IBD, I have found similar patterns, as well as, surprisingly, a higher propensity for reactions to raw and fibrous vegetables and fruit. I seriously would not have believed salad and blueberries could cause such distress as they do in some people with IBD and IBS until I did a deep dive into the mechanism of action behind this.

I've also found that fatty foods, caffeine, alcohol, and food additives can be major triggers for some. I haven't found many research studies that fully support my observations. Many of the studies are over twenty years old, and some are inconclusive. For example, one study suggested that soy would be beneficial for people with IBS, while others suggest it could be a problem. For me personally, soy lecithin was a *huge* IBS trigger. According to Liz Lipski, PhD, CCN, IFM educator, and the author of *Digestive Wellness*, the most common foods that trigger IBS are wheat, corn, dairy, coffee, tea, citrus, and chocolate.

While looking at studies of food allergies, sensitivities, and intolerances, I've come to the conclusion that we often become sensitive to what we eat the most. It's interesting that I don't think I have ever seen a case of someone reacting to mango or celery in the United States, yet they're common allergens in China and parts of Europe, respectively.

This is why personalization through elimination diets and targeted testing (vs. avoiding the food your friend from Philadelphia said helped her) seems to produce better results in most people with IBS.

Let's review some of the most common reactive foods in IBS (according to my observations and the published research), the reasons why they might cause issues in an individual, how to tell which foods trigger you, and what you can do about it.

Gluten and Wheat

Wheat bread has been called "the staff of life" because it's such a prevalent food in many cultures. Unfortunately, this common staple is also the most common trigger for digestive distress in people with IBS. People can have reactions to various components of wheat, including gluten, and there are multiple proposed mechanisms and reasons why one may react to wheat-based products.

Gluten is a protein found in wheat, barley, and rye—it's found in bread, cereals, and pasta, but also hidden in many processed foods, medications, and even personal care products. It's made up of several proteins, with gliadin being the main culprit behind the immune reactions seen in celiac disease, which can be the root cause of IBS in up to 25 percent of cases.

Celiac Disease

Celiac disease is the most severe form of gluten sensitivity, affecting those with IBS four times more often compared to the general population. Celiac disease has earned the nickname "the great imitator" due to its wide range of symptoms, from anemia to infertility, digestive issues, and other autoimmune conditions, and it is often misdiagnosed as IBS.

When someone with celiac disease consumes gluten, their immune system attacks the gut lining, destroying the villi—tiny projections that absorb nutrients. This damage leads to malnutrition and digestive issues and creates opportunities for pathogenic bacteria to thrive, perpetuating inflammation. Gluten also triggers zonulin, a protein that opens up the tight junctions in the gut lining, leading to intestinal permeability ("leaky gut"), allowing toxins and microbes to leak into the bloodstream, fueling the immune response.

If untreated, celiac disease can have serious long-term effects. That's why it's crucial to rule it out when diagnosing IBS. Unfortunately, many doctors still overlook it.

Testing for Celiac Disease

Celiac disease, sometimes called an autoimmune reaction to gluten, may be the cause behind 25 percent of cases of IBS, and I believe that if you have IBS symptoms, getting tested for celiac disease is critical. In people with celiac disease, gluten causes a severe and long-lasting Type IV hypersensitivity reaction, also known as a delayed reaction, that typically occurs forty-eight to seventy-two hours after eating the offending foods. The reaction to eating even a tiny bit of gluten can last for weeks or months. Because it's a delayed and long-lasting reaction, celiac disease is often missed, so testing is very important. It can also inform us as to how intensely we should avoid gluten.

The risk for celiac disease increases if you have a family history of the disease, European ancestry, and/or a personal history of other autoimmune disorders.

However, testing isn't perfect, and many tests require you to be consuming gluten during the testing period for accurate results. Blood tests, such as the tissue transglutaminase IgA (tTG-IgA), deamidated gliadin peptide (DGP), and endomysial antibody (EMA), are commonly used, but a biopsy of the small intestine is the gold standard for diagnosis. Elevated antibodies and inflammation in the gut lining typically confirm celiac disease.

If you've already gone gluten-free, a genetic test for HLA-DQ2 and HLA-DQ8 can indicate celiac disease susceptibility without requiring a gluten challenge. Thirty percent of all people have these genes, and the genes only predict *susceptibility*, not whether the celiac disease is expressed.

What to Do If You Have Celiac Disease

- A strict, lifelong gluten-free diet is the main treatment for celiac disease.

- Gluten can hide in sauces, gravies, beer, soups, salad dressings, processed meats, fried foods, and even some unexpected places like fruit wax, cutting boards, and utensils. Nonfood items such as medications, supplements, and personal care products (like lipstick or shampoo) may also contain gluten, so it's essential to check labels carefully. Even art supplies and rubber gloves can have gluten, making handwashing important to avoid accidental ingestion.

- In some cases, eliminating additional foods may be necessary, as it's common for those with celiac disease to have secondary food sensitivities. For example, damaged villi can cause lactose intolerance, known as secondary lactose intolerance. There's also potential for cross-reactive reactions, where proteins in other foods trigger the same immune response as gluten. Amaranth, egg, sesame, buckwheat, hemp, sorghum, chocolate, millet, soy, coffee, oats, tapioca, corn, potato, teff, dairy proteins, rice, and yeast are potential gluten–cross reactive foods. My book *Hashimoto's Food Pharmacology* contains over one hundred recipes and resources for going gluten-, dairy-, and soy-free!

- Treating gut infections may be required for full symptom resolution. People with celiac disease are at greater risk of gut infections that can perpetuate digestive symptoms, despite eating a gluten-free diet. Pathogenic parasites including *Giardia lamblia, Ancylostoma duodenale, Entamoeba histolytica, Cyclospora cayetanensis, Hymenolepis nana, Cryptosporidium, Cyclospora,* and *Isospora belli* have all been reported to be more common in celiac disease and can be drivers of symptoms. Addressing these triggers is key to feeling 100 percent better. For more, see chapter 10.

- You may also need to consider Systemic Nickel Hypersensitivity as a contributor.

Non-Celiac Gluten Sensitivity (NCGS)

Some people react to gluten without having celiac disease. Known as non-celiac gluten sensitivity (NCGS), this condition causes celiac disease–like symptoms but without the typical antibodies or gut damage. This immune-mediated food sensitivity has been identified and scientifically validated, despite being pooh-poohed as a source of digestive issues by mainstream medicine (though many patients and functional medicine practitioners have been aware of it for many years). Research suggests that about 6 percent of the U.S. population has NCGS, though the real number may be higher.

In one study, 71 percent of people with diarrhea-predominant IBS improved on a gluten-free diet, even without a celiac disease diagnosis. In people with diarrhea-predominant IBS, gluten increases bowel movement frequency and small bowel permeability, and people with IBS who reintroduced gluten after excluding it for four weeks significantly worsened their symptoms within one week.

Testing for NCGS and What to Do If You Have It

While there's no test for NCGS, an elimination diet remains the best way to identify this sensitivity. Trust your body—if gluten triggers symptoms, it's worth avoiding.

Non-Celiac Wheat Sensitivity (NCWS)

The protein gluten isn't the only potential troublemaker when it comes to wheat-based foods. Some people react to alpha-amylase/trypsin inhibitors (ATIs), non-gluten proteins that trigger immune responses and gut inflammation. Modern types of wheat have shown higher ATI inflammatory activity than older variants and may contribute to the rise in non-celiac wheat sensitivity (NCWS), which is estimated to affect up to 10 percent of the population.

Testing for NCWS and What to Do If You Have It

IgG sensitivity testing can identify if wheat is a reactive food for you. In my experience, removing wheat for three to six months while following gut-healing protocols to address underlying triggers that increase the risk of food reactions (gut infections, nutrient deficiencies, intestinal permeability, intestinal overgrowths, dysbiosis) and addressing circulating immune complexes (CICs) can resolve most IgG reactions. For more on IgG testing and next steps, see the box on page 102.

Other Causes of Gluten/Wheat Reactions

Reactions to wheat and gluten can also stem from other factors, such as:

- Nickel sensitivity: Nickel sensitivity, affecting about 8.6 percent of people worldwide, can cause reactions to wheat due its high nickel content.

- Dysbiosis: Leccioli and colleagues have proposed that the root cause of gluten sensitivity may be a decrease in the gut bacteria *Firmicutes* and/or *Bifidobacteria*, which produce the anti-inflammatory, gut-healing, short-chain fatty acid butyrate.

- SIBO and fructan content: Fructan is a fermentable oligosaccharide found in wheat and has been identified as one of the carbohydrates that isn't properly absorbed in the intestines of those with SIBO, one potential cause of IBS.

- Histamine overload: Some people struggle with high intolerance, due to having too much histamine in their body or a poor ability to break it down. Eating foods high in histamine or histidine (a precursor to histamine) can trigger symptoms. Theories suggest wheat can be an issue because it contains histidine and that wheat can trigger the release of histamine from cells.

- Glyphosate content: Because wheat products in the United States are treated with the pesticide glyphosate, and glyphosate exposure can lead to damaged microvilli, decreased enzyme activity, and dysbiosis, some have theorized that it's the glyphosate, not the wheat, that's problematic for our digestion.

While science continues to evolve, I believe we should listen to our bodies, not headlines. If gluten or wheat doesn't agree with you, it's worth paying attention to those signals and making adjustments.

Is It Just American Bread?

Many Americans say they can eat bread in Europe, but not in the United States, leading them to believe that "American wheat" is the problem.

But being somewhere on the gluten intolerance spectrum is not just an American phenomenon. The prevalence of celiac disease in a large sample of the European population (Finland, Germany, Italy, and the UK) was found to be about 1 percent, similar to the rates in

> the United States. Additionally, the prevalence of celiac disease and gluten sensitivity worldwide does seem to be increasing.
>
> Having lived in both the United States and Europe myself and having worked with clients residing in Europe, Asia, Australia, South America, and Africa, I can tell you that people with Hashimoto's thyroiditis, autoimmunity, and IBS tend to feel better when off wheat, regardless of where they live.
>
> However, the experience of being able to tolerate wheat in a foreign country is valid. Wheat proteins vary by region, so the immune system may not immediately recognize foreign proteins as problematic when traveling, creating what I call the "gluten honeymoon phenomenon." You might be able to tolerate wheat abroad for a while (on average, two weeks), but the reaction usually catches up eventually.

Dairy

If ice cream is more pain than pleasure, it may be a sign of dairy sensitivity. Dairy is another common reactive food for people, and it contains a few different elements that may cause reactions, including lactose and the dairy proteins casein and whey. In some cases, people may also react to dairy fats, such as butter and ghee.

Lactose Intolerance

Lactose intolerance can make dairy difficult to digest because of a deficiency in the lactase enzyme, which breaks down the milk sugar lactose, leading to bloating, gas, and diarrhea. Experiencing digestive symptoms soon after consuming dairy products is a very good indication you may be deficient in lactase. Signs and symptoms such as gas, bloating, stomach pain, cramping, and diarrhea usually appear about thirty minutes to two hours after eating lactose-containing foods. Lactose intolerance can increase with age and is very common, affecting up to 65 percent of people worldwide after infancy. Ethnicity matters, too. People of European descent are more likely to retain lactase enzyme activity into adulthood, whereas 70 to 100 percent of people of East Asian descent may be lactose intolerant. Recent research on lactose and IBS concluded that most patients with the initial diagnosis of IBS were actually lactose intolerant.

Testing for Lactose Intolerance
You can test for lactose intolerance with a hydrogen breath test or a glucose blood test, which can be ordered by most doctors.

What to Do If You Have Lactose Intolerance
A lactose-free diet has been found to improve symptoms in a significant proportion of people with IBS. Ways to address IBS symptoms due to lactose intolerance include:

- Eliminating all dairy
- Continuing to eat dairy while supplementing with the lactase enzyme to help with symptoms. Options include Lactaid (caplets and chewables) and Seeking Health lactase drops.
- Eating low-lactose dairy products, lactose-free dairy products, and/or dairy products with added lactase.

If you've already tried lactase supplements but are still experiencing symptoms from dairy products, you may have a reaction to other components of dairy, including the proteins casein and/or whey, which are sadly not digested by lactase. See the entry on whey and casein sensitivity for more guidance.

Lactase deficiency may also occur due to damage of the lactase-producing brush border from any condition that damages the mucosal lining of the small intestine such as SIBO, *Giardia* and other parasitic infections that impact the small intestine, celiac disease, ulcerative colitis, and Crohn's disease.

An imbalance of gut flora may also contribute. Without enough of certain types of bacteria, including *Lactobacillus* and *Bifidobacteria*, the production of lactase and the ability to digest and absorb the lactose contained in dairy products is compromised.

Low-Lactose and Lactose-Free Dairy Products

Low-Lactose Cheeses	Muenster, Camembert, Brie, cheddar (mild and sharp), provolone, Gouda, blue cheese, Parmesan, Swiss
Low-Lactose Yogurt	Greek-style yogurt, especially full fat
Low-Lactose Dairy	Fermented dairy products like kefir
Lactose-Free Milk Options	Green Valley Creamery, Horizon Organic, Organic Valley, Lactaid Milk

Whey and Casein Sensitivity

Beyond lactose, people may react to the proteins in dairy—whey and casein. Unlike lactose intolerance, which is enzyme-related, these sensitivities are immune-mediated. This means that consuming dairy products like milk, cheese, yogurt, or ice cream can trigger digestive issues and inflammation in those who are sensitive. For people with lactose intolerance, avoiding high-lactose foods or using lactase supplements may be enough, but those with protein sensitivities often need to avoid all dairy products, as these proteins are present in almost all forms of dairy, including many protein powders!

Furthermore, once a person becomes sensitized to the dairy proteins in one species of ruminants (usually cows), they may have a cross-reaction to other types of milk (including goat's milk and sheep's milk), because the proteins in goat's and sheep's milk are very similar to cow's milk proteins (with about 60 to 75 percent rate of cross-reactivity).

The one possible exception is camel milk. It does not contain beta-lactalbumin (a certain type of whey protein) and has a different structure of casein compared to cow's milk. One study on those with an allergy to cow's milk found only 18 percent had camel milk cross-reactivity.

Some argue that raw milk is less problematic than pasteurized milk, as pasteurization can alter the structure of dairy proteins, potentially making them more likely to trigger an immune response. This could potentially be true if a person spent their entire life drinking only raw milk. However, most of us have already been sensitized to the pasteurized cow's milk proteins and will likely react to the raw milk dairy proteins.

Testing for Whey and Casein Sensitivity

IgG sensitivity testing can identify if dairy proteins are reactive for you. For more on IgG testing, see the box on page 102.

What to Do If You Have Dairy Sensitivity

Dairy sensitivity is a common trigger for IBS and also a reactive food for up to 80 percent of people with Hashimoto's thyroiditis, so I have a ton of experience with it. A common question I get is "Do we need to be dairy-free forever, or can we reintroduce dairy after some time?"

In my experience, eliminating gut infections, supporting proper digestion, and using systemic enzymes are critical parts of resolving most Type III food sensitivities, but dairy was a reaction that stumped me for the longest time and persisted for me, despite addressing infections and taking systemic and digestive enzymes.

Back in 2018, I started using carnitine and alfalfa together while breastfeeding, as both are supportive nutrients for breastfeeding moms recommended by my son's pediatrician and a lactation consultant (separately). I am not quite sure as to why, but the synergy of these two particular supplements made my dairy sensitivity go away within three days of starting them. I've given those supplements to a few additional guinea pigs and they, too, have reported that their dairy sensitivity resolved! In my personal observations, loss of dairy tolerance is often due to low carnitine or infections (especially *H. pylori* infections).

Another set of clients reported that camel milk helped them eliminate cow milk sensitivities. Yosef Shabo, an Israeli doctor, reported a study of eight children with various levels of food reactions (allergies and sensitivities) to cow's milk dairy. Camel milk was not only well-tolerated by the children, it also appeared to reduce or eliminate their food sensitivities, even to cow's milk! The effects in some of the children were permanent when the camel milk was discontinued; in others, the reactions returned after stopping camel milk.

Interestingly, I wonder if camel milk's high carnitine content and antimicrobial effects against *H. pylori* might be part of the reason why.

IgG Food Sensitivities

Testing

IgG food sensitivities are known as delayed reactions under the category of Type III hypersensitivity reactions. They are notoriously difficult to discover because symptoms can appear over the course of hours or days after eating an offending food! These inflammatory responses cause gastrointestinal distress and IBS-like symptoms but don't trigger the type of intestinal damage found in celiac disease.

With continued consumption of foods we are sensitive to, the body's immune response becomes less specific and more chronic, often leading to systemic inflammation and sensitivity to more and more foods over time. IgG sensitivities are often a forgotten cause of food reactions, yet my experience and research have found that eliminating foods based on IgG antibodies may be effective in reducing IBS symptoms.

In an IgG-guided elimination diet, foods that came up problematic on a blood IgG test are eliminated. A 2021 study found an IgG-food-antibody-guided elimination diet was more effective than the low FODMAP diet for IBS symptoms in women with mixed IBS. Studies comparing the IgG-guided elimination diets to sham diets found the IgG-guided diets to be more effective. The tricky part is that not all IgG tests are created equal.

Let me say this again: Not all IgG food sensitivity tests are created equal. The tests are considered experimental, and they're not standardized, so the methodology between labs can vary greatly. For example, one lab may use cooked foods to do the test, while another one may use raw foods . . . I have reviewed hundreds of food sensitivity tests over the last ten-plus years, and the one company that has produced accurate and reproducible IgG food sensitivity tests results time and time again is Alletess Lab.

Alletess Lab offers various IgG food sensitivity panels, and I most often recommend the 96 or 184 food panel. It tests for common reactive foods in IBS including gluten, dairy proteins, soy, grains, nuts, seeds, and various fruits and vegetables. I like using tests in people who have already eliminated the "usual suspects" but are still symptomatic. Tests have shown that random foods like pineapple, peaches, and ginger can be digestive triggers for some people.

What to Do If You Have IgG Food Reactions

Removing the reactive foods often causes symptom resolution on so many fronts, and it's often the first step, but please don't think the foods causing your IgG reactions are evil and should be banished for all of eternity. In my experience, after a three-to-six-month elimination and some gut healing (ahem, the focus of this book), most IgG reactions go away. I have also come across another way to reduce IgG food sensitivities quickly while working on identifying your triggers and healing: addressing circulating immune complexes (CICs)!

CICs result from IgG antibodies binding to reactive foods. They come together to form a blob that floats around and can be deposited into joints or kidneys, leading to a lot of inflammation. I think of CICs as the equivalent to Wild West sheriffs carrying Wanted posters of outlaws everywhere.

Systemic enzymes, sometimes called proteolytic enzymes, are a type of enzyme taken on an empty stomach that can help break down CICs, leading to less inflammation and fewer reactive foods. I think of systemic enzymes as a cleanup crew that can help lower overall inflammation in the body.

The key thing to remember about these enzymes is that they are not to be taken with food; rather they should be taken on an empty stomach, at least forty-five minutes before a meal, or one and a half hours after a meal. Otherwise, they will get used up in the process of digestion instead of getting into the bloodstream to act on CICs.

Various formulations of proteolytic enzymes are available and may consist of ingredients such as protease, trypsin, chymotrypsin, serratiopeptidase, and/or nattokinase. High-quality options include Rootcology Systemic Enzymes, Wobenzym, Designs for Health Inflammatone, and Pure Encapsulations Systemic Enzyme Complex.

Eggs

In people with IBS, eggs are one of the top three common triggers for symptoms alongside dairy and wheat. One reason is an IgG reaction, but I believe another potential reason is that egg whites are considered histamine liberators, and this may trigger symptoms in some. Sulfur intolerance is another mechanism that may explain why some people react poorly to eggs. Eggs are high in sulfur, and if someone has a sensitivity to it, they may experience excess gas and bloating.

Testing for Egg Sensitivity and What to Do If You Have It

IgG sensitivity testing can identify if eggs are a reactive food for you. In my experience, removing eggs for three to six months while following gut-healing protocols to address underlying triggers that increase the risk of food reactions (gut infections, nutrient deficiencies, intestinal permeability, intestinal overgrowths, dysbiosis) and addressing circulating immune complexes (CICs) can resolve most IgG reactions. For more on IgG testing and next steps, see the box on page 102.

Additionally, you may wish to try my protocol for healing sulfur intolerance (see below) if you react to eggs, garlic, onions, and cruciferous vegetables or sulfur-containing supplements such as N-acetyl cysteine (NAC).

Protocol for Healing Sulfur Intolerance

If you react to eggs, garlic, onions, and cruciferous vegetables or sulfur-containing supplements such as N-acetyl cysteine (NAC), you might have sulfur intolerance due to a metabolic buildup of sulfur caused by SIBO (see chapter 9). In that case, you would need to clear the overgrowth in order to restore your tolerance, but you can also support the processing of "backlogged" sulfur by limiting the intake of sulfur-containing foods and supplements and providing nutrients and cofactors required for proper sulfur metabolism. Generally speaking, people see results in a few days to a few weeks.

- Limit your intake of high-sulfur foods (eggs, garlic, onions, and cruciferous vegetables) and supplements (NAC, alpha-lipoic acid [ALA], bromelain and papain, chlorella, cysteine, dimethyl sulfoxide [DMSO], dimercaptosuccinic acid [DMSA], extracts of sulfur-rich foods, garlic oil, glutathione, methionine, and turmeric) for four weeks.

- Take sulfur cofactor supplements including L-carnitine, butyrate, molybdenum, thiamine, hydroxycobalamin, and B_{12}.

- Boron, dandelion tea, lysine, magnesium citrate, strontium, vitamin E, and zinc may also help.

Soy

In my experience, I've found that soy is one of the most common IgG reactive substances. Soy can be hard to avoid, as it's found not only in foods such as edamame beans, soy milk, tofu, tempeh, miso, and soy sauce, but also in many processed foods and even supplements. Many processed gluten-free products contain soy, as do dairy-free processed foods and vegan foods, which can be one reason why people who go "gluten free" to help digestive symptoms don't always feel better. Ingredients to look out for include soy lecithin, bean curd, hydrolyzed soy protein, soybeans, edamame, natto, okara, yuba, tamari, olestra (Olean), gum arabic, carob, and hydrolyzed vegetable protein.

Testing for Soy Sensitivity and What to Do If You Have It

IgG sensitivity testing can identify if soy is a reactive food for you. In my experience, removing soy for three to six months while following gut-healing protocols to address underlying triggers that increase the risk of food reactions (gut infections, nutrient deficiencies, intestinal permeability, intestinal overgrowths, dysbiosis) and addressing circulating immune complexes (CICs) can resolve most IgG reactions. For more on IgG testing and next steps, see the box on page 102.

What About Food Allergies?

IgE allergies, also known as Type I hypersensitivities, are often labeled as "true allergies," but I prefer not to use this term—it implies that other reactions aren't as real or significant, which isn't true! These reactions are known for being immediate, usually occurring within minutes of consuming a reactive food. Symptoms can range from mild, like an itchy rash (hives), to severe, including throat swelling, shortness of breath, vomiting, dizziness, low blood pressure, or even digestive issues like nausea, diarrhea, cramping, and abdominal pain. In some cases, these reactions can be life-threatening. Peanuts, tree nuts, and shellfish are the most common triggering foods.

Research shows that food allergies can contribute to IBS symptoms when a person also has an atopic condition, such as asthma, eczema, or allergic rhinitis.

IgE Food Allergies Testing

If you have atopy and IBS, it makes sense to do an IgE food allergy test to see which foods are triggering your IBS symptoms via the IgE pathway. However, if you have IBS but don't have any of the conditions associated without atopy, IgE testing won't be particularly useful in pinpointing IBS food triggers. I wish I'd shared that with my friend Craig—he didn't have atopy but spent a lot of time and money on inconclusive allergy tests!

If you have IBS and atopy, seeing an allergist or immunologist for testing can help identify IBS food triggers. Testing options include the classic skin prick test (or what I affectionately call the "itchy back test") and blood tests that look for IgE antibodies specific to certain foods.

What to Do If You Have IgE Food Allergies

Avoidance of allergic foods and desensitization strategies such as immunotherapy are usually the mainstay recommendation for people who have IgE-driven food allergies. Immunotherapy can be a helpful (though very lengthy) road to recovery and involves exposure to tiny, controlled amounts of the allergic food with increasing doses over time. This can take months, sometimes years, and the end goal is for the person to become desensitized to the foods over time, so the immune system will no longer react to them, even when they're eaten in regular amounts.

Immunotherapy is usually done via injections, typically called "allergy shots," but there are three additional types of immunotherapy methods that have recently become more available: oral immunotherapy (OIT); sublingual immunotherapy (SLIT), in which the allergen is taken under the tongue; and epicutaneous immunotherapy (EPIT), when the allergen is applied to the skin.

According to the Cleveland Clinic, up to 80 percent of people see significant improvement in allergy symptoms with allergy shots, but the treatments need to be used for three to five years in order to stick.

The methods of eliminating and desensitizing can work well for all types of IgE-type allergies, but people with IBS-D may find that the oral medication cromolyn sodium provides more rapid results and does not require food abstinence.

In 1995, a group of Italian researchers compared the effects of an elimination diet vs. using oral cromolyn sodium 1,500 mg/day for one month in 428 people with IBS-D and food allergies. They found that the oral cromolyn sodium was more effective for resolving symptoms compared to the elimination diet, especially in people who had positive skin prick tests for food allergies. Cromolyn

> sodium is a mast cell stabilizer typically used for allergies available as a prescription for oral use. Old-school compounding pharmacists and integrative physicians in my circle have known about it for decades, yet for some reason, it's rarely used. Another medication that acts as a mast cell stabilizer and antihistamine, ketotifen, is a potential option for the prevention and treatment of food allergies.

High-Nickel Foods

Some people may react to seemingly random foods, such as wheat, rye, oats, millet, buckwheat, cocoa, chocolate, tea, gelatin, baking powder, soy products, red kidney beans, peas, lentils, peanuts, chickpeas, dried fruits, as well as canned foods and beverages. What do all of these foods have in common? They're high in nickel! A small study compared the rates of nickel hypersensitivity in people with IBS and healthy controls and found that nickel hypersensitivity was present in 40 percent of the IBS group and 17.5 percent of the control group. Interestingly, as many as 20 percent of Europeans have nickel hypersensitivity, and some estimates put it at 30 percent or more of the general population.

Nickel hypersensitivity, also known as nickel allergy or systemic nickel allergy syndrome (SNAS), is a Type IV hypersensitivity reaction that results from an adverse immune response to nickel exposure.

If you've ever heard of nickel allergy, you may associate it with people getting red, burning rashes on their earlobes after wearing a pair of cheap metal earrings, or rashes on their wrists from cheap metal bracelets. However, it doesn't just affect skin. If the tissues of the digestive system come into contact with nickel through certain foods, they can also become inflamed, leading to abdominal pain, heartburn, constipation, diarrhea, gas, and other digestive problems.

Even though nickel sensitivity is widespread and more prevalent in people with IBS, particularly women, many gastroenterologists are unfamiliar with it and not trained to consider it as a potential root cause of digestive symptoms. Innovative health care professionals, such as registered dietitian Suzie Finkel, MS, RD, CDN, are trying to change that by raising awareness of this overlooked condition and how it can mimic some of the symptoms of IBS. "Doctors who treat IBS patients [who are not responding to treatment] need to consider the possibility that they have SNAS and send them for testing," she has said regarding her work. "If they come back positive, simple dietary changes can address it."

Testing for Systemic Nickel Allergy Syndrome (SNAS)
SNAS is a delayed, long-lasting, Type IV hypersensitivity to nickel and often results in gastrointestinal symptoms such as nausea, diarrhea, abdominal pain, and constipation.

Because nickel is present in our soil and water and we can ingest nickel through a number of different foods and even via our cooking utensils, it may be tricky for people to pinpoint offending foods. If you suspect you may be dealing with a nickel hypersensitivity, the MELISA (Memory Lymphocyte Immunostimulation Assay) test is a whole-blood test to detect hypersensitivity to metals, including nickel, mercury, copper, and lead.

Note, while wheat is a high-nickel food, studies suggest that people who have celiac disease and are nonresponsive to a gluten-free diet and those with NCGS and NCWS may also have nickel hypersensitivity.

What to Do If You Have Systemic Nickel Hypersensitivity
Limiting exposure to nickel by eating a low-nickel diet (see the box on page 111) has been found to reduce the number of inflammatory cytokines in sensitive people, thus lowering inflammation overall and helping to ease symptoms.

Limiting your exposure to nickel in other ways may also help. The most common sources of exposure are medical devices (mesh used in hernia repair, surgical clips used in gallbladder surgeries, IUD devices, orthodontic appliances, and dental crowns and bridges), cookware (stainless steel pans), and electronic devices (iPhones, household appliances). Choosing nickel-free stainless steel, bamboo, or wooden cooking utensils and 100 percent ceramic-coated cookware (Xtrema has been shown to not leach any metals) may also help. If your nickel sensitivity is caused by a nickel-containing implant of some sort, removing it could be helpful in resolving your symptoms. A study found that in twenty-eight patients with mesh implants who also presented with symptoms, 68 percent had an improvement and/or resolution of their symptoms within the first month after mesh removal.

Several studies have shown that oral hyposensitization therapy to be helpful in increasing nickel tolerance. A 1998 clinical trial found that 85 percent of nickel-allergic patients experienced a subjective improvement in their skin reactions after undergoing sublingual (under the tongue) oral hyposensitization therapy.

Additionally, nickel can be removed from the body by sweating it out through activities like hot yoga or sauna therapy. Studies have found that certain heavy metals such as nickel are more concentrated in sweat than in urine when they are excreted from the body. Supplementing with cofactors such as vitamin C, zinc, iron, riboflavin, selenium, and vitamin E can also help. Curcumin may also support clearance of various metals from the body, including nickel.

Low-Nickel Diet

Avoiding and/or limiting your intake of foods high in nickel may help reduce the daily total amount of ingested nickel, which in turn may reduce or eliminate nickel-related symptoms and flares. The low-nickel diet eliminates or limits the following: whole wheat, whole grain, rye, oats, soy products, millet, buckwheat, cocoa,

> chocolate, tea, gelatin, baking powder, legumes (peas, lentils, peanuts, red kidney beans, soya beans, chickpeas), dried fruits, canned foods, licorice, spinach, alcoholic beverages (beer, red wine), coffee, shellfish, certain fish species (salmon, mackerel, tuna, herring), certain seeds/nuts (sunflower seeds, linseeds, hazelnuts, marzipan, walnuts), tomato, onion, garlic, raw carrots, lettuce, raspberries, and processed foods.

High-Fiber Foods

In my early work with digestive issues, I was shocked at how one of my client's diarrhea seemed to be flared up by lettuce! And then various clients reported that consuming more fiber, the standard recommendation for IBS, made their symptoms significantly worse! Since that time I have learned that yes, difficulty digesting fibrous foods such as beans, cabbage, lentils, raw vegetables, and fruits is one potential IBS pattern.

While these foods are generally considered to be healthy foods, they can cause digestive distress for some—as many of us learned in elementary school, "Beans, beans, they're good for your heart! The more you eat, the more you fart!"

However, conventional wisdom always recommends more fiber, and in some cases, indeed, consuming more dietary fiber can help both constipation and diarrhea by encouraging regular, well-formed, and easy-to-pass stool.

Because of this, I wondered why so many of my clients were reacting negatively to fiber. In doing more research, I learned that humans don't digest fiber in the same way we digest protein, carbohydrates, and fats because we don't have specific "fiber digestive enzymes"; rather, we get by with a little bit of help from our friends in the gut microbiome.

There are two types of fiber: soluble and insoluble fiber. Soluble fiber—found in beans, oats, peas, apples, and citrus fruits—dissolves in water and is fermented by beneficial gut bacteria, producing gut-supporting fatty acids. A healthy microbiome will do a beautiful job of helping us digest soluble fiber, but dysbiosis (an imbalance in the gut microbiome), SIBO, gut inflammation (including IBD), and/or parasitic infections within our microbiome can make it difficult to properly break it down, leading to gas, bloating, and constipation. In some cases, especially in conditions such as IBD, certain microbes that normally help digest fibers may be lacking, leading to inflammation. Studies show that specific types of fiber, like oligofructose, can trigger inflammatory responses in those missing the right microbes.

Insoluble fiber, which doesn't dissolve and remains unchanged as it moves through the digestive tract, can cause mechanical irritation in sensitive individuals. Found in foods like leafy greens, celery, and bell peppers, this roughage can help with bowel regularity in the right amounts but may also lead to loose stools and diarrhea if consumed excessively. Bloating and abdominal discomfort after consuming vegetables and fruits and undigested plant fibers in stool are the most telltale signs that fibrous foods may be triggering for you. Additional symptoms include hemorrhoids, gas, constipation, acne/skin breakouts, loss of appetite, nausea and vomiting, fever, and fast heartbeat.

FOODS HIGH IN SOLUBLE FIBER	FOODS HIGH IN INSOLUBLE FIBER
Beans (black, lima, kidney)	Beans (black, garbanzo, lentils, split peas)
Brussels sprouts	Artichoke
Broccoli	Cauliflower
Carrots	Green beans
Cauliflower	Potatoes (white and sweet)
Green beans	Carrots
Green leafy vegetables	Apples
Root vegetables (sweet potatoes, turnips)	Apricots
Avocado	Citrus fruit
Pears	Pears
Figs	Strawberries

IBS

FOODS HIGH IN SOLUBLE FIBER	FOODS HIGH IN INSOLUBLE FIBER
Nectarines	Raspberries
Apricots	Nuts (almonds, walnuts)
Apples	Seeds (sunflower, sesame, flax, quinoa)
Guavas	Whole grains
Fruit skins (if well-tolerated)	Whole-wheat flour
Flaxseeds	Wheat bran
Sunflower seeds	Oat bran
Hazelnuts	
Oats	
Barley	

Testing for Fiber Digestion Issues

Stool tests that look at your microbiome, such as the Vibrant Wellness Gut Zoomer 3.0, Enbiosis, and Viome Gut Intelligence Test, may offer clues as to why you have fiber digestive issues. (For more, see chapter 7.)

What to Do If You Have Fiber Digestion Issues

One of the reasons I am so passionate about what I do is because I'm tired of cookie-cutter approaches that suggest "everyone" should eat the same diet (i.e., "more fruits and vegetables")! If you are the person who gets flared up by blueberries, lettuce, raw fruit, and fibrous vegetables, you will likely benefit from a short exclusion of them, diet modifications, and/or targeted digestive enzymes, rather than eating more of them! Please note that in contrast to some well-meaning approaches of using diet for long-term symptom management without further investigation, most exclusions I recommend are temporary to help manage symptoms while addressing the causes.

Cook and purée raw vegetables: The process of cooking and/or puréeing vegetables softens some of the tough fibers, making them more easily absorbed. Enjoy soups and stews and other well-cooked foods. Once these are tolerated, you can try to work your way back to raw vegetables. First, start by adding in some raw, peeled, and puréed vegetables, then progress to raw, peeled fruits and vegetables, and eventually try the raw and unpeeled variety.

Drink smoothies or vegetable juice: By blending or juicing the vegetables we consume, the fibers are broken down or extracted for easier digestion. Be sure to "chew" your smoothies to start the process of digestion.

Consume fermented vegetables: The fermentation process is similar to how the body digests food, so these foods are essentially "predigested" and more readily absorbed.

Fiber digestive enzymes: Supplementing with fiber digestive enzymes can help minimize IBS symptoms by supporting the breakdown of soluble fiber (leaving less food for pathogenic microbes) and reducing IBS flares from insoluble fiber.

Here is a list of key enzymes that can greatly help with the breakdown of fiber:

- Alpha-Galactosidase: This enzyme helps break down galactooligosaccharides (GOS), a type of nonabsorbable fiber found in beans, root vegetables, and some dairy products.
- Beta-Glucanase: This enzyme helps break down beta-glucans, which can be found in a variety of grains like barley and oats, mushrooms, algae, and yeast.
- Phytase: Phytase helps break down phytic acid, found in nuts, seeds, grains, and legumes. Phytic acid can bind iron and zinc and make them unusable.
- Cellulase: Cellulase helps break down cellulose, found in the walls of plant cells.
- Hemicellulase: This enzyme breaks down hemicellulose, a specific form of cellulose.

I formulated Rootcology Broad Spectrum Enzymes specifically to help those who have trouble digesting fiber. Other high-quality brands that contain similar ingredients include Designs for Health Plant Enzyme Digestive Formula and SFI Health Ther-Biotic Vital-Zymes Complete.

Certain bacterial strains such as *Bifidobacteria* are more likely to digest fiber and make beneficial by-products, so a trial of these probiotics may help.

Fructose Intolerance

If fruit turns your tummy into a ticking time bomb, you might have fructose intolerance. Fructose is found in most fruits (especially apples, bananas, figs, grapes, jackfruit, mangoes, pears, and watermelon) and some vegetables (peas, artichokes, asparagus, onion, mushrooms, tomato products, and red peppers) as well as in high-fructose corn syrup, honey, agave, molasses, and coconut sugar. It is everywhere in the modern Western diet, from soda and fruit juices to breads, sauces, and many packaged foods.

Dietary fructose intolerance occurs when cells in the intestine don't absorb fructose as they should, leading to unpleasant digestive symptoms from bacterial fermentation in the large intestine, such as bloating, abdominal pain, gas, and diarrhea. Research suggests that about 22 percent of people with IBS have fructose intolerance, with some studies finding the incidence to be higher, affecting 30 to 40 percent of people with IBS.

There are two main types of fructose intolerance. (1) Hereditary fructose intolerance (HFI) is a rare genetic disorder caused by a deficiency of the enzyme aldolase B, which is necessary for metabolizing fructose in the liver. This condition is usually diagnosed in infancy when fructose-containing foods are introduced, and not usually relevant for people with IBS, but worth mentioning for the sake of completeness. (2) The second type of fructose intolerance is sometimes called fructose malabsorption.

Testing for Fructose Intolerance

Hereditary fructose intolerance (which is rare) can be confirmed by a genetic test, while a fructose breath test is used to measure the amount of methane and hydrogen exhaled after ingesting fructose. High levels may indicate a difficulty digesting fructose.

What to Do If You Have Fructose Intolerance

Because fructose is primarily absorbed in the brush border of the small intestine via the GLUT5 transporter, in many cases, fructose intolerance may be secondary to other issues impacting the brush border of small intestine, such as SIBO, a protozoal infection of the small intestine (such as *Giardia*), celiac disease, and IBD, which can lead to malabsorption in the small intestine. For me, dietary fructose intolerance is a red flag for SIBO or *Giardia*, with one study showing that 26.5 percent of affected people had a *Giardia* infection.

Reducing fructose intake for several weeks can help relieve symptoms. Foods can be reintroduced slowly to determine how much fructose is well tolerated. Additionally, taking the enzyme xylose isomerase, which converts fructose into glucose, while working on resolving small intestinal infections/overgrowths can be helpful.

By taking this enzyme supplement, people with fructose malabsorption can often tolerate higher amounts of fructose, as glucose is more readily absorbed by the small intestine without the need for transporters.

Xylose isomerase (also known as glucose isomerase) is an enzyme that is not normally produced in the small intestine but is produced primarily by certain bacteria in the gut, including *Bacillus coagulans*, which is available as a soil-based probiotic (see chapter 7). Supplementing with the probiotic can be helpful, as well as supplementing with the digestive enzyme directly. Brands containing xylose isomerase include

Omne Diem Fructose Digest and Fructaid. Some FODMAP digestive formulations, such as Microbiome Labs FODMATE Digestive Enzymes, will also contain this enzyme.

Sucrose Intolerance

If sugar makes your stomach feel sour instead of sweet, you may just have sucrose intolerance. Sucrose occurs naturally in some foods and is the main component of table sugar. Any foods containing sugar (as well as maple syrup, beans, lentils, apricots, bananas, grapefruit, apples, cantaloupe, peaches, pineapple, and mango) will contain sucrose. Symptoms of dietary sucrose intolerance have a huge overlap with IBS symptoms and include postprandial cramping, bloating, gas, and diarrhea. Sucrose intolerance is caused by a deficiency of the enzyme sucrase-isomaltase and may be more common than is recognized, with recent studies finding over a third of people with IBS-D may have sucrose intolerance. Reasons for sucrose intolerance include a rare condition known as congenital sucrase-isomaltase deficiency (CSID) and damage to the brush border, which produces carbohydrate-digesting enzymes.

Testing for Sucrose Intolerance

The gold standard test for determining sucrose intolerance is an intestinal biopsy. However, this is a very invasive test. Most doctors will do a sucrose hydrogen breath test. After ingesting 50 grams of sucrose, the breath is measured for hydrogen levels, and if there is a sufficient rise, this may suggest sucrase deficiency.

What to Do If You Have Sucrose Intolerance

In one study, people who tested positive for sucrose intolerance were able to experience a symptom reduction in 60 percent through dietary modifications and/or enzyme replacement.

- Low-sucrose diet: Reducing sucrose intake for several weeks may be helpful in reducing digestive symptoms. Foods can be reintroduced slowly to determine how much sucrose is tolerated.

- Enzyme replacement therapy: Supplementing with sucrase (usually called invertase) may be helpful in alleviating symptoms in cases due to damage to the brush border. I have not seen any stand-alone sucrase/invertase supplements other than liquids used for candy making, which I don't believe should be used. That said, I don't see the harm in using a source of invertase that also contains additional enzymes. Rootcology Broad Spectrum Enzymes, SFI Health Ther-Biotic Vital-Zymes Complete, Pure Encapsulations Digestive Enzymes Ultra, Transformation Enzymes Digest, and SFI Health Ther-Biotic SIBB-Zymes all contain invertase. If you have the genetic condition CSID, there is a prescription enzyme replacement therapy called Sucraid that contains sacrosidase.

High FODMAP Foods

Lactose, fructose, and sucrose are three common sugars that can wreak havoc on the digestive tract, but there are also a few more to consider. FODMAPs are a collection of short-chain carbohydrates (sugars) that occur naturally in a variety of foods. The term "FODMAP" is an acronym for the categories of carbohydrates that have proven to be problematic in some people with IBS (in particular those with SIBO and those with damage to the villi in the small intestine).

- Fermentable: These carbs are fermentable by gut bacteria. Fermentation is the process through which they feed on undigested carbohydrates, converting them to intestinal gases.

- Oligosaccharides: These are soluble plant fibers, or prebiotics, which feed the good bacteria in the gut. They include fructans and GOS (galacto-oligosaccharides or galactans), which can be found in foods such as wheat, rye, onions, garlic, and legumes.

- Disaccharides: Lactose, found in dairy products like milk, soft cheeses, and yogurt.

- Monosaccharides: Fructose, found in honey, high-fructose corn syrups, and many fruits, such as apples and pears.

- Polyols: These are sugar alcohols, such as sorbitol and mannitol, found naturally in some fruits and vegetables and used as artificial sweeteners.

In people with SIBO and certain intestinal disorders, carbohydrates (specifically FODMAPs) aren't properly digested due to a lack of digestive enzymes. Undigested FODMAPs move from the small intestine to the large intestine, where they pull water into the colon, causing diarrhea. Bacteria in both the small and large intestines ferment these FODMAPs, producing gas and other by-products that lead to symptoms like bloating, flatulence, abdominal pain, and altered gut motility (diarrhea or constipation). It's possible to react to one or more of these.

Testing for FODMAP Reactions

A relatively new device called the FoodMarble AIRE is the world's first handheld hydrogen breath testing device you can use at home. There are two versions of this device. One measures hydrogen only, and the other measures both hydrogen and methane, providing instant feedback about your body's reactions to foods. This can help individuals determine which FODMAPs are contributing to fermentation in the gut and triggering their symptoms, so they can modify their diet accordingly.

What to Do If You React to the Remaining FODMAPs

Following the low FODMAP diet can be helpful for symptom management! That said, please note the diet acts more as a Band-Aid if the cause of the SIBO is not addressed. Previous assumptions were that the low FODMAP approach would starve the SIBO bacteria and could be used as treatment for SIBO or after using antimicrobials for SIBO to prevent recurrence, but recent research suggests otherwise; the diet may actually worsen dysbiosis and bacterial diversity. For this reason, the highly restricted FODMAP diet is not a long-term solution but rather a short-term way to manage symptoms while treating SIBO with targeted therapies (see chapter 9).

Additionally, SIBO can lead to digestive enzyme disturbances in the small intestine, the place where carbohydrates are digested, so using digestive enzymes that support the digestion of FODMAP foods individually or as one formulation such as Microbiome Labs FODMATE Digestive Enzymes can help lessen symptoms (see chapter 5).

> ### Getting Started with a Low FODMAP Diet
>
> The low FODMAP diet is specifically designed for individuals with SIBO and has been shown to alleviate IBS symptoms in 50 to 80 percent of cases. By removing carbohydrates that are high in fermentable sugars, the diet reduces symptoms by starving the gut bacteria that may be causing problems.
>
> The strict elimination phase of the low FODMAP diet lasts between two to six weeks. During this time, you remove all high FODMAP foods to give your gut a chance to reset. Afterward, you'll begin to reintroduce foods slowly to see which ones you tolerate well. This helps create a personalized version of the diet that works for your digestive system.

The three stages of the low FODMAP diet are as follows:

1. Elimination (two to six weeks): During this phase, all high FODMAP foods are removed from your diet. You'll focus on low FODMAP foods that are less likely to cause fermentation in the gut. Many people feel symptom relief in this stage, which is a sign you're ready to move forward.

2. Reintroduction: You'll begin reintroducing one category of high FODMAP foods at a time over three-day intervals. This allows you to determine your tolerance for each food and gauge how much (if any) you can handle. Some people may find they can eat small amounts of certain foods, while others may need to avoid specific groups entirely.

3. Personalization: Once you've completed the reintroduction phase, you'll have a clear idea of which high FODMAP foods trigger your symptoms. At this point, you'll personalize your diet, avoiding trigger foods and reintroducing others that are safe in moderate amounts. Over time, as your gut heals, you may even be able to reintroduce, in small amounts, foods previously not tolerated.

It's important to remember that while the diet can be effective, following a strict low FODMAP plan for long periods can reduce gut bacterial diversity. Therefore, it is intended to be a temporary tool for healing the gut. The Monash University FODMAP app is a valuable resource, offering lists of low and high FODMAP foods and recipes to help you stay on track during the process.

Foods High in Histamines, Salicylates, and Oxalates, Oh My!

The three most common metabolic intolerances that can be potential drivers of IBS symptoms include histamine intolerance, oxalate intolerance, and salicylate intolerance. Some professionals recommend limiting these foods indefinitely, but in my clinical experience, an intolerance to these three food types is often caused by some sort of microbial overgrowth or infection that overproduces histamines, salicylates, and oxalates. This overgrowth, coupled with a deficiency in the cofactors needed to break them down, can lead to innocent foods containing these compounds becoming inflammatory. Treating the microbes and replenishing nutrients have resolved these food reactions for many of my clients.

Histamine Intolerance

Foods that are either high in histamine themselves or cause mast cells in the body to release more histamine include: fermented foods and drinks, alcohol, chocolate, dairy, wheat, cured meats, soured foods, most cheeses, seafood (canned or smoked), bone broth with collagen, honey, nuts, pork, some fruits (e.g., bananas, papayas, strawberries), and some fresh vegetables (e.g., tomatoes, spinach, nightshades, fava beans, mushrooms). Associated symptoms include asthma; eczema; flushing; hives; heart arrhythmia; stomach pain; cramping; nausea; vomiting; headaches and migraines; low blood pressure; runny, stuffy nose; swelling in the face, mouth, or throat; fatigue; heavy menstrual cramping; constipation; and itchiness.

Testing for Histamine Intolerance

I have found that certain gut infections, such as *H. pylori, Candida, Blasto, Dientamoeba fragilis,* and mold colonization can lead to issues with histamine. Some integrative practitioners have been trained to use whole blood histamine levels as a marker. This can give some insight but is not often used. The Diagnostic Solutions GI-MAP test can indicate levels of microbes that may be producing excess histamine, and the Organic Acids Test (OAT) can show markers that could indicate high histamine levels in the body.

What to Do If You Have Histamine Intolerance

Histamine intolerance often occurs when we have too many histamine-producing microbes and not enough substances on board that clear out histamine. Treating mold, yeast, *H. pylori,* and various histamine-producing bacteria can help resolve histamine intolerance. While working on finding and treating the microbes, following a low-histamine diet can help. You may also wish to avoid histamine-producing probiotic strains, including: *Lactobacillus buchneri, Lactobacillus helveticus, Lactobacillus hilgardii, Lactobacillus reuteri,* and *Streptococcus thermophilus.*

Furthermore, taking the diamine oxidase (DAO) enzyme, which breaks down histamines from food, and avoiding DAO blockers such as alcohol and green and black tea, can ensure histamine is cleared out properly. An additional, very helpful, yet often overlooked protocol to support the metabolic breakdown of histamine is vitamin B_6 (I prefer the P5P form), zinc picolinate (30 mg per day), and methionine or SAMe.

Oxalate Intolerance

High oxalate foods associated with oxalate sensitivity include: dark leafy greens (spinach, kale, chard), root vegetables (beets, sweet potatoes), nuts/seeds (almonds, walnuts, cashews), legumes (navy beans, lentils), soy products, grains (buckwheat, brown rice, wheat berries), rhubarb, rice bran, dates, cocoa powder, okra, and raspberries. Associated symptoms include: joint pain, pain in the body, burning with urination, burning with bowel movements, intestinal permeability, depression, and kidney stones.

Testing for Oxalate Intolerance

Oxalate buildups that are nongenetic are usually caused by *Candida* colonization, mold colonization, and sometimes an overactive glyoxylate pathway. An Organic Acids Test (OAT) can indicate if you're dealing with excess oxalates, as well as the reason they're overproduced.

What to Do If You Have Oxalate Intolerance

To reverse oxalate buildup, a low-oxalate diet, combined with addressing the root cause, is key. The goal is to lower intake to under 100 mg of oxalates per day, and, ideally, under 50 mg. However, it's important to lower oxalates gradually to avoid "oxalate dumping," which can cause unpleasant symptoms such as rashes, mood changes, and fatigue.

If mold or *Candida* colonization is present, treating the mold and *Candida* colonization is the key to resolving oxalate sensitivities, but lowering intake of dietary oxalates and supporting oxalate metabolism can help symptoms. If the glyoxylate pathway is overactive (per the OAT test), stopping supplements such as glycine, glutamine, or glycinate can help slow down the internal production of oxalates.

Eating oxalate-containing foods along with magnesium citrate or calcium citrate can help with preventing the absorption of oxalates. Probiotics that contain oxalyl-CoA decarboxylase, such as *Bifidobacterium lactis* (found in SFI Health Ther-Biotic Complete and Rootcology ProB 50) or *Enterococcus faecali* (found in Dr. Ohhira's brand of probiotics) can help break down oxalates. (Note, Dr. Ohhira's brand uses fermented soy in the development of the probiotics, but most people with soy reactions should be able to tolerate it.) Additionally, taking 50 mg or so per day of P5P (the active form of vitamin B_6) can help with the breakdown and tolerance of oxalates while working on the causes.

Salicylate Intolerance

Salicylate is rarely discussed as a potential cause of IBS-D, but a relevant one, as some recommendations for IBS utilize high salicylate substances such as peppermint tea, CBD, or hemp, which would make a person with salicylate intolerance feel worse. Salicylate sensitivity was initially described by Dr. Benjamin Feingold, who noticed some of his young and hyperactive patients seemed to be triggered by salicylate, which can be found in food additives and naturally occurs in fruits and vegetables. High salicylate foods include most fresh fruits (exceptions include apples, pears, papayas, and rhubarb, which are low in salicylates), nightshade vegetables, condiments and spices (e.g., Worcestershire sauce, vinegar, curry, cayenne, dill, aniseed), most commercial sauces, jams and dressings, some vegetables (e.g., alfalfa sprouts, chili, olives, hot peppers, zucchini, mushrooms, gherkins, radishes), honey, and mint. In addition to attention deficit hyperactivity disorder (ADHD), symptoms may include diarrhea, a stuffy nose, nasal polyps, asthma, and hives. In some cases, people may also report allergies to aspirin and peppermint (both are salicylates). Though the consensus on what causes salicylate intolerance is still out, in my experience, this condition occurs due to a buildup of salicylates, potentially due to salicylate-producing bacteria in the gut (including some types of SIBO).

Testing for Salicylate Intolerance

An Organic Acids Test (OAT) can indicate excess salicylates, which may be overproduced by the microbiome or due to a deficiency in cofactors.

What to Do If You Have Salicylate Intolerance

Avoiding high-salicylate foods can be incredibly helpful for symptoms, but like all metabolic intolerances, the issue stems from a buildup and poor processing. It's been suggested that various microbes produce salicylates, though I can't confirm which ones. Unlike Dr. Feingold, who initially recommended lifelong avoidance of salicylate foods, I have found that pausing intake of high-salicylate foods, medications, and supplements along with improving salicylate metabolism by supplementing with the amino acid glycine can eliminate salicylate sensitivity.

I could write a whole book on resolving metabolic intolerances! For a detailed guide on reversing sulfur, histamine, oxalate, and salicylate issues, please go to ibsrootcause.com/bonus.

High-Salicylate Medications and Supplements

Medications: Aspirin (acetylsalicylic acid), Pepto-Bismol (bismuth subsalicylate), Alka-Seltzer, topical pain relievers (such as Bengay, Icy Hot), methyl salicylate–containing liniments and balms, diflunisal, salsalate, magnesium salicylate.

Supplements: White willow bark, wintergreen supplements, herbal supplements derived from high-salicylate plants (e.g., turmeric, peppermint, rosemary), hemp, CBD.

Essential Oils: Wintergreen essential oil, peppermint essential oil, clove essential oil, eucalyptus essential oil, rosemary essential oil, spearmint essential oil, thyme essential oil, lavender essential oil.

Alcohol, Caffeine, and Other Mechanical Triggers

Alcohol, caffeine, and other "mechanical triggers" such as food additives that can be irritating to people with IBS are unrelated to an immune-system response and seemingly unconnected to an enzyme deficiency or metabolic buildup. They could be reactive due to the microbiome or perhaps an infection, but the reason could be simply the mechanism of the substance and taking it in excess, so limiting them is the best strategy for success that I know of. An elimination diet can help identify if these foods are an issue for you.

Alcohol

Alcohol consumption increases our risk for health problems and disease, and for some with IBS, it is a mechanical trigger that will cause a flare in their symptoms. In an observational study on women with IBS, researchers found that binge drinking (defined as four or more drinks per day) had the greatest effect on GI symptoms such as diarrhea, nausea, stomach pain, and indigestion the next day. This association was stronger for women with IBS-diarrhea than for IBS-constipation or IBS-mixed. Light to moderate drinking was either not associated or weakly associated with IBS symptoms. There are several ways alcohol consumption impacts the gut and can potentially result in IBS symptoms. Alcohol and its metabolites have been shown to decrease gastric motility and increase intestinal permeability. People who drink regularly exhibit malabsorption of carbohydrates, fat, proteins, and xylose, which can contribute to symptoms. Lastly, regular drinking has been shown to alter the microbiome, reducing the variability of bacteria in the gut.

Caffeine

When it comes to IBS, caffeine is a double-edged sword. For some people, caffeine is a mechanical trigger that can make diarrhea worse, and others may rely on it to relieve their constipation. This is because caffeine stimulates the production of several key gut hormones including gastrin and cholecystokinin (CCK), which stimulate contractions in the gut.

A 2021 study found individuals who drank caffeine regularly were more likely to have IBS, specifically an increased chance of IBS-C, possibly due to the diuretic effects of caffeine leading to dehydration. More specifically, people who drank the most caffeine (more than 106 mg per day) had a 47 percent higher chance of having IBS than those who drank less than 69 mg per day. There was a stronger association between caffeine intake and IBS in women and those who were overweight or obese.

> ## Why Does Coffee Help You Poop?
>
> While it's a commonly reported experience that coffee helps many people poop, the research isn't totally clear why. The caffeine in coffee may be responsible for the urge to have a bowel movement. Caffeine stimulates the production of gastrin and cholecystokinin (CCK), two hormones that play a role in gut motility. Research has found that caffeinated coffee is 60 percent more effective than water in stimulating contractions in the gut and 23 percent more effective than decaf coffee. There may also be compounds in coffee independent of caffeine that stimulate bowel movements, as decaf coffee still does influence bowel movements. For example, coffee stimulates the release of gastrin, which promotes colonic activity.
>
> The caffeine in black tea (and really any caffeinated beverage) may also help stimulate a bowel movement (good if you have constipation, not so good when you have diarrhea), while certain herbal teas, such as slippery elm and fennel, may help ease digestive symptoms and constipation. For more on herbal teas, see the box on page 147.

Carbonated Beverages

Any sort of carbonated beverage like soda or sparkling water, and even those "healthy" fizzy drinks that are supposed to be good for your gut health, can be a mechanical trigger for IBS symptoms. A 2012 study found that a higher intake of carbonated beverages was associated with a higher incidence of symptoms, especially in IBS-D. This may be because the carbonation itself can cause gas and bloating, or it could be due to the number of other ingredients like caffeine, artificial sweeteners, and preservatives commonly found in many carbonated drinks.

Citrus

The high acidity of lemons, limes, oranges, grapefruits, and other citrus fruits can irritate the esophagus, aggravating acid reflux and the lining of the stomach, contributing to indigestion, heartburn, and stomach pain.

Spicy Foods

Turning up the heat with hot peppers (chili, habanero, cayenne) can irritate the gastrointestinal tract and trigger abdominal pain, indigestion, and diarrhea, and consumption of spicy foods is directly associated with IBS, particularly in women. One study found that people who consumed spicy foods more than ten times per week were 92 percent more likely to have IBS compared with those who never consumed spicy foods, and women who consumed spicy foods more than ten times per week were two times more likely to have IBS compared with those who never consumed spicy foods.

Capsaicin, the active ingredient in hot peppers, irritates the tissue lining the gut and is the source of the burning sensation you may feel. It activates receptors that tell the brain the body is overheating, triggering the release of endorphins and dopamine—why we sometimes experience a "high" from eating spicy foods—and a speeding up of gut motility to get rid of the threat resulting in diarrhea. Capsaicin can also induce intestinal permeability.

Food Additives

Could eating too many gummy bears send you running to the nearest bathroom with sphincter-screaming explosive diarrhea, toxic flatulence, and cramps, sweating, and bloating that makes a bout of food poisoning feel like a walk in the park? Sure can! Just ask the poor souls sent sprinting to the bathroom with "an 'intestinal powerwash'" or "Gummy Bear 'Cleanse'" after the Haribo candy company replaced their usual sweetener with the sugar alcohol maltitol. One woman described her daylong experience on the toilet after eating twenty candies as her "worst nightmare," with a "torrential flood of 100 percent flammable liquid, like Napalm, spewing from her backend." "There was stuff coming out of me that I ate at my wedding in 2005!" she shared. (Haribo has since changed the recipe.)

Certain food additives, including sweeteners such as sugar alcohols, can act as mechanical triggers for IBS-like symptoms, especially diarrhea. Additives are used to improve the taste, texture, freshness, and shelf life of packaged foods. Researchers have even proposed that the increased consumption of processed foods containing an array of food additives—found in more than 50 percent of food products—could be the reason for the increase in cases of IBS and IBD.

The emulsifiers polysorbate 80 and carboxymethyl cellulose (CMC), noncaloric artificial sweeteners such as sucralose and saccharin, maltodextrin, titanium dioxide, ethylenediaminetetraacetic acid (EDTA), carrageenan, erythritol, and microbial transglutaminases have all been linked to IBD.

Most people can tolerate food additives in small amounts and won't feel their effect until they consume too much in one sitting, but some people may be hypersensitive and feel their negative effects even after a small dose. Either way, dialing back on food additives is a good way to go. Packaged foods usually contain more than one additive, and there's a lot we still don't know about how they interact with one another and with the body over time.

Food additives can trigger the following symptoms:

- Diarrhea: Sugar alcohols draw water into the colon, acting like a laxative. A little can ease constipation, but too much can result in loose stools and diarrhea. Disaster pants.

- Alterations in the gut microbiome: Additives like sugar alcohols, preservatives, and emulsifiers alter gut bacteria, leading to dysbiosis and inflammation. Emulsifiers, for example, can alter the amount of sulfate-reducing bacteria, increase gut permeability, and trigger visceral pain.

- Inflammation: Studies have associated the increased and prolonged consumption of food additives with the development of colitis, inflammation of the colon. Chronic consumption of emulsifiers, in particular carrageenan, can erode the protective mucus lining of the gut. Food colorants and preservatives have also been linked to a pro-inflammatory response.

There are over three thousand food additives on the market, but these are some of the most common additives known to cause digestive problems:

Sugar alcohols

As a society, many of us have become aware of the harm of the artificial sweeteners sucralose and saccharin. However, there's another set of not-so-sweet substances that has become popular in recent years. Sugar alcohols, also known as polyols (the P in FODMAPs), are low-calorie sweeteners that won't spike blood sugar and have become popular sugar substitutes in many sugar-free/no-sugar options such as chewing gum, cough drops, beverages, baked goods, and foods marketed as keto-friendly and diabetic-friendly.

Sugar alcohols are poorly absorbed in the small intestine, and the undigested portions reach the colon, where bacteria ferment them, leading to gas, bloating, and abdominal pain. They also draw water into the colon, causing loose stools and sudden diarrhea. Well-known as effective laxatives, sugar alcohols such as maltitol are sometimes prescribed by doctors to ease constipation. While smaller amounts are added to foods, and foods that contain the sugar alcohols sorbitol and mannitol must include a warning label that "excess consumption may have a laxative effect," "excess consumption" may vary per individual.

Common sugar alcohols include:

- Erythritol: Commonly found in processed "keto" foods and snacks, unfortunately this low-calorie sweetener seemed to trigger my husband to have ulcerative colitis, so it's worth being mindful of its effect on your digestive issues.

- Maltitol: Found in no-sugar-added candies and chocolates, but also used as a laxative.

- Mannitol: Its laxative effect is so strong that mannitol is used to clear the bowels before bowel surgery!

- Sorbitol: If you've ever wondered why prunes are recommended to keep you regular, sorbitol is the answer. Prunes and prune juice are high in sorbitol, and this sugar alcohol has one of the highest laxative effects out of all of the sugar alcohols.

- Xylitol: While it has some positive side effects, such as reducing harmful bacteria in the mouth—this is why it's often found in toothpastes—xylitol may also contribute to gut dysbiosis.

Thickeners
In addition to maltodextrin and titanium dioxide, thickeners such as guar gum and xanthan gum are used in many foods, including yogurt, coconut milk, condiments, gluten-free breads and cakes, soups, sauces, and puddings, and can cause bloating, gas, and diarrhea and may shift the microbiome, increase inflammation of the colon, and exacerbate symptoms for people with IBS.

Emulsifiers

In addition to polysorbate 80 and carboxymethyl cellulose, soy lecithin is one of the most frequently used food additives today. Soy lecithin is a popular emulsifier, giving salad dressing and chocolate their smooth, blended texture and appearance. It's often used in nonstick cooking sprays and even found in dietary supplements. Though it may contain only trace amounts of soy protein (the trigger for allergies and sensitivities), this amount may still trigger a response in those who are highly soy sensitive. Furthermore, soy lecithin can shift the microbiome toward dysbiosis and has been linked to colitis, intestinal permeability, and IBS. In excess amounts, soy lecithin can cause cramps, pain, nausea, a feeling of fullness, and diarrhea. This was the main driver of my explosive diarrhea when I was in pharmacy school!

Carrageenan

Carrageenan helps make foods "gel" and is often found in vegan foods as a substitute for gelatin and dairy. It can cause loose stools and diarrhea and has been associated with altering the microbiome, damaging the gut lining, and increasing inflammation, which may contribute to the development of IBD.

MCT Oil

Thinking of adding a splash of MCT oil to your morning coffee just like Emma Stone and Kourtney Kardashian? Start low and go slow! MCT oil, made from a fatty acid found in coconut oil, may help increase energy and focus because it is so easily absorbed by the body, but too much, too soon, can send you running for the nearest toilet, or worse, leave you with an embarrassing case of "disaster pants," as dubbed by Bulletproof Coffee and Danger Coffee founder Dave Asprey. Large doses can irritate the gut and trigger a response to flush it out as quickly as possible.

Testing for Sensitivity to Food Additives

While explosive diarrhea after eating too many gummy bears is a hard-to-miss sign that you have a reaction to food additives, you may also wish to do some testing. I have searched far and wide and have found one potential test. Vibrant Wellness Food Additives Test is an experimental test for immune reactivity to food additives. Though I don't have much experience with it, it may be helpful to your journey.

Fatty Foods

Surveys have found that approximately 50 percent of people with IBS identify fatty foods as a trigger for diarrhea, gas, bloating, nausea, heartburn, and stomach pain. A deficiency in fat digestive enzymes, such as pancreatic enzymes, poor or inadequate bile flow, and/or bile malabsorption, can make it extra difficult to digest and absorb fats. See the next chapter for more.

Foods High in Protein

People who struggle with bloating, acid reflux, low energy, and IBS symptoms from foods high in protein, such as steaks and other meats, often have deficiencies in stomach acid, which helps to digest protein-containing foods. See the next chapter for more.

FOOD REACTION	TESTING	TREATMENT
Food allergy	IgE skin and blood testing	-Elimination, desensitization, oral cromolyn sodium (IBS-D), ketotifen
Celiac disease	Celiac testing	-Gluten-free diet -Gut infection treatment
Non-celiac gluten sensitivity (NCGS)		-Three-to-six-month elimination with gut-healing protocols -Systemic (proteolytic) enzymes
Non-celiac wheat sensitivity (NCWS)	IgG food sensitivity testing	-Three-to-six-month elimination with gut-healing protocols -Systemic (proteolytic) enzymes

IBS

FOOD REACTION	TESTING	TREATMENT
Lactose intolerance	FoodMarble AIRE hydrogen breath test and glucose blood test	-Low lactose or lactose-free diet -Lactase enzyme -SIBO treatment -Parasitic infection treatment -Balance gut flora
Whey and casein (the proteins in dairy) sensitivity	IgG food sensitivity testing	-Carnitine and alfalfa -Camel milk
Eggs	IgG food sensitivity testing	-Three-to-six-month elimination with gut-healing protocols -Systemic (proteolytic) enzymes -Sulfur intolerance protocol (refer to page 105)
Soy	IgG food sensitivity testing	-Three-to-six-month elimination with gut-healing protocols -Systemic (proteolytic) enzymes
High-nickel foods	MELISA test	-Low-nickel diet -Limited exposure from other sources (medical and electronic devices, cookware, implants) -Oral hyposensitization therapy -Activities to sweat it out (yoga, sauna) -Vitamin C, zinc, iron, riboflavin, selenium, vitamin E, and curcumin
High-fiber foods, raw foods	Vibrant Wellness Gut Zoomer 3.0, EnbiosiS, and Viome Gut Intelligence Test	-Exclusion (temporary, for symptom management) -Food prep modifications -Fiber digestive enzymes -Probiotics
Fructose intolerance	FoodMarble AIRE hydrogen breath test and sucrose breath test	-Low-fructose diet (temporary, for symptom management) -SIBO treatment -Parasitic infection treatment -Xylose isomerase enzymes
Sucrose intolerance	FoodMarble AIRE hydrogen breath test and sucrose breath test	-Low-sucrose diet (temporary, for symptom management) -Sucrase (invertase) -SIBO treatment -Parasitic infection treatment

FOOD REACTION	TESTING	TREATMENT
High FODMAP foods	FoodMarble AIRE hydrogen breath test	-Low FODMAP diet (temporary, for symptom management) -SIBO treatment -Parasitic infection treatment -Digestive enzymes
Histamine intolerance	Diagnostic Solutions GI-MAP test and Mosaic Diagnostics Organic Acids Test (OAT)	-Low histamine diet (temporary, for symptom management) -Mold, yeast, *H. pylori,* and/or various histamine-producing bacteria treatment -Diamine oxidase (DAO) enzyme -Avoid DAO blockers -Vitamin B_6, zinc picolinate (30 mg per day), and methionine or SAMe
Oxalate sensitivity	Mosaic Diagnostics Organic Acids Test (OAT)	-Low-oxalate diet (temporary, for symptom management) -Mold or *Candida* treatment -Magnesium citrate or calcium citrate with oxalate-containing foods -Probiotics that contain oxalyl-CoA decarboxylase -P5P (50 mg or so per day)
Salicylate intolerance	Mosaic Diagnostics Organic Acids Test (OAT)	-Low-salicylate diet and avoidance of high-salicylate medications and supplements (temporary, for symptom management) -Glycine
Alcohol, caffeine, carbonated beverages, citrus, spicy foods, and other irritants or mechanical triggers		-Limit intake
Food additives	Vibrant Wellness Food Additives Test (experimental)	-Limit intake

FOOD REACTION	TESTING	TREATMENT
Fatty foods		-Digestive enzymes -Support bile flow -Bile acid sequestrants (to relieve symptoms of bile acid malabsorption) (see chapter 5 for more)
Protein		-Support stomach acid (see chapter 5 for more)

Chapter Summary

- Removing reactive foods can significantly improve symptoms of IBS in most people—it's a game changer!

- Foods can cause reactions for a variety of reasons . . .

- In some cases, eliminating the offending food can resolve IBS symptoms within just a few short days. In most cases (except celiac disease), removal of the triggering food is only for a period of time while the gut heals.

- In the case of atopy, consider an IgE skin test, and if allergies are identified, avoidance of allergic foods and desensitization strategies.

- IgG food sensitivity tests can be helpful in identifying food sensitivities, but not all tests are created equal. I have found Alletess Lab IgG food sensitivity tests to produce the most accurate and reproducible results.

- Systemic enzymes can help with IgG food reactions.

- An elimination diet eliminating gluten, dairy, soy, corn, sugar, spicy foods, alcohol, and caffeine provides an individualized way to determine your unique food triggers.

Visit https://ibsrootcause.com/bonus for notes on this chapter.

CHAPTER 5

Digestion and Digestive Enzymes

Hippocrates, the ancient Greek philosopher who was also a physician, is quoted as saying, "Poor digestion is the root of all evil," and I have to agree (especially when it comes to irritable bowel syndrome)!

After all, we are not just what we eat but what we *digest*.

The gut performs an all-important role of digesting and absorbing nutrients we take in and need for energy, cell growth and repair, and numerous other important functions that keep our bodily systems running and us feeling our best.

While we don't often think about it and it sort of just occurs behind the scenes, digestion is a multistep process that involves numerous organs working together. In a well-functioning digestive system, the body produces the appropriate enzymes to break down larger complex molecules of food into smaller molecules to be used as fuel. What we don't realize is that because the process of digestion is so intricate and multifaceted, there are plenty of things that can go wrong and lead to digestive distress.

An imbalance in just one key enzyme can mean disaster for our digestive system. The symptoms of digestive enzyme deficiency sound a lot like irritable bowel syndrome and include constipation, gas, bloating, abdominal pain, and diarrhea.

In addition to digestive symptoms, enzyme deficiencies can also lead to malabsorption, resulting in a diminished ability to absorb proper nutrients from the food we eat, including protein, fat, and/or starches and fiber, each potentially resulting in seemingly unrelated symptoms such as dry hair, hair loss, anemia, fatigue, and weight loss (depending on the enzyme that's deficient).

Supporting our digestive process can be a game changer in resolving IBS symptoms (and often many other weird residual symptoms as well). In this chapter, we will focus on lifestyle changes as well as broad-spectrum and targeted enzyme supplementation for relief of IBS symptoms. We will also cover bile acid malabsorption, a common yet underappreciated cause of diarrhea.

What Can Go Wrong With Our Digestion?

There are various types of digestive system issues that can lead to IBS symptoms, including:

- low stomach acid, leading to protein digestive issues
- low levels of pancreatic enzymes, leading to issues with digestion of starches, fats, and protein
- deficiencies in bile production/secretion, leading to fat malabsorption
- bile acid malabsorption due to overproduction of bile or poor absorption, leading to issues with fat digestion and also straight-up diarrhea, no matter what you eat
- low levels of brush border enzymes in the small intestine, leading to carbohydrate digestive enzyme deficiencies, including lactose intolerance
- imbalance of colonic bacteria, leading to poor digestion of fiber

You may benefit from some broad-spectrum ways of supporting digestion, or you may need specific targeted interventions for one or more digestive enzymes. Let's start with some broad-spectrum digestive recommendations before we dive into ways to support specific enzymes.

Broad-Spectrum Ideas

If you know that a certain type of food triggers you, you may benefit from following a plan targeted to boost the enzymes needed to digest that particular food. If you don't know which food triggers your digestive issues, that's OK, too. There are broad-spectrum measures that can be undertaken, including broad-spectrum enzymes. (Some individuals may need one type of digestive enzyme. Others may need multiple types.)

Best Practices to Support Digestion

Incorporating a few best practices to promote healthy digestion can help relieve symptoms by making the entire digestive process run more smoothly and efficiently as well as make mealtime more satisfying and enjoyable:

Lifestyle Support for Optimizing Digestion
Relax While You Eat

Have you heard of the autonomic nervous system (ANS)? It sounds a little bit like automatic nervous system, and it's a helpful way of remembering its function. Our ANS helps with doing background jobs in our day-to-day life, such as digestion. It has two main settings, the sympathetic and parasympathetic setting. The sympathetic setting is activated when we sense danger or stress and is focused on fight, flight, and freeze. Digestion slows to conserve energy. The parasympathetic is our setting focused on resting and digesting. Eating while we're relaxed supports optimal digestion. Taking a few deep breaths or a moment to calm yourself if you are feeling emotional, hurried, angry, or upset before starting a meal can make a huge difference.

The Steps of Digestion

1. The digestive process starts with chewing! When food enters the mouth, teeth start tearing and chewing food into smaller pieces while digestive enzymes in saliva, such as amylase and lipase, get to work breaking down food into smaller particles.

2. Next, food travels down the esophagus.

3. It passes into the stomach, where a protein digestive enzyme known as pepsin is activated by stomach acid (made of hydrochloric acid) and, with the help of several other powerful enzymes, the digestive process continues.

4. When the semisolid contents of the stomach, known as chyme, are processed enough, the chyme proceeds into the small intestine, where additional enzymes take action. The small intestine releases its own enzymes from the intestinal brush border, including dextrinase, glucoamylase, maltase, sucrase, and lactase, and is also the action site for enzymes released by the pancreas, including trypsin and chymotrypsin to aid with protein digestion, amylase to support carbohydrate digestion, and lipase to help with digesting fats.

To finish off fat digestion, we need bile to break down fats into fatty acids. Bile is produced by the liver and stored in the gallbladder, but like much of our digestive process, its site of action is the small intestine.

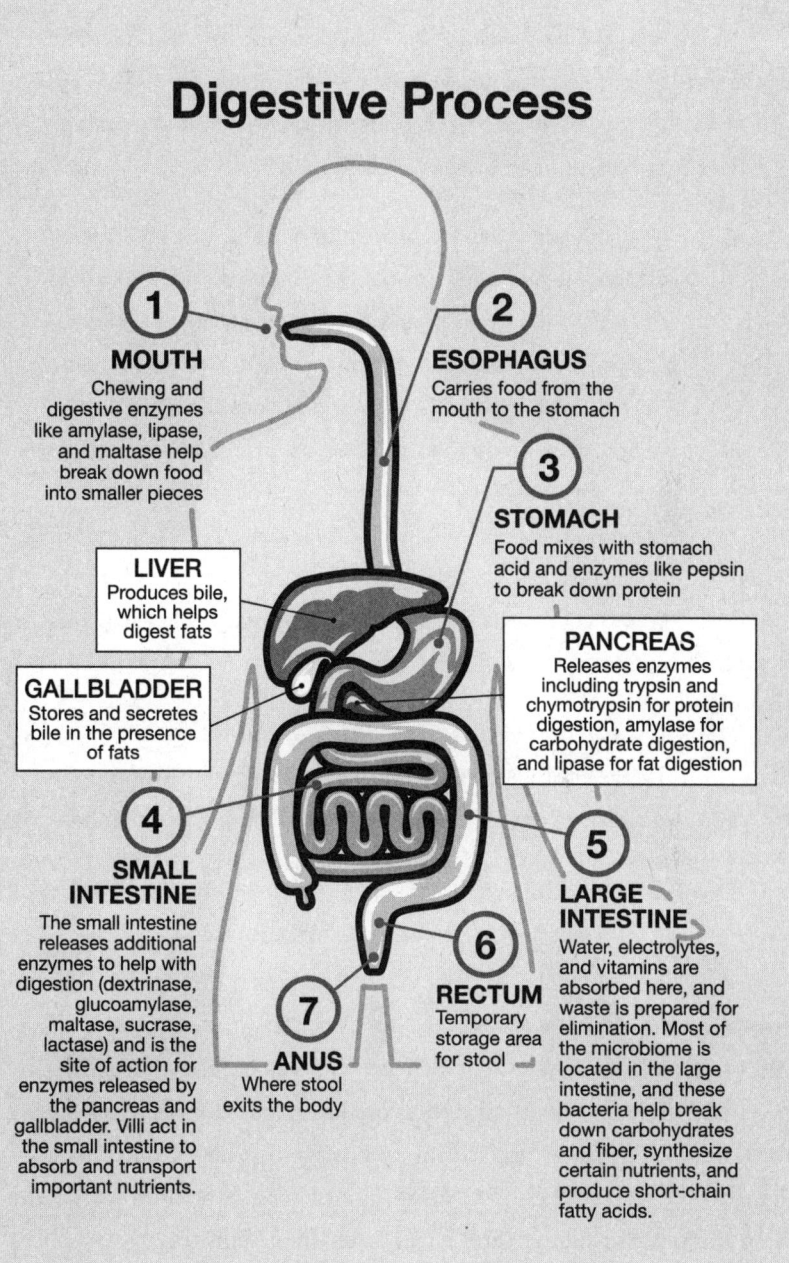

Once food is fully digested, villi—tiny fingerlike bristles found on the intestinal wall of the small intestine—grab onto any usable nutrients and drop them into the bloodstream and lymphatic system, where they can be used by the rest of the body.

(5) After the nutrients have been absorbed, the liquid food residue and any waste products from the digestive process move on to the large intestine, or colon. Millions of gut bacteria, also known as the gut microbiome, live in the colon and aid the further digestion and absorption of nutrients, including the breakdown of fiber to produce gut-protective short-chain fatty acids (SCFAs), as well as help regulate the immune system and hormone levels, synthesize mood-supporting neurotransmitters such as serotonin, and protect against harmful bacteria, among many other valuable functions.

(6) As waste passes through the colon, it is prepared for elimination until it is ultimately released through the rectum and anus (7) as a bowel movement. This is how poop happens.

Slow Down When You're Eating

One of my colleagues spoke of a client who was suffering digestive distress. The client frequently ate McDonald's in his car while on breaks from his work and was not willing to change his diet or take any supplements. After some consideration, my colleague recommended the client simply slow down and savor each bite. Amazingly, the client came back and said that after twenty years, his digestive stress was completely gone. By slowing down, he also realized he didn't actually enjoy the taste of McDonald's and ended up changing his diet on his own accord. The body provides important messages when we slow down to listen!

Do a Lot of Chewing

Chewing kicks off the digestive process, and the more you chew, the more thoroughly your food will be broken down, lowering the risk of gas, bloating, constipation, indigestion, and other digestive issues. The number of chews you need per food depends on the texture of the food, with softer textures generally requiring less chewing—twenty or so chews per bite of food may suffice—while harder textures like nuts and meat may require forty or more chews per bite. Don't forget to chew liquid foods such as smoothies or blended soup for optimal digestion.

Experiment to See How Beverages Affect Your Digestion

Some people believe drinking liquids with meals can dilute digestive juices. However, there isn't any research to back up this claim. That being said, anecdotally some people say avoiding drinking liquids such as cold beverages at meals improves their digestion, while others find sipping on warm beverages such as digestive teas before, during, and after eating can help digestion.

Exercise

Physical activity can help relieve stress and promote rest-and-digest mode while also supporting healthy digestion by promoting gut motility, increasing transit time, and encouraging regular and easier-to-pass bowel movements. Researchers have found that less active people are more likely to have IBS than people who are more physically active. Scientists (and dog walkers) believe that the physical motion of bending, twisting, or bouncing as well as increased breathing and increased heart rate can stimulate intestinal muscle contractions. Regular exercise can increase the number of beneficial species in the gut and may increase digestive enzyme production.

You don't need to do anything intense to feel the benefits. Just committing to three hourlong sessions of yoga or walking per week can work wonders for gut support.

(Please note that too much exercise, such as ultra-marathon running, can increase the likelihood of diarrhea—if you've ever gone on a run and suddenly had to poop, you know what I mean! If this is you, see the information on glutamine in chapter 6.)

Food as Medicine

Foods that can help with digestion include:

Hot Lemon Water

Drinking the juice of one lemon in a cup of hot water first thing in the morning can help boost the secretion of stomach acid. If desired, you can even add some sweetener like stevia or maple syrup to taste. Do not use if you have an ulcer or gastritis. To protect teeth enamel, drink lemon water through a straw, or rinse your mouth with water and baking soda after drinking. And of course make sure it's not too hot to drink!

Apple Cider Vinegar

One teaspoon of apple cider vinegar in one glass of cold water can also increase stomach acid. Do not use if you have an ulcer or gastritis, and please don't drink it straight.

Fermented Foods

Fermented foods such as sauerkraut, kimchi, yogurt, kefir, and kombucha can help boost stomach acid and contain probiotics that are beneficial for digestion. Eating these foods regularly can increase the number of beneficial bacteria that help with digestion. Please note that introducing fermented foods too quickly can result in digestive distress as the gut microbiome changes. A reaction to fermented foods could also indicate SIBO or an infection of histamine-producing microbes in the gut. See chapter 9 for more on bacterial overgrowths and chapter 10 for infections.

Bone Broth

Gelatin-rich bone broth stimulates the production of stomach acid and draws fluid into the intestine, improving gut motility and supporting healthy bowel movements. (See more on page 244.)

Bitter Foods and Spices

Eating bitter foods and spices triggers the production of gastrin, which stimulates gastric acid production. Many digestive tinctures and formulations include a number of bitter herbs, but many foods fall into this category as well. Coffee, cocoa, green tea, cruciferous vegetables, dark leafy greens, and citrus peel are all considered bitter foods.

Digestive Teas

Herbal teas have been used for thousands of years to support healthy digestion and treat digestive issues including nausea, constipation, gas, and indigestion. Try out some of the suggested options in the Digestive Teas box (see below)—hot or cold—to find ones that suit you best.

Digestive Teas

- **Anise:** Anise may soothe the gastrointestinal tract and help reduce gas and stomach upset.
- **Catnip:** The compound nepetalactone in catnip acts as a sedative, lending this herb its calming, stress-reducing qualities. It's also known for relieving cramps, gas, and indigestion.

- Marshmallow and slippery elm: Their mucilaginous properties help to soothe an inflamed intestinal tract.

- Peppermint: Peppermint oil is known for its ability to relax the muscles of the gastrointestinal tract, which can help alleviate bloating and gas.

- Ginger: Ginger has anti-inflammatory and digestive properties that can help reduce bloating and soothe the digestive system.

- Fennel: Fennel seeds and tea are often used to alleviate bloating and support digestion.

- Chamomile: Chamomile tea has a calming effect on the digestive system and may help relieve bloating and discomfort.

For a comprehensive guide to digestive teas, please go to ibsrootcause.com/bonus.

Supplementing Digestive Enzymes

In some cases, you may need more targeted support, including digestive enzymes. While conventional medicine largely ignores digestive enzymes (with the exception of extreme cases), digestive enzymes are a key feature of the integrative, alternative, and functional medicine approaches to health.

A 2008 study published in *Alternative Medicine Review* found that supplementing with digestive enzymes provided a safe and effective treatment for various digestive issues, including lactose intolerance, celiac disease, and other digestive malabsorption disorders. This is likely because supplementing with the proper digestive enzymes:

- Increases nutrient absorption, which can help address underlying nutrient deficiencies contributing to poor gut health, among other benefits.

- Allows the body to focus its resources on healing, instead of working overtime to break down foods when an enzyme deficiency is present.

- Helps reverse intestinal permeability, as undigested food particles may damage the intestinal lining.

- Reduces food sensitivities—when food particles are poorly digested, we are more likely to become sensitive to them.

- Reduces inflammation and the autoimmune process. Poorly digested molecules of food can feed problematic bacteria that live in the gut, as well as enter the intestinal lining and become absorbed into the bloodstream, resulting in inflammation and autoimmunity.

Let's take a closer look at how taking the appropriate digestive enzymes to assist your body in processing food and absorbing nutrients could get at the root of your symptoms.

Broad-Spectrum Enzymes

Broad-spectrum enzymes contain a variety of ingredients that promote the breakdown of a wide range of nutrients, including fiber, starch, fat, and protein. Some digestive enzyme supplement formulations provide us with replacement enzymes to do the digestive work on our behalf, while other enzyme formulations support the body's own digestive pathways. Broad-spectrum options include digestive bitters, which *stimulate* our own production of digestive enzymes, and multi-ingredient enzyme formulations that *replace* enzymes.

Digestive Bitter Supplements

Digestive bitter supplements boost our own endogenous enzymes by stimulating the bitter receptors in our mouth, tongue, stomach, gut, liver, and pancreas. Using bitters helps us restore our enzyme levels over time.

Common ingredients in digestive bitters supplements include:

- Angelica (*Angelica archangelica*): Angelica has traditionally been used in European countries to relieve digestive problems, including heartburn, gas, bloating, and upset stomach.

- Burdock: Burdock is known as a diuretic, supporting digestion by helping flush waste from the body, and is a powerful anti-inflammatory.

- Chinese rhubarb: Rhubarb protects intestinal barrier function and promotes peristalsis (the wavelike motions that propel food through the digestive tract).

- Dandelion: Dandelion root supports proper timing of the digestive process so food does not pass too quickly or too slowly through the GI tract and stimulates the healthy flow of bile supporting fat digestion.

- Fennel: Fennel enhances natural digestive enzyme activity in the small intestine, reducing stomach discomfort and bloating, and supports bowel regularity.

- Gentian: Gentian supports bile flow, which can relieve occasional upset stomach or heartburn after eating and reduce flatulence and feeling full after eating.

- Ginger: Gingerols in ginger are known to ameliorate occasional indigestion, bloating, belching, and discomfort after meals.

- Lemon balm: Lemon balm helps calm occasional discomfort associated with indigestion, gas, and bloating, through supporting the parasympathetic nervous system, responsible for the "rest and digest" mode.

- Valerian: This medicinal herb has been used for centuries to treat digestive issues and insomnia, and can increase the amount of the neurotransmitter GABA (gamma-aminobutyric acid) in the body, associated with calming, sedative, and pain-relieving effects. Valerian can also speed up the digestive system (good for relieving constipation) and act as a carminative, preventing and relieving gas.

Digestive bitters can be purchased as stand-alone versions or as blends. High-quality blended options include:

- Wellena Liver and Digestive Bitters Kit, pre- and post-meal digestive support in liquid formulations containing angelica, burdock, gentian, fennel, and ginger.
- Quicksilver Scientific Dr. Shade's Bitters No. 9, a liposomal liquid containing burdock and dandelion.
- Nature's Way NatureWorks Swedish Bitters, a liquid herbal formula containing angelica, Chinese rhubarb, and valerian.

Multi-Ingredient Digestive Enzyme Formulation
Another option for digestive enzyme support is using supplements that contain a variety of enzymes to support the healthy breakdown and

digestion of the macronutrients (fat, protein, carbohydrates) in a wide range of foods.

Broad-spectrum digestive enzyme formations often include enzymes that target:

- Starches such as amylase
- Sugars such as lactase, sucrase, and maltase
- Vegetables and fiber such as cellulase, phytase, beta-glucanase, alpha-galactosidase, and galactomannan
- Proteins such as protease
- Fats such as lipase

Each company has a unique formulation, and you may need to try different ones to find the combination of enzymes that works best for you.

High-quality options include:

- Rootcology Broad Spectrum Enzymes
- SFI Health Ther-Biotic SIBB-Zymes
- SFI Health Ther-Biotic Vital-Zymes Complete
- Pure Encapsulations Digestive Enzymes Ultra
- Transformation Enzymes Digest

Beyond Broad-Spectrum Support

For some people with IBS, the broad-spectrum recommendations for digestive support just might do the trick, but others may need to do deeper digestive digging. Some individuals may have significant deficiencies in specific digestive enzymes and may require targeted doses of them. Others may have imbalances in the digestive process that need to be addressed to restore healthy digestive function.

Low Stomach Acid

If you often feel like food is sitting in your stomach for hours, struggle with acid reflux, or feel bloated after eating high-protein meals like steak, you might have low stomach acid. Other clues include B_{12} or iron deficiency, hypothyroidism, frequent antacid use, or a sensation of fullness shortly after eating, or as some might say "I feel like the food just sits there. Like a rock in my stomach." If your energy levels drop postmeal and you feel like your body is using too much energy to digest your food, low stomach acid could be behind it.

I personally experienced this when eating red meat, which led to discomfort and digestive issues. For others, these symptoms may show up with dairy, gluten, eggs, or other proteins. I initially eliminated red meat, gluten, and dairy, which helped. But it wasn't until I supported my stomach acid that I saw a major improvement in my digestion and food reactions.

Low stomach acid prevents the enzyme pepsin from properly breaking down proteins, which is often the root cause behind protein digestion issues. If you've ever experienced acid reflux, you may be under the assumption that excess stomach acid is problematic; however, inadequate stomach acid (known as hypochlorhydria) or absent stomach acid (achlorhydria) makes it difficult to digest protein and can actually be the cause behind acid reflux! People with IBS are four times more likely to experience acid reflux, and according to one study, up to 50 percent of people with IBS also have acid reflux. Low stomach acid doesn't just lead to acid reflux, though. It is also a contributing factor to IBS symptoms, food sensitivities, gut infections, and gut dysbiosis. Low stomach acid is one of the driving factors behind SIBO as well!

Age, stress, and deficiencies (such as thiamine) can reduce stomach acid levels, and *Helicobacter pylori* infections are another common culprit. Medications such as PPIs (e.g., Nexium, Prilosec) or H2 blockers (e.g., Pepcid) can also cause long-term digestive issues by suppressing stomach acid production.

If you're considering stopping acid-suppressing meds, it's essential to taper off slowly to avoid rebound effects. For a detailed weaning guide, check out my resources at ibsrootcause.com/bonus.

You can test stomach acid levels via the Heidelberg pH test (which is somewhat invasive), but oftentimes functional medicine practitioners recommend a Betaine with Pepsin Challenge to determine whether a person would benefit from stomach acid support.

Supporting Stomach Acid

Supplementing with betaine with pepsin can be highly effective for supporting low stomach acid and improving protein digestion. Betaine, derived from beets, helps increase stomach acidity, which is crucial for activating pepsin—a digestive enzyme that breaks down protein into smaller, absorbable components. This combination is essential for absorbing important nutrients such as protein, calcium, B_{12}, and iron. Pepsin, often sourced from pigs, ensures that proteins are properly digested so the small intestine can absorb them efficiently. This duo can make a big difference for those struggling with low stomach acid and related digestive issues. High-quality brands include: Rootcology Betaine with Pepsin, Pure Encapsulations Betaine HCl Pepsin, Xymogen GastrAcid, Nutridyn HCl Support, and Ortho Molecular Betaine & Pepsin.

To determine your proper dose, take the Betaine with Pepsin Challenge (see opposite page). Please note that each manufacturer may use varying amounts of betaine and pepsin in their formulation, so if you switch brands of supplements, your dose may need to be adjusted.

While most digestive enzymes are well tolerated by most people, betaine with pepsin should be avoided by individuals with active ulcers and those taking NSAID medication. Using acid-blocking medications will also negate the effects of betaine with pepsin, so I often recommend weaning off acid suppressants before using it.

Betaine with Pepsin Challenge

Betaine with pepsin should be taken after a protein-rich meal, starting with one capsule per meal. The dose should be increased by one more capsule at each meal, until symptoms of too much acid are felt, such as burping, burning, and warming in the stomach region. At that point, you will know that your dose is one capsule less than what resulted in symptoms. (Drinking a mixture of 1 teaspoon of baking soda in a glass of water can reduce these temporary symptoms.)

Titration Sample Schedule to Start Your HCl Therapy

- Meal No. 1: Took one capsule, didn't feel symptoms

- Meal No. 2: Took two capsules, didn't feel symptoms

- Meal No. 3: Took three capsules, didn't feel symptoms

- Meal No. 4: Took four capsules, felt symptoms

- Target dose: Three capsules (one capsule less than what resulted in symptoms)

Additional Methods for Supporting Stomach Acid

In addition to following the broad-spectrum digestive best practices (page 141) that promote the optimal release of stomach acid, including chewing food thoroughly (especially important for "tough" foods such as steaks) and utilizing apple cider vinegar or hot lemon water and digestive bitters, you may wish to do the following:

Add a High-Quality Source of Sodium

Stomach acid is composed of chloride, and salt (sodium chloride) is a good source. Sprinkle high-quality sea salt, a better choice than more processed options like iodized table salt, on foods and beverages to support digestion.

Consider Thiamine

Thiamine deficiency is an important yet often overlooked cause of low stomach acid. For more on replenishing thiamine levels, see chapter 6.

> ## Betaine and the MTHFR Gene Mutation
>
> If you have the MTHFR gene mutation, betaine with pepsin can be particularly beneficial for relieving digestive symptoms, as well as issues with pain, mood, and fatigue. The mutation can lead to higher levels of homocysteine, which disrupts methylation—a process vital for optimal body function. Elevated homocysteine has been linked to heart disease, pregnancy complications, and impaired detoxification.
>
> Betaine helps break down homocysteine while improving protein digestion and nutrient absorption, especially for those who may be deficient in trimethylglycine due to the mutation. In addition to betaine with pepsin, supplements like Rootcology MTHFR Pathways or Pure Encapsulations Homocysteine Factors (which contain riboflavin, B_6, folate, and B_{12}) can further support methylation.

Pancreatic Enzyme Deficiency

Pancreatic enzyme deficiencies can cause digestive issues that often seem unrelated to specific foods. However, fat digestion is commonly impacted. Fat digestion problems can show up as greasy, shiny stools, or stools that are light in color and foul-smelling. If you experience diarrhea or bloating two to four hours after meals, particularly after eating fatty foods, you might be low in pancreatic enzymes or bile (see page 156). Symptoms like dry skin, unexplained weight loss, and deficiencies in vitamins A, D, E, and K are also common. Research shows that 5 percent to 13 percent of people with IBS have insufficient pancreatic enzyme production, which may also contribute to diarrhea and abdominal pain in IBS-D.

While pancreatic enzyme insufficiency is more commonly associated with conditions like cystic fibrosis, it can also be due to non-pancreatic causes such as villous atrophy, SIBO, gut infection, celiac disease, Crohn's disease, and gallstones. Mold exposure, hypothyroidism, autoimmune conditions, a history of alcoholism, and chronic stress also increase the risk.

Exocrine pancreatic insufficiency (EPI) is a more severe deficiency in enzymes, primarily of the lipase enzyme, resulting in fat malabsorption and steatorrhea (greasy stools). Chronic pancreatitis is the main cause of EPI, with as many as eight in ten adults with pancreatitis developing EPI, but there are other causes as well, such as alcohol use, IBD, SIBO, celiac, stress, or heavy metal toxicity. In non-pancreatic cases of EPI, the loss of the intestinal brush border proteins of the villi is thought to be the primary driver. Studies suggest that 5 percent of people with IBS-D meet the criteria for EPI.

A simple stool test of fecal elastase, an enzyme produced by the pancreas, can be tested as a stand-alone or part of a comprehensive stool analysis (CSA) to determine if one has pancreatic enzyme deficiencies. Anything less than 200 μ/g is considered insufficiency and generally does require supplementation. A healthy, well-functioning digestive tract should have levels greater than 500 μ/g, and thus a level between 200 μ/g and 500 μ/g may already indicate a decrease in pancreatic output and may benefit from supplementation. Stool tests that measure fecal elastase include Diagnostic Solutions GI-MAP, Vibrant

Wellness Gut Zoomer 3.0, Genova Diagnostics GI Effects, Mosaic Diagnostics Comprehensive Stool Analysis, and Doctor's Data GI360.

Supporting Pancreatic Enzymes

In my experience, pancreatic enzyme deficiencies can be reversed about 50 percent of the time with a few weeks to a few months of supplementing with pancreatic enzymes. In other cases, people may need to take the enzymes long term and do more detective work to identify why they are deficient in pancreatic enzymes. Supplementing with pancreatic enzymes may also reduce bile acid malabsorption (see page 162).

Research indicates that pancreatic enzyme therapy might relieve abdominal pain and diarrhea in people with IBS-D and can significantly improve stool frequency, consistency, abdominal pain scores, distension, and IBS severity scores in people with EPI.

Pancreatic enzymes are available as prescriptions and as supplements (in many countries including the United States). The prescription enzymes are derived from animals and are bioidentical to the enzymes the body makes.

Commercial pancreatic enzymes contain a mixture of the enzymes amylase, lipase, and protease, and they are sometimes referred to as pancreases, pancrelipase, and/or pancreatin.

Prescription options include Creon, Pancreaze, Zenpep, Ultresa, Viokase, and Pertzye

Pure Encapsulations Pancreatic Enzyme Formula Supplement: This formula contains a blend of lipase, amylase, and protease and is my preferred go-to when people need a higher dose of pancreatic enzymes but not as high as prescription versions.

Dosing pancreatic enzymes: Prescription pancreatic enzymes are dosed by weight and meal size, while supplemental versions usually provide a starting dose on the package (which may be enough for many cases of mild fat digestive issues but may need to be increased to your individual needs).

Our pancreas works, along with our liver and gallbladder, to break down and absorb fats in the small intestine. If using pancreatic enzymes alone doesn't help, consider adding bile supportive supplements such as ox bile to pancreatic enzymes. Supplement options with pancreatic enzymes and ox bile combined include Rootcology Pancreatic Enzymes Plus and Designs for Health PaleoZyme.

If pancreatic enzymes don't solve the problem after one to two months, and if fat malabsorption is ongoing, consider turning to additional liver and gallbladder support measures to ensure that they are producing and secreting bile effectively.

Additional Strategies for Supporting Pancreatic Enzymes

Reduce Alcohol Intake and Cease Smoking
Both are risk factors for pancreatitis.

Consider Adjusting Your Eating Habits
Eating smaller frequent meals may help with better absorption, while adding digestive herbs to meals can help stimulate digestive enzymes. For example, curcumin increases lipase activity by 80 percent, and coriander, turmeric, red chili, black pepper, cumin, and ginger have all been shown to enhance pancreatic enzymes and bile flow. While fats are essential to our survival and we never want to be on a "fat-free" diet, we may need to be mindful of the kinds of fats we eat. Some may benefit from incorporating easier-to-digest fats such as coconut oil.

Poor Bile Flow

Low bile flow can make it tough to digest fats properly, leading to issues like diarrhea, bloating, and gas after meals. Food might sit too long in the digestive tract, triggering symptoms like SIBO and food sensitivities, both of which can contribute to IBS. Sluggish bile production can be caused by medications (like antibiotics or contraceptives), hormonal imbalances (like estrogen dominance), or nutrient deficiencies (vitamins A and D and amino acids like taurine).

Mold toxicity has also been linked to poor bile flow, as mold's endotoxins block bile formation. Insufficient bile flow is often a sign that the gallbladder and/or liver is malfunctioning, which can cause abdominal pain (upper right side or middle), pain after eating, cramping, and diarrhea. Studies have shown that people with IBS are three times more likely to undergo gallbladder removal (cholecystectomy). Hypothyroidism can further slow bile flow, making fat digestion even more challenging.

Supporting Bile Flow and Fat Digestion

If you're struggling with fat digestion or gallbladder issues, there are several key strategies that can help improve bile flow and overall fat metabolism.

Limit or Avoid Gallbladder-Unfriendly Foods

Onions, milk, pork, poultry, coffee, nuts, corn, tomatoes, and oranges have been found to cause gallbladder/fat digestion issues. Gluten has also been linked to gallbladder issues. You might want to avoid these, at least until your fat digestion improves.

Consider Cholagogues

Cholagogues are substances that help increase bile flow/production and include:

- Artichoke extract has prokinetic benefits, supporting the passage of food through the digestive tract—and can help stimulate bile production and flow from the liver.

- Taurine is an amino acid that is a major constituent of bile. It protects the body from both toxicity and oxidative stress and can naturally improve bile production.

- Herbs including gentian, ginger, fennel, and dandelion—which can be used as stand-alone supplements, as teas, or as part of a digestive bitters supplement—have been found to help increase bile flow.

- Milk thistle contains silymarin, a liver-protective compound with antioxidant and potential anti-inflammatory effects. It has been shown to stimulate bile production in the liver and improve pancreatic function after exposure to toxic agents.

- L-methionine is an amino acid can improve liver function and bile flow by preventing excess fat buildup in the liver and by breaking down histamines.

- Inositol is a sugar has been shown to improve bile acid secretion as well as reduce oxidative stress.

Consider Supplemental Bile Acids
Supplementing with bile acids can provide extra bile and increase bile flow to aid fat digestion.

Ursodiol
Available by prescription, ursodiol is a capsule or tablet that contains ursodeoxycholic acid, a naturally occurring bile acid found in human bile and the bile of certain species of bears that is now produced synthetically by pharmaceutical companies. It increases bile flow by stimulating the production of bile by the liver and decreases the cholesterol content of bile, reducing sludge and preventing the formation of gallstones.

Ox Bile
Bile salts (the building blocks of bile acid) from oxen have been shown to increase bile flow and support fat digestibility in animal studies. Ox

bile can be found in combination products such as Rootcology Liver and Gallbladder Support or as a stand-alone supplement—for example Allergy Research Group Ox Bile. I recommend working with a practitioner to determine your ideal dose.

TUDCA (Tauroursodeoxycholic Acid)
A specific form of bile acids derived from the amino acid taurine. A high-quality option is Cellcore Advanced TUDCA.

Consider Additional Support
Supplementing with carnitine to support fat transport and fat-soluble vitamins (see the box on page 187 in chapter 6) can also be helpful.

Bile Acid Malabsorption

Bile acid malabsorption (BAM) is another key issue that can lead to digestive distress, particularly in people with IBS-D symptoms. Bile acid malabsorption has been found in approximately 10 to 35 percent of people with IBS-D type symptoms, and it may be a treatable cause behind diarrhea in up to 30 percent of cases of IBS-D! Normally, bile is reabsorbed after doing its job in digestion, but when this doesn't happen, excess bile moves into the colon, causing watery diarrhea. Symptoms may include watery diarrhea multiple times per day; vomiting bile; malabsorption of food; painful, urgent, watery, or smelly stools; yellow stools; stomach cramps; bloating; weight gain or loss; and nausea.

Dr. Saad F. Habba first described this and called it "Habba syndrome" in 2011, and since that time, other researchers have also made the connection between IBS-D and BAM.

BAM occurs when either too much bile is produced or the body isn't absorbing it properly. There are four main types of BAM:

1. Type 1 is linked to damage in the ileum (small intestine), often due to surgery or conditions like Crohn's disease.

2. Type 2 involves overproduction of bile by the liver, usually due to disrupted communication between the liver and intestines.
3. Type 3 is triggered by other GI diseases, like celiac disease, pancreatitis, or SIBO, or gallbladder removal.
4. Type 4 occurs due to elevated triglycerides or certain medications, such as Metformin.

Testing is available, though not always widely accessible, with fecal bile acid excretion and serum 7αC4 tests being the most common. In many cases, doctors may recommend a therapeutic trial with bile sequestrant medications like cholestyramine or colesevelam to manage symptoms and confirm BAM. A ten-day trial of cholestyramine, at a dose of 4–36 grams per day, has been suggested as a potential screening test. Fani and colleagues from the University of Pisa suggest, "In patients with symptom improvement, the treatment may be stopped, and, if the BAM symptoms reappear after seven days, the test is considered positive."

Relieving Symptoms of Bile Acid Malabsorption
Using bile acid sequestrants for BAM is the best-studied approach to relieve symptoms, and I am not aware of other therapies that are as effective at this time.

Bile sequestrant medications work by blocking bile acid in the stomach and include:

- Cholestyramine: 4 grams per day, or up to 4 times daily
- Colestipol: 4 grams per day, or up to 4 times daily
- Colesevelam: 1,875 mg up to twice daily

That said, if the cause of BAM has been identified, that may also lead to symptom resolution. As a pharmacist, I can't hold back from talking about stopping/finding an alternative to metformin if that's the cause (ahem, look into berberine). Additionally, high triglyceride levels can be normalized with 4 grams of fish oil per day (see chapter 6).

Furthermore, some research ties the gut microbiome to BAM, and increasing *Bifidobacteria* while lowering *E. coli* may help (bacteriophage supplements often do both). *Lactobacillus-* and *Bifidobacteria-*based probiotics may also reduce the amount of bile acids that reach the gut.

There are also some complementary medicine options that can alleviate symptoms a bit while you are investigating root causes or waiting to find a doctor who can provide testing or a prescription for one of the above.

Diet

Dietary fibers, including the soluble fiber pectin, can bind to secondary bile acids and aid their elimination, while resistant starch found in foods like cooked, then cooled rice, green bananas, and potatoes can support proper bile acid metabolism and rebalance the gut flora. Certain vegetables are also helpful for binding bile, including beets, okra, and asparagus. Compared to cholestyramine (the gold standard), the relative effectiveness of binding bile acids for beets is 54 percent, for okra it is 34 percent, and for asparagus it is 13 percent.

Enzyme Supplements

In those lacking pancreatic enzymes, supplementing with them can help with BAM. Anecdotally, a few people reported symptom relief of BAM with Rootcology Liver and Gallbladder Support, potentially due to the bile-thinning properties that make the bile easier to reabsorb.

Lecithin

Lecithin, derived from soy or sunflower, contains phosphatidylcholine, which can help thin out bile, making it easier to absorb. NOW Foods Sunflower Lecithin is one option.

Activated Charcoal

Activated charcoal binds to bile so it doesn't bring more water into the intestines, reducing diarrhea. Please note that excess use can lead to constipation. A high-quality option is Integrative Therapeutics Activated Charcoal.

Brush Border Enzyme Deficiency

If high-carb or FODMAP-rich meals make you feel bloated and gassy, or if you wake up with a flat stomach that looks five months pregnant by evening, a brush border enzyme deficiency might be at play. Other signs can include acne flare-ups and inconsistent bowel habits like diarrhea alternating with constipation.

Brush border enzymes are the enzymes produced by the plasma membrane that lines the microvilli of the small intestine, also known as the "brush border." These enzymes are primarily responsible for digesting carbohydrates and proteins. Carbohydrates, consisting of fiber, starch, and sugar, are one of the three macronutrients found in many different foods. The body turns these carbohydrates into glucose for energy. Complex carbohydrates are found in fruits, vegetables, and whole grains, while sugar and refined grain products are considered simple carbohydrates. There are several different types of sugars found in foods, including glucose, fructose (found mainly in fruit), sucrose (found mainly in table sugar), lactose (found mainly in dairy), and maltose (found mainly in grains and some fruits). Carbohydrates are primarily digested by enzymes that break them down into simpler sugars that are easier to digest. The following are the main enzymes involved in carbohydrate digestion. They are all secreted by the brush border in the small intestine except for amylase, which is produced by the salivary glands and the pancreas.

- Amylase: Amylase is an enzyme that breaks down complex carbohydrates, such as starch, into simpler sugars like maltose.

- Maltase: Maltase is an enzyme that further breaks down maltose into glucose.

- Sucrase: Sucrase is responsible for breaking down sucrose (table sugar) into glucose and fructose.

- Lactase: Lactase is needed for the digestion of lactose, the sugar found in milk. It breaks lactose into glucose and galactose.

Brush border enzymes work in synergy with amylase to help break down complex carbohydrates such as starch into simple sugars that the body can absorb and use for energy. When someone doesn't have enough brush border enzymes, they might experience bloating, stomach pain, nausea, flatulence, and diarrhea, especially after eating carbohydrate-rich foods or dairy products.

Damage to the brush border can also result in exocrine pancreatic insufficiency, leading to digestive symptoms and nutrient deficiencies.

A few of the most common carbohydrate digestive issues are lactose intolerance (deficiency of the lactase enzyme), fructose intolerance (usually a malabsorption issue due to damage of the brush border), and sucrose intolerance (deficiency of the enzyme sucrase-isomaltase). As all three of these are common digestive triggers, they were covered in detail in chapter 4.

Not All That Flattens the Villi Is Celiac Disease

The villi, small fingerlike structures in the intestines, are crucial for nutrient absorption. When they flatten, or atrophy, due to damage, nutrient absorption decreases, leading to deficiencies, diarrhea, and weight loss. While celiac disease is responsible for most cases of villous atrophy, other factors can damage the villi, too.

> Certain medications have been linked to villous damage, including mycophenolate mofetil, azathioprine, methotrexate, nonsteroidal anti-inflammatory drugs (NSAIDs), and olmesartan.
>
> Conditions such as common variable immune deficiency (CVID), collagenous sprue, tropical sprue, Whipple's disease, viral infections (HIV, norovirus, rotavirus, adenovirus, and astrovirus), and protozoal infections (such as *Giardia*) can also be culprits.
>
> Additionally, the following can contribute to villous atrophy: nutrient deficiencies including L-glutamine, toxic burden (including mold exposure), chronic stress, gastric pH imbalances, bacterial overgrowth, food allergies, and any chronic inflammation of the gut (Crohn's disease).

How Do You Know If You Have Digestive Enzyme Deficiencies?

Symptoms that may suggest you have digestive enzyme deficiencies include many of the symptoms of IBS, such as bloating after meals, diarrhea, and/or constipation, abdominal discomfort, and seeing undigested food in stool. (Except corn! It never ceases to aMAIZE me that no matter how perfect our digestion is and how much we chew it, corn always makes an appearance in our poop! Apologies for the "corny" joke.) I've also found that some people may experience acid reflux, feeling like food is stuck in their stomach, or fatigue after eating as a main symptom.

Some people with digestive issues may find they are seemingly triggered by the texture of certain foods. Others may find they don't do well with lactose, excess fruit, raw vegetables, or fiber, others with fats, and yet others with dense protein foods such as steaks. (I have had the pleasure of experiencing all of these at various points in my life.) Each of these is a clue that a part of your digestive process needs help. In contrast, BAM presents with a pretty unique profile of multiple bouts of diarrhea per day.

> ### What About Fiber Digestion?
>
> Trouble with fiber digestion often presents as bloating or constipation after eating high-fiber foods or raw vegetables. If you notice undigested food, particularly vegetable fibers, in your stool or struggle with hemorrhoids, your gut microbiome might be out of balance. See strategies in chapters 4 and 7.

How Do You Know Which Enzyme Is Out of Balance?

Recognizing the signs of enzyme deficiencies can be tricky, as they often overlap with other digestive issues, but there are some telltale symptoms for specific types of enzyme deficiencies.

Testing and trials can also help determine what particular deficiency you may have. I have created a guide to help identify some of the standout patterns and symptoms that may suggest one particular enzyme deficiency over another.

Please note that I have included pancreatic enzymes and bile together. Both are needed for fat digestion and it's difficult to tease out the individual enzyme with symptoms alone, but fecal elastase testing can identify a pancreatic enzyme deficiency over a bile issue. When it comes to BAM, diarrhea multiple times each day is a telltale symptom.

Symptoms of Digestive Enzyme Deficiencies

	LOW STOMACH ACID	PANCREATIC ENZYMES/BILE DEFICIENCY	CARBOHYDRATE ENZYME DEFICIENCIES	FIBER/ DYSBIOSIS
Diets that make you feel better	Vegan, vegetarian diets	Low-fat diet or not really sure	Low-carb, sugar-free, limited fruit, low FODMAP	Paleo, carnivore, keto diet, well-cooked diet
Diets that make you feel worse	Animal protein rich, tough meats like steaks	Fatty foods/keto diet	High-sugar, fruit, high FODMAP	High-fiber, raw vegetables and/or fruit
Telltale signs	B_{12} or iron deficiency, taking antacids, acid reflux, feels like food sits in your stomach, low energy, pain	Bleeding tendency, vitamin deficiencies in A, D, E, K, unexplained weight loss, dry skin, gallbladder pain, adult acne, symptoms 2 to 4 hours after eating	Bloating, stomach looks flat in the morning but five months pregnant in the evening	Acne/skin breakouts
Co-occurring	SIBO, parasites, frequent food poisoning	Protozoan infections	SIBO, celiac disease, *Candidiasis*, protozoa	Dysbiosis
Poop	Diarrhea or constipation, or mixed	Diarrhea, or alternating constipation/diarrhea; fatty, greasy, or shiny stools; light-colored, yellow, foul-smelling poop that floats; stool poorly formed; three or more large BMs per day	Diarrhea or constipation, or mixed	Vegetable fibers in stool; hemorrhoids; mostly constipation

Recommended Brands of Enzymes to Support Digestion

- Broad-spectrum digestive enzyme support:
  » Digestive bitters: Wellena Liver and Digestive Bitters Kit, Quicksilver Scientific Dr. Shade's Bitters No. 9, Nature's Way NatureWorks Swedish Bitters, Designs for Health CarminaGest
  » Multi-ingredient enzymes: Rootcology Broad Spectrum Enzymes, SFI Health Ther-Biotic SIBB-Zymes, SFI Health Ther-Biotic Vital-Zymes Complete, Pure Encapsulations Digestive Enzymes Ultra, and Transformation Enzymes Digest
- Protein digestion support: Rootcology Betaine with Pepsin, Pure Encapsulations Betaine HCl Pepsin, Xymogen GastrAcid, Nutridyn HCl Support, Ortho Molecular Betaine, and Pepsin
- Fat digestion support:
  » Pure Encapsulations Pancreatic Enzyme Formula
  » With ox bile: Rootcology Pancreatic Enzymes Plus, Designs for Health PaleoZyme
  » Prescription options: Creon, Pancreaze, Zenpep, Ultresa, Viokase, Pertzye
- FODMAP digestion support: Microbiome Labs FODMATE Digestive Enzymes
- Lactose digestive enzymes: Seeking Health Lactase Drops, Lactaid
- Fructose digestive enzymes: Omne Diem Fructose Digest, Fructaid, Microbiome Labs FODMATE Digestive Enzymes
- Sucrose digestive enzymes: Rootcology Broad Spectrum Enzymes, SFI Health Ther-Biotic SIBB-Zymes, SFI Health Ther-Biotic

> Vital-Zymes Complete, Pure Encapsulations Digestive Enzymes Ultra, Transformation Enzymes Digest
>
> • Fiber digestive issues: Rootcology Broad Spectrum Enzymes, Designs for Health Plant Enzyme Digestive Formula, SFI Health Ther-Biotic Vital-Zymes Complete

Chapter Summary

- Supporting our digestive process with lifestyle changes to encourage a parasympathetic rest-and-digest mode (relax and slow down while eating) and optimize digestion (chew well, move regularly) as well as broad-spectrum and targeted digestive enzyme supplementation to help the body break down food are powerful ways to relieve IBS-related symptoms.

- Broad-spectrum digestive support practices include using food as medicine (hot lemon water, apple cider vinegar, fermented foods, bone broth, bitter foods and spices, herbal digestive teas) and supplementing with digestive bitters and multi-ingredient enzyme formulations.

- Low stomach acid, low levels of pancreatic enzymes, bile deficiency, bile acid malabsorption, low levels of brush border enzymes in the small intestine, and an imbalance of colonic bacteria are digestive system issues that can lead to IBS symptoms.

- While there is a big overlap in symptoms among these deficiencies, testing and trials can help determine whether you have a particular deficiency, as can the standout patterns and symptoms in the chart on page 169.

- Though the specifics depend on the particular enzyme deficiency, there are simple lifestyle strategies and supplement options for each type that can help restore and optimize healthy digestion.

Visit https://ibsrootcause.com/bonus for notes on this chapter.

CHAPTER 6

Depletions

Whether you have diarrhea or constipation, nutrient deficiencies can be a very important root cause of IBS symptoms and can be a stand-alone cause of IBS or a consequence of enzyme deficiencies, SIBO, and other causes.

Macronutrients (protein, fats) and micronutrients (vitamins) are necessary for optimal digestive health. Without enough gut-supporting nutrients on board, a range of uncomfortable symptoms—depending on which nutrient (or nutrients!) are deficient—will persist and worsen.

There are many reasons you may be experiencing nutrient deficiencies, including our current farming practices and eating the Standard Western Diet.

Additionally, gut inflammation, an imbalance of gut flora, and digestive enzyme deficiencies can prevent the proper extraction of nutrients from our food, and overgrowths and infections can intercept nutrients so that we never actually receive them! Various types of medications, including acid blockers, which are widely used by those with acid reflux and other IBS-related symptoms, and health conditions such as hypothyroidism can also deplete valuable nutrients.

Ironically, restrictive diets utilized for IBS, such as the low FODMAP diet and gluten-free diet, can potentially lead to nutrient depletions.

Growing up in the 2000s, I received most of my "nutrition education" from Subway commercials, and it's sad to note that most health care professionals are not properly trained in nutrition—even my doctorate program in pharmacy taught me very little about proper nutrition! After years of continuing education, I know now that it's best to avoid processed foods that are stripped of nutrients and stick to real, whole foods as often as possible.

Is Your Diet Providing the Nutrients You Need?

While mainstream media will have you believe that you can get all your nutrients from food, I have found that is simply not the case. Eating a diet rich in a diversity of whole foods, proper enzyme supplementation, and targeted nutrient supplementation is the best way to ensure we are taking in a healthy array of nutrients and preventing depletions, especially with digestive issues! We covered digestive enzymes in the previous chapter, and we will do a deep dive on supplementation here, but for now, let's focus on the impact of diet. People following a restrictive diet may find that they are not consuming all of the nutrients their body needs to function properly.

DIET TYPE	NUTRIENTS DEPLETED
Gluten-free diet	Vitamins A, B_1, B_2, B_3, B_5, B_6, B_7, B_9, B_{12}, and D, calcium, copper, iron, magnesium, phosphorus, selenium, and zinc
Grain-free diets	Selenium, thiamine, iron, and zinc
Vegan and vegetarian diets	Vitamin B_{12}, calcium, chromium, copper, iodine, iron, magnesium, manganese, omega-3 fatty acids, and zinc

DIET TYPE	NUTRIENTS DEPLETED
Low FODMAP diet	Calcium and fiber
Low-fat diets	Vitamins A, D, E, and K and omega-3 fatty acids
High-protein diets	Vitamins B_1, B_6, B_7, D, and E, calcium, chromium, folate, iodine, iron, magnesium, and molybdenum
Dairy- and lactose-free diet	Vitamins D and B_1 and calcium
Low-carbohydrate diets	Vitamins B_2, B_6, and B_9, calcium, fiber, iron, magnesium, and potassium
Carnivore diets	Fiber and vitamins and minerals found in plant foods
Standard American Diet	Vitamins A, D, E, and K, calcium, iodine, magnesium, omega-3 fatty acids, potassium, and zinc

Are Nutrient Deficiencies the Chicken or the Egg?

People with IBS are often deficient in numerous nutrients, but which nutrient deficiencies *cause* IBS symptoms and which nutrient deficiencies are a *consequence* of IBS symptoms? I suppose if you're trying to optimize your health it doesn't necessarily make a difference, but in this chapter we will focus on specific nutrients that tend to be needle movers for resolving IBS symptoms.

Glutamine, zinc, and vitamins A and D can help resolve diarrhea, while thiamine, magnesium, fatty acids, vitamin C, and potassium can help resolve constipation. Please note that in excess, vitamin D can cause constipation.

Long-term IBS often leads to nutrient deficiencies, possibly due to a combination of malabsorption, restrictive diets, or gut infections. A 2022 review showed that people with IBS tend to have lower levels of vitamins B_2, D, calcium, and iron. Exclusion diets, commonly used for symptom management, can also reduce intake of vitamins B_1, B_2, calcium, iron, and zinc.

In addition to the nutrients mentioned earlier, I would also consider testing and optimizing vitamin B_{12} levels and addressing the fat-soluble vitamins E and K for anyone with IBS. Vitamin B_{12} deficiency is often a consequence of low stomach acid, SIBO, and gut infections, and vitamins E and K are commonly depleted due to fat malabsorption, which usually manifests as diarrhea. Furthermore, thiamine deficiency can also result from prolonged diarrhea and lead to constipation.

While it's hard to say whether nutrient deficiencies are the cause or result of IBS, addressing them is essential for improving symptoms and overall health. Some nutrients can be safely supplemented without testing, but others do require lab work to ensure proper levels (see below for guidance).

Test or Guess?

While some nutrients are safe to supplement with, even in higher doses, there are some nutrients that can build up in the body and become toxic to us. The questions are: When should we test and is it OK to guess? It depends on the nutrient, and the dose you are supplementing.

- Best to test: vitamin B_{12}, iron/ferritin, and vitamin D. Iron and vitamin D can lead to problems when they're both too low or too high, so I always recommend testing before supplementing and monitoring levels while supplementing. Low B_{12} levels may indicate pernicious anemia, a condition where oral B_{12} supplements are not effective and B_{12} injections or sublingual administration may be required, so it's super important to monitor whether treatment is effective.

- Depends on dose: Zinc is generally safe to supplement without testing at up to 30 mg per day, but doses higher than that can lead to copper depletion, so if you choose to supplement with higher doses, I recommend testing both zinc and copper levels.

- OK to guess: Most of the other nutrients I discuss in this chapter are generally safe and well tolerated. Furthermore, tests are not as readily available.

Nutrients for Resolving Diarrhea

Glutamine, zinc, and vitamin A can help resolve diarrhea and are often well tolerated and generally safe to supplement without testing.

Glutamine

Glutamine is essential for a healthy gut barrier and immune system. L-glutamine, the form used by the body and found in foods and supplements, has been researched for various digestive issues such as Crohn's disease, celiac disease, IBS, and intestinal infections.

It is the most studied substance for healing intestinal permeability, a common feature of IBS-D (see chapter 8). Glutamine serves as fuel for gut and immune cells, preventing bacteria from leaking out of the gut.

A deficiency can lead to gut inflammation, intestinal lining damage, villous atrophy, mucosal ulcerations, and higher susceptibility to infections. Supplementing with L-glutamine has been shown to reduce gut inflammation and repair the damage to the gut lining caused by NSAIDs or surgery.

L-glutamine is particularly helpful for IBS-D, often resolving diarrhea quickly—even leading to constipation if dosed up too quickly—whether caused by post-infectious IBS-D, SIBO, infections, or exercise-induced diarrhea. In one study, 15 grams per day improved IBS symptoms for those on a low FODMAP diet.

While the body can produce glutamine, chronic stress, intense exercise (such as ultra marathon running), infections, food allergies, and inflammatory conditions like IBS, IBD, and celiac disease can deplete it. Major injuries, infections, chemotherapy, and radiation can also increase glutamine needs, as can being in a catabolic state (when the body is breaking down muscle for energy).

Symptoms of glutamine deficiency can be hard to pinpoint, but if you have IBS-D, cravings, blood sugar issues, or exercise-induced diarrhea, you might benefit from a glutamine trial. It's safe, well-tolerated, and has a pleasant taste. Vegans and vegetarians are at a higher risk for deficiency, since glutamine is primarily found in animal protein.

The Catabolic State

When the body is in a catabolic state (due to chronic inflammation, illness, or infection), it starts breaking down muscle for fuel. This is the opposite of the healthier anabolic state, where the body builds and repairs muscle, leaving you feeling strong and healthy.

In a catabolic state, you may notice muscle loss, increased body fat (some people call this "skinny fat"), fatigue, pain, infections that linger, poor sleep, digestion issues, cravings, depression, or anxiety. Physical activities—both intense and light—may become more difficult.

To move your body from a catabolic state to an anabolic state, you'll want to support your body with amino acids, including L-glutamine, optimize thyroid hormone levels, ensure you're eating enough protein (and digesting it), support your stress response, address underlying infections, address nutrient deficiencies such as carnitine, magnesium, and zinc, and incorporate lower-intensity exercise like yoga, Pilates, and weight training (versus intense cardio).

Replenishing Glutamine

Glutamine-Rich Foods

Beef, chicken, and fish are high in L-glutamine (1.2–1.7 g per 100 g). Bone broth and gelatin are also great sources and easier to digest. That said, to truly move the needle in IBS-D, an L-glutamine supplement in a therapeutic dose may be needed.

L-Glutamine Supplement

Research has shown supplementing up to 0.65 gram per kilogram of body mass is well tolerated. For a 150-pound person, that equates to about 44 grams. Start with 5 grams per day, working up to 45 grams (divided into three doses).

For best results, you may wish to combine L-glutamine with other gut-healing ingredients such as zinc carnosine and mucilaginous herbs (see chapter 8). For IBS-D, supplementing for two to six months is generally helpful. Various companies make stand-alone L-glutamine powders (such as Pure Encapsulations L-Glutamine), and L-glutamine is a common ingredient in gut-healing powders such as Rootcology Gut R&R and Designs for Health GI Revive.

What If You Can't Tolerate Glutamine?

Some people experience brain fog, anxiety, and irritability from supplementing with glutamine due to histamine intolerance or an excess conversion to glutamate, an excitatory neurotransmitter. This is often caused by a vitamin B_6 deficiency. Vitamin B_6 is necessary for the metabolism of glutamate and the breakdown of histamine.

Supplementing with B_6, in the active form known as P5P, can help with tolerating L-glutamine. To resolve glutamine reactions,

> you may wish to supplement with P5P (Rootcology P5P is a high-quality option) for one to two weeks before starting L-glutamine.
>
> Additional substances that over-convert to glutamate in the presence of a B_6 deficiency include glycine, glycinate, GABA, and alpha-ketoglutarate. If you continue to have an adverse reaction to glutamine, you may need to continue with the P5P for a longer period of time or address other potential issues such as histamine intolerance (see chapter 4). Please note that some practitioners use L-glutamine depletion to starve cancer cells, so be sure to check with your doctor if you have a history of cancer.

Zinc

Though the body needs only small amounts of this trace mineral, zinc is a major player in gut health. Research has found that those with IBS have significantly higher copper-zinc ratios, suggesting zinc deficiency. A recent study found that people with IBS-D had serum levels of zinc that were much lower, and this was associated with higher levels of zonulin, an indication of impaired intestinal barrier function. Zinc also plays an important role in our susceptibility to infections and reduced detoxification of bacterial toxins.

Replenishing zinc has been shown to repair intestinal permeability and have a beneficial impact on gut inflammation. Studies have also found that it promotes the growth of probiotics such as *Lactobacillus* spp., inhibits the growth of pathogenic *Escherichia coli*, and prevents diarrhea.

Because zinc is not stored in the body, a daily intake is recommended, even for the general population.

Celiac disease, prolonged diarrhea, and other malabsorption syndromes can impair the gut's ability to absorb zinc. Depletions can also be caused by other root causes associated with IBS symptoms such as low stomach acid; hypocortisolism; certain medications, such as PPIs (proton pump inhibitors); and various gut infections, such as *Giardia*.

Some of the most common symptoms of zinc deficiency include poor wound healing, dandruff, eczema or other skin rashes, skin issues (acne, canker sores, foot fungus), poor appetite, diarrhea, impaired smell/taste, white spots on nails, and frequent colds or respiratory infections (weakened immune system).

I don't often recommend testing before supplementing with zinc (a dose up to 30 mg can be safely trialed by most people), but a zinc plasma test can be helpful for monitoring zinc status and when using zinc supplements above 30 mg. Please note that reference ranges can vary. Quest Diagnostics uses the reference range of 60–130 mcg/dL, and the ideal levels indicating zinc sufficiency are 120–130 mcg/dL. Additionally, low alkaline phosphatase levels [usually part of a CBC (complete blood count) test] can indicate zinc deficiency.

Replenishing Zinc
Foods High in Zinc

High amounts of zinc are found in animal products such as oysters and red meats, though zinc supplements are what I typically recommend to move the needle in IBS.

Zinc Carnosine

Zinc carnosine, a combination of zinc and the amino acid L-carnosine, is my preferred form of zinc for gut health. It stays intact in the acidic environment of the stomach and adheres effectively to gut wounds, where it separates into zinc and L-carnosine to heal gut tissue. It has powerful mucosal-protective and anti-ulcerative properties, supports the intestinal lining, and helps maintain tight junctions. Some great stand-alone zinc carnosine supplements include Integrative Therapeutics Zinc Carnosine, Pure Encapsulations Peptic-Care, and Seeking Health Zinc Carnosine. I've also formulated Rootcology Gut R&R,

which combines zinc carnosine, L-glutamine, and other gut-healing herbs in one delicious supplement.

For those seeking alternative forms of zinc, I recommend zinc picolinate (from Pure Encapsulations), oyster supplements, and compounded topical zinc. Topical zinc is particularly useful for individuals who have difficulty swallowing or absorbing zinc orally.

Vitamin A

Vitamin A is vital for gut health, supporting the growth and maintenance of the gut lining and mucus layer. A deficiency can lead to intestinal permeability, gut dysbiosis, and inflammation, especially in those with IBS or fat malabsorption.

It also plays a key role in the immune system, helping produce T cells that fight infections and lower inflammation. A deficiency in vitamin A has been linked to higher levels of pro-inflammatory molecules and can cause skin issues, vision problems, poor wound healing, and increased susceptibility to infections.

Since the body can't produce vitamin A, it must come from the diet. The most bioavailable form, retinol, is found in animal foods like liver, egg yolks, and seafood, making vegans and vegetarians more prone to deficiency. Plant-based sources contain beta-carotene, but only 55 percent of people can efficiently convert it to retinol. For the 45 percent (myself included) with a genetic variation in the BCMO1 gene, this conversion is impaired, requiring us to rely more on animal sources.

Vitamin A depletion may be more common in those with fat malabsorption due to bile issues, chronic pancreatitis, and exocrine pancreatic insufficiency.

Symptoms of deficiency can include skin disorders, acne, cystic acne, vision problems (especially night blindness), poor wound healing, dry skin, dry eyes, fertility issues, and frequent infections. While testing for vitamin A isn't routine, you can self-order a vitamin A test through Ulta Labs. Low fecal elastase on a stool test may also suggest a deficiency, especially in those with pancreatic insufficiency.

Replenishing Vitamin A
Foods Rich in Vitamin A

If you're not sure about your genes, the best way to make sure you're getting enough vitamin A is to eat a variety of foods high in vitamin A (or its precursors), including beef liver, the richest source of retinol (aim for one serving one to two times per week), wild-caught salmon, sweet potatoes, spinach, yellow peppers, carrots, and broccoli.

Supplementation

Consider vitamin A drops, like SFI Health Micellized Vitamin A Liquid or Seeking Health Vitamin A Drops, or high-quality cod liver oil from brands like Pure Encapsulations.

I recommend working with a practitioner to evaluate your need to supplement with vitamin A, as too much can lead to toxicity (irritability; vomiting; peeling skin; dry, rough skin; and eyebrow hair loss are signs of toxicity). Prolonged intake of high levels of vitamin A can result in damage to the liver, the bones, and the central nervous system.

Vitamin D: Implicated in Both Diarrhea and Constipation

Vitamin D helps maintain the integrity of the gut lining, protecting against intestinal permeability, and supports a healthy gut microbiome by increasing its diversity. It also acts as a powerful antioxidant, reducing inflammation and the risk of infections. Vitamin D is vital for gut health and immune balance, yet many of us are deficient, especially if we spend a lot of time indoors. Low vitamin D levels are common in those with IBS and correlated with symptom severity. Studies have linked vitamin D deficiency to both constipation and diarrhea, yet more research needs to be done to determine if vitamin D deficiency is causing these issues or if chronic constipation or diarrhea due to fat malabsorption is causing low vitamin D. Either way, it's important to make sure you are getting sufficient vitamin D.

While vitamin D is present in foods like fatty fish and fortified dairy, it's hard to get enough from diet alone, particularly if you have fat malabsorption or gut conditions like Crohn's disease, ulcerative colitis, or celiac disease. The most effective way to get vitamin D is through sunlight exposure, but those of us who don't work as lifeguards in Southern California generally don't get enough sunlight exposure. As a result, at least 35 percent of U.S. adults are vitamin D deficient.

Signs of deficiency include fatigue, muscle and bone pain, frequent infections, poor wound healing, depression, hair loss, and conditions like osteoporosis or autoimmune diseases. Since vitamin D is fat-soluble, it's important to test your levels before supplementing.

The 25(OH)D test is preferred, and while most labs flag levels under 30 ng/mL as deficient, I have found that optimal levels are typically between 60 and 80 ng/mL.

Replenishing Vitamin D

Diet

Include foods like wild salmon, cod liver oil, and eggs in your diet, though keep in mind these may not be enough, especially if you have fat malabsorption.

Sunlight

Regular sun exposure is one of the best ways to boost vitamin D. Aim for 10 to 20 minutes of midday sun daily, as tolerated by your skin type. Apps like D-Minder can help track safe sun exposure as determined by our skin type and location. For those in less sunny climates, a beach vacation might be the perfect prescription! Please note, in cases of severe deficiency, getting adequate vitamin D levels would require you to spend four to six hours exposed on a sunny beach . . . for seven days straight. As lovely as that sounds, that's simply not possible for many of us.

Supplements

Vitamin D_3 supplements can help those of us who can't take an extended beach vacation or live in climates that do not provide us with adequate amounts of sun exposure year-round. Research suggests supplementing with vitamin D can improve symptoms, including abdominal pain and gas. A typical dose is 1,000–5,000 IU per day for mild to moderate deficiency, and up to 10,000 IU daily or 50,000 IU weekly for severe deficiency, under a practitioner's guidance. Take supplements with a meal to boost absorption by 30 to 50 percent. Please note that in excess, vitamin D can be toxic and may cause constipation, so recheck your levels in three to six months. High-quality options include Pure Encapsulations Vitamin D_3.

Nutrients for Resolving Constipation
Omega-3 Fatty Acids

Essential fatty acids (EFAs), such as omega-3s, are powerful allies for the healthy functioning of the digestive tract. They enhance intestinal barrier integrity and can help resolve constipation by stimulating intestinal motility and lubricating the intestinal walls. EFAs are needed to synthesize prostaglandins, hormonelike compounds in the body that help regulate the contractions of the smooth muscles lining the GI tract that influence gut motility and transit time. They also support a smooth transit of food through the digestive tract.

Omega-3s support a healthy microbiome by increasing the diversity and abundance of beneficial gut microbiota such as *Bifidobacteria*, which in turn promotes the production of anti-inflammatory SCFAs (short-chain fatty acids). The anti-inflammatory effects of omega-3s have been shown to improve inflammation-related conditions such as constipation, pain, intestinal permeability, and IBD and can prevent relapse of rheumatoid arthritis and Crohn's disease, among others.

EFAs are naturally occurring fats that the body cannot produce; therefore they must be obtained from foods or supplements. The body requires about a 1:1 ratio of omega-3 and omega-6 fats, but today many of us, especially those on the Standard American Diet, get too many omega-6s and not enough omega-3s because we consume meat and fish from animals fed grain, soy, and other foods that are not part of their natural diet, and processed foods made with oils high in omega-6s, such as sunflower and canola. In some cases, the ratio is as high as 1:25. This can be a problem because omega-3 fatty acids reduce inflammation, while omega-6 fatty acids can promote the inflammation associated with many gut disorders including constipation, intestinal permeability, and IBD.

Depletions can also be caused by a low-fat diet, fat malabsorption issues, certain medications (such as female hormones found in oral contraceptives and hormone replacement therapy), or deficiencies in thiamine (vitamin B_1), vitamin B_6, zinc, and magnesium, the nutrients required to convert the short-chain omega-3 fatty acid ALA into the long-chain omega-3s EPA and DHA.

Symptoms of fatty acid deficiency include constipation; light colored, hard, or foul-smelling stool; soft, cracked, or brittle nails; dry, itchy, scaling, or flaking skin; hard earwax; chicken skin (tiny bumps on the backs of arms or on the trunk); dandruff; aching or stiffness in the joints; thirst most of the time; poor mood; difficulty paying attention and/or memory loss; and premenstrual syndrome.

It is generally safe to supplement without testing. If any of the symptoms apply to you, supplementing with fish oil is usually recommended.

Replenishing Omega-3 Fatty Acids
Foods Rich in Omega-3 Fatty Acids

While wild-caught fresh fish can be an excellent source of omega-3 fatty acids, use caution when consuming increased amounts of fish. Numerous studies (including the National Health and Nutrition Examination Survey, or NHANES) have concluded that eating fish is the primary driver of elevated levels of mercury in the body. However, even regularly consuming low-mercury, wild-caught seafood, such as salmon, sardines, and shellfish, might not provide therapeutic amounts of the EPA and DHA that the body requires to reduce inflammation. Grass-fed meats also include a good amount of these omega-3 fatty acids, and freshly ground flaxseeds, chia seeds, and walnuts are great sources of ALA.

Fish Oil

Look for a professional quality fish oil supplement that has been molecularly distilled and filtered. This process ensures purity and helps eliminate contaminants including heavy metals, pesticides, solvents, and PCBs. Consider 1 to 4 grams of Pure Encapsulations EPA/DHA Essentials daily. Cod liver oil provides another option that combines EPA and DHA with vitamins A and D. Nordic Naturals Arctic Cod Liver Oil and Pure Encapsulations Cod Liver Oil are high-quality options. Consider 1 teaspoon daily. For optimal absorption, take fish oil with a meal containing quality fats. Additionally, Seacure, made from the flesh of whitefish, provides omega-3 fatty acids along with gut-supporting amino acids.

Supplementing with Fat-Soluble Vitamins A, D, E, K, and Fish Oil

If you're deficient in one fat-soluble vitamin due to fat malabsorption, it's likely you may also be deficient in other fat-soluble vitamins and fatty acids. If you have fat malabsorption, you may wish to cover your bases and supplement with fish oil and all four fat-soluble vitamins (A, D, E, and K). A few multi-ingredient formulas containing fat-soluble vitamins are DaVinci Labs ADK and Designs for Health ADK Evail.

> Please note that taking vitamin D when vitamin K is deficient can lead to arterial issues. Taking vitamin K along with vitamin D helps direct calcium to the bones and prevents arterial calcification. While vitamin K deficiency isn't routinely tested, signs include easy bruising, excess bleeding, and heavy periods.

Thiamine

Thiamine (vitamin B_1) deficiency can be at the root of several IBS-related symptoms, including constipation. Thiamine deficiency inhibits the release of stomach acid, significantly decreases the amount and potency of digestive enzymes and brush border enzymes, and reduces bile flow, all of which compromise the proper breakdown and absorption of fats, proteins, and other nutrients and slow the progress of food through the digestive tract.

Thiamine also is essential for the synthesis of acetylcholine, the main neurotransmitter used by the vagus nerve to help regulate gut motility. Deficiency can cause low vagal tone and impaired gut contractility in the stomach and small intestine. In studies, supplementing with thiamine has been shown to improve gut motility.

A lack of thiamine can also contribute to an imbalanced gut microbiome, including an increased susceptibility to SIBO and gut infections. According to nutritional researcher Elliot Overton, thiamine deficiency is one of the most overlooked causes of SIBO and IBS-C.

In pharmacy school, I learned about beriberi, a disease caused by severe thiamine deficiency that included symptoms of shortness of breath, rapid heart rate, and decreased muscle function caused by alcoholism or a diet focused on mostly refined carbohydrates such as rice. However, mild to moderate thiamine deficiency can occur in people with diarrhea, malabsorption, celiac disease, IBD, and various autoimmune conditions. On my own healing journey, I was personally shocked that I had thiamine deficiency despite eating a varied diet and abstaining from alcohol.

Furthermore, certain food products, such as black tea, coffee, raw fish, and shellfish, contain thiaminases, enzymes that destroy thiamine. Consuming large quantities of these foods and eating them alongside other thiamine-containing foods can inhibit our ability to absorb adequate levels of thiamine.

While several of the causes of thiamine deficiency such as alcohol use disorder indicate a high risk for thiamine deficiency, signs of mild deficiency are subtle and can be missed via blood tests and by most physicians.

Symptoms of milder forms of thiamine deficiency include fatigue, irritability, depression, constipation, abdominal discomfort, low blood pressure, adrenal issues (the adrenal glands produce hormones that help regulate the body's response to stress), trouble digesting carbohydrates, acid reflux, slowed gastric motility and emptying (gastroparesis), bloating, and gas.

Long-term thiamine deficiency can lead to various symptoms, including brain fog, difficulty breathing, and heart damage. It can also lead to toxic levels of buildup of lactic acid and pyruvic acid, leading to symptoms like fatigue, muscle cramps, nausea, and even mental health issues.

Unfortunately, standard blood tests for thiamine deficiency will only flag severe deficiencies. If you've been struggling with constipation, low stomach acid, carbohydrate intolerance, fatigue, and other symptoms associated with thiamine deficiency, you may benefit from extra thiamine intake. Generally, most people can supplement without prior testing.

Replenishing Thiamine
Thiamine Supplementation

In my experience, mega-doses of thiamine, such as 600 mg per day, are required to move the needle with fatigue and digestion. Thus I typically recommend supplements instead of thiamine-containing foods.

Thiamine supplements can be made as a water-soluble or fat-soluble form.

- Thiamine mononitrate and thiamine hydrochloride are synthetic water-soluble forms that are commonly used in supplements.

- Fat-soluble derivatives of thiamine, such as allithiamine and benfotiamine, are better absorbed by the body and may have additional brain benefits. I have had the most success and experience with benfotiamine. High-quality options include Rootcology Benfotiamine, Pure Encapsulations BenfoMax, and Life Extension Benfotiamine at doses of 600 mg or so per day. An allithiamine option is Thiamax Thiamine.

Magnesium

Magnesium deficiency is a common cause of gut motility issues and constipation, and it is estimated that 50 percent of the U.S. population is not getting enough. Constipation is a red flag for magnesium deficiency, one of the most commonly reported IBS-related symptoms. One study of over three thousand Japanese women linked low magnesium levels to a higher prevalence of constipation. Magnesium supports healthy gut motility by helping draw water into the intestines to soften stool, which makes it easier to pass and stimulates muscle contractions in the digestive tract. Magnesium also supports the mitochondria, optimizing the production of energy and healthy muscle tone required for proper peristalsis, the wavelike muscle action that moves food through the gastrointestinal system.

Magnesium is fundamental to a healthy stress response, and chronic stress can significantly compromise magnesium levels. Other potential causes of deficiency include age (the ability to absorb magnesium in the gut is reduced with age, while the excretion of magnesium through the kidney increases), chronic diarrhea, diabetes, hypothyroidism, alcohol use (alcohol can double, or even quadruple, our excretion of magnesium), and certain medications. These include proton pump inhibitors (Nexium, Prilosec, omeprazole, Protonix), female hormones (oral contraceptives and hormone replacement therapy), and antibiotics.

Magnesium is used for various metabolic processes and is depleted by stress, and so I always say that magnesium deficiency is so common in our modern world that if you have constipation and are not supplementing with magnesium, you're likely magnesium deficient.

Additional common symptoms of deficiency include menstrual cramps, leg cramps or cramps anywhere else in the body, hormonal issues, sensitivity to loud noises, joint pain, depression, irritability and anxiety, frequent headaches or migraines, trouble swallowing, acid reflux, fatigue, muscle twitching, trouble falling and/or staying asleep, hand cramps, premenstrual syndrome, and heart flutters, skipped beats, or palpitations. I generally don't test people for magnesium deficiency, as it is generally safe to take magnesium without testing.

Replenishing Magnesium
Magnesium Supplements

Different forms of magnesium can serve different purposes, and each will have different amounts of elemental magnesium and will need to be dosed slightly differently. If you're constipated, the two most helpful versions are:

- Magnesium citrate: Generally the preferred form because it tends to be more effective at raising magnesium levels in the body, it is also a relatively gentle and generally well-tolerated osmotic laxative that in some cases can get things moving in as few as one to four hours. High-quality magnesium citrate options include Rootcology Magnesium Citrate Powder, Designs for Health's MagCitrate Powder, or Pure Encapsulations Magnesium (Citrate). The usual starting dose for magnesium citrate is 400 mg at bedtime, but magnesium can be dosed to bowel tolerance, meaning you can increase your dosage until your bowel movements become regular, better formed, and easy to pass.

- Magnesium oxide: This form is known for its strong laxative effects and is often used to treat constipation. Typical doses are between 310 and 420 mg.

- Epsom salt bath: It can boost magnesium levels and relieve constipation, especially for those who are not absorbing nutrients well due to gut issues.

Epsom Salts for Constipation?

Epsom salts are marketed for constipation use if taken internally, but I don't recommend using them for that purpose because they don't taste great and dosing can be tricky, leading to GI distress. Rather, I prefer using Epsom salts for soaking in warm baths. You can absorb magnesium through your skin, so Epsom salt baths can be an effective way to boost magnesium levels and to relieve constipation. They can provide quick relief of stomach and muscle cramps and can help reduce stress and constipation. Add 1 cup of Epsom salts to a warm bath and soak for 20 minutes for maximum benefit.

Vitamin C

Vitamin C deficiency can cause constipation by inhibiting the wavelike movements that push food through the gut and aid in healthy bowel movements. Research has found vitamin C speeds transit time. Vitamin C also acts as an osmotic laxative, pulling water into the intestines and increasing the water content of stool, making it softer and easier to pass.

Vitamin C is necessary for the production of collagen, the main structural support protein used to make connective tissue throughout the body, and necessary to maintain the integrity and proper functioning of the gut lining. Collagen is associated with reduced intestinal permeability and inflammation and increased levels of beneficial SCFAs in the gut microbiome, such as butyrate.

Vitamin C is an essential micronutrient that the body doesn't make and needs to get regularly from outside sources to prevent deficiency, which affects about 6 percent of adults in the United States, though evidence suggests many people may have low levels. It's found in a range of fruits and vegetables, such as citrus fruits, berries, potatoes, tomatoes, and leafy greens.

A diet lacking in vitamin C–rich foods, low-carbohydrate diets, malabsorption disorders (IBD, celiac disease), food sensitivities, certain medications (aspirin and NSAIDs; acid blockers including PPIs such as Prilosec, Nexium, and omeprazole; H2 receptor blockers such as Pepcid; and female hormones found in oral contraceptives and hormone replacement therapy), alcohol use disorder, smoking, and eating disorders are risk factors for vitamin C deficiency.

Signs of vitamin C deficiency include dry and splitting hair; inflamed and bleeding gums; rough, dry, scaly skin; corkscrew-shaped body hair; easy bruising and slow wound healing; painful, swollen joints; nosebleeds; and decreased ability to ward off infection. It is generally safe to supplement without testing. If any of the symptoms apply to you, supplementing with vitamin C may be beneficial. The body excretes vitamin C it doesn't need in urine, so getting too much is unlikely to be harmful, but large doses of vitamin C supplements can cause diarrhea and stomach cramps.

Replenishing Vitamin C

Vitamin C–Rich Foods

Foods high in vitamin C include citrus fruits, strawberries, camu camu, acerola cherries, kiwi, cantaloupe, bell peppers, broccoli, cauliflower, sweet potatoes, kale, spinach, and Brussels sprouts.

Vitamin C Supplements

A total daily intake of 500–3,000 mg of vitamin C is generally recommended, as tolerated. If you take too much and experience a loose stool, decrease the dose. My favorite way to boost vitamin C is through an electrolyte blend powder, such as Rootcology Electrolyte Blend or Designs for Health Electrolyte Synergy. This powder contains 1,734 mg of vitamin C, along with other vital nutrients and minerals to support hydration. Some people may also benefit from a stand-alone vitamin C supplement, such as NOW Foods Chewable C-500. In cases of extreme deficiency, a blood test may be done to check for anemia (vitamin C helps with iron absorption). Vitamin C, like magnesium, can be dosed to bowel tolerance, meaning you can increase your dosage until your bowel movements become regular, better formed, and easy to pass.

Potassium

Low levels of potassium, an electrolyte that helps maintain fluid balance within the body, slows gut motility and contributes to constipation. Our muscles need potassium to work properly, and deficiency can leave the muscles lining the digestive tract weak and unable to contract, inhibiting the movement of fecal matter. Additionally, potassium helps draw water into the colon and soften stool. Low levels can mean dry, difficult-to-pass poop.

Potassium levels in the body can become low due to excessive loss caused by laxatives, diuretics, vomiting, and/or diarrhea. Other common causes include dehydration and stress.

Signs of potassium deficiency include constipation, fatigue, frequent urination, muscle weakness and spasms, heart palpitations, and low blood pressure.

If you experience a collection of these symptoms, you may benefit from experimenting with increasing potassium to see if it helps to improve your symptoms.

Please note that electrolyte imbalances may be compounded by intense exercise, living in a hot or dry climate, and drinking caffeine or alcohol. If any of these are true for you, you may need more water and electrolytes than you think.

While a blood test can measure potassium levels, results will be abnormal only in the case of a severe imbalance. Some may have "subclinical imbalances" that are less severe and not present on blood tests, yet can still impact digestive health.

Replenishing Potassium

Potassium-Rich Foods

High-potassium foods include: bananas, sweet potatoes, potatoes, coconut water, avocados, winter squash, beans, dried apricots, prunes, raisins, yogurt, spinach, artichoke, and beet greens.

Proper Hydration

It is important to focus on drinking enough water to maintain balanced electrolyte levels. To determine the precise amount of water your body needs, calculate half your body weight in pounds, then aim to drink that number of ounces of water per day. For example, a 150-pound person would aim to drink 75 ounces of water per day. Consider this hydration blend to boost potassium:

1 quart coconut water
¼ to ½ teaspoon sea salt (white, gray, or pink)

Electrolyte Supplement

An electrolyte supplement like the Rootcology Electrolyte Blend contains potassium along with other electrolytes, such as sodium, chloride, and magnesium, and other digestive-supporting ingredients such as vitamin C. Other high-quality blends include Designs for Health Electrolyte Synergy and Pure Encapsulations Electrolyte/Energy Formula.

Commonly Co-Occurring Deficiencies: B_{12} and Ferritin

In addition to addressing nutrient deficiencies to resolve diarrhea or constipation, people with IBS may benefit from supporting B_{12} and ferritin (iron storage protein) levels. They may be deficient in both due to triggers such as SIBO, parasitic infections, low stomach acid, and *H. pylori*, which can lead to malabsorption of these nutrients and some of the non-gut symptoms that commonly occur in people with IBS, such as fatigue and mood issues. Addressing these deficiencies may not *resolve* IBS, but it can resolve many associated symptoms.

Vitamin B_{12} Deficiency

Vegans and vegetarians are at higher risk of B_{12} deficiency, since it's found only in animal products. Even meat-eaters can be deficient due to low stomach acid, *H. pylori* infections, or pernicious anemia (which prevents B_{12} absorption).

Vitamin B_{12} is water-soluble, so the risk of overdose is low. I recommend testing B_{12} levels (optimal range: 700–800 pg/mL). If levels are below 700 pg/mL, supplementation is necessary. In cases of low stomach acid or pernicious anemia, sublingual or injectable forms of B_{12} are more effective than oral supplements.

I recommend methylcobalamin, adenosylcobalamin, or hydroxocobalamin over cyanocobalamin.

Sublingual dosing:

- 5,000 mcg daily for 10 days to start
- 5,000 mcg once per week for four weeks
- 5,000 mcg monthly for maintenance

High-quality options include Pure Encapsulations B_{12} Liquid, Seeking Health Hydroxo B_{12} lozenges, and Designs for Health Vitamin B_{12} lozenges.

Please note, low stomach acid, acid reflux, B_{12} deficiency, and autoimmune pernicious anemia can all be linked to *H. pylori* infection. Addressing this infection may help resolve these issues (see chapter 10 for more information).

Iron Deficiency/Low Ferritin

Vegans, vegetarians, and those with IBS-related conditions like SIBO or low stomach acid are at higher risk of iron deficiency anemia. Ferritin is a key test, with optimal levels at 90 to 110 ng/mL.

For individuals with gut issues, absorbing iron from food or supplements may be challenging, and oral iron can worsen gut problems by causing constipation and supporting pathogenic biofilms. In these cases, lactoferrin or iron infusions may be more effective. Lactoferrin not only raises serum iron, hemoglobin, and ferritin levels more effectively than ferrous sulfate but also reduces gastrointestinal distress, acts as a biofilm buster, and binds iron for our use while depriving microbes of it. Iron infusions bypass the gut and can restore iron levels in minutes!

> Conversely, too much iron can be toxic and may trigger or exacerbate IBD. Elevated ferritin levels may indicate iron overload, and blood donations can be beneficial in these cases. Regularly retesting ferritin levels ensures your body is not overloaded with iron.

Chapter Summary

- Nutrient deficiencies can be a stand-alone cause of IBS symptoms or a consequence of other root causes.

- Glutamine, zinc, and vitamin A can help resolve diarrhea and are often well tolerated and generally safe to supplement without testing.

- Vitamin D deficiency has been implicated in both diarrhea and constipation—and excess vitamin D can cause constipation.

- Fatty acids, thiamine, magnesium, vitamin C, and potassium deficiency have been implicated in constipation and replenishing levels can help.

- It is best to test vitamin B_{12}, iron/ferritin, and vitamin D before supplementing and monitoring levels while supplementing.

Visit https://ibsrootcause.com/bonus for notes on this chapter.

CHAPTER 7

Deficiency of Beneficial Bacteria, Excess Pathogenic Bacteria

The gut is home to trillions of bacteria, known collectively as the gut microbiome. The microbiome affects the body's ability to digest food and absorb nutrients, regulate hormones and the immune system, and balance mood.

In a healthy microbiome, we have an abundance of beneficial bacteria (that help us digest foods and extract nutrients and keep the peace in the gut), a limited amount of opportunistic bacteria (that can become problematic when stressed), and few to none pathogenic microbes (that can cause *a lot* of trouble).

Dysbiosis occurs when one or more of these elements are out of balance. As Dr. Vincent Pedre, author of *Happy Gut* and *The GutSMART Protocol*, has defined it, "Dysbiosis is an imbalance between favorable and unfavorable microorganisms in the gut that tips the scales toward unfavorable ones."

Gut dysbiosis can cause numerous digestive problems including gas, bloating, diarrhea, constipation, malabsorption of foods, and abdominal pain as well as increase intestinal permeability.

It's important to note that an out-of-balance microbiome can lead to a whole host of other health consequences, including increasing the risk of developing autoimmune conditions, celiac disease, and rheumatoid arthritis.

Scientists continue to identify the role of individual microbes using state-of-the-art DNA analysis and have concluded that greater microbiota diversity (many different species abundantly distributed) is necessary for optimal health.

Lower diversity in your microbiome is generally a marker of dysbiosis, which has been associated with the onset and progression of disease states including indigestion, colitis, metabolic disorders (obesity, insulin resistance, diabetes), and inflammatory bowel diseases, as well as depression and autoimmune conditions.

When the microbiome is out of balance, so is everything else! Restoring balance can not just significantly help to resolve IBS-associated symptoms but may also improve and/or prevent many autoimmune issues, hormonal imbalances, and health conditions, and even help us reach a healthier weight.

In this chapter, we'll focus on addressing what I call a "dysbiosis of deficiency," or simply put, when there are not enough beneficial bacteria. A deficiency of beneficial bacteria leads to an excess of opportunistic microbes, such as *Bacillus*, *Staphylococcus*, and *Streptococcus*, and may co-occur with pathogens. We'll cover clearing out the bad guys of bacterial overgrowths and pathogenic microbes in chapters 9 and 10.

Dysbiosis Patterns Seen in IBS

When it comes to IBS, dysbiosis, or an imbalance in your microbiome, is one of the key causes, but it's not always a straightforward picture. Research has shown that many people with IBS have increased levels of potentially harmful bacteria while beneficial bacteria tend to be significantly reduced. Additionally, their microbiome may have lowered diversity.

However, the data as to which specific microbes are implicated can be conflicting! Some research has noted increased levels of *Firmicutes, Lactobacillus,* and *Ruminococcus,* alongside decreased *Erysipelotrichaceae* in people with IBS, while others mentioned an increase. Findings on *Prevotella, Bifidobacteria,* and *methanogens* are also mixed, with some studies suggesting an increase and others showing a decrease in these bacteria.

There's also an ongoing debate about the ratio between *Firmicutes* and *Bacteroidetes,* two dominant phyla in the gut. Some studies suggest that an increased ratio might be tied to IBS, while others show no significant difference at all. The variation in findings could stem from differences in study populations, regions of the gut sampled, or even the specific subtype of IBS being investigated. An individual's microbiota is shaped by their genetics, environment, and lifestyle, with notable differences based on geography and ethnicity. Furthermore, these variations are largely influenced by diet.

When we look at IBS subtypes, the patterns shift slightly. For IBS-D (diarrhea-predominant), there's often an increase in *Enterobacteriaceae* and *Proteobacteria,* and a reduction in *Firmicutes* and *Fusobacteria.* Meanwhile, IBS-C (constipation-predominant) tends to show a higher prevalence of methane-producing bacteria, particularly *Methanobacteriales,* which are thought to slow gut motility.

Some studies have observed increased levels of harmful bacteria such as *Veillonella, Clostridium coccoides,* and *Pseudomonas aeruginosa* in those with IBS, which could further contribute to the condition's symptoms.

The challenge in researching IBS-related dysbiosis lies in the inconsistencies across studies. The variations in sampling methods, population differences, and analytical techniques make it difficult to draw concrete conclusions, but it's clear that balancing the gut microbiome is one key for managing IBS.

Bacteria "earn" their labels as good or bad citizens in part due to the roles they take on within the gut environment and the substances they produce, which can either benefit or harm their host.

The Good, the Potentially Bad, and the Ugly

Some of the dominant bacteria found in the human gut (representing about 90 percent of gut bacteria) include gram-positive bacteria from the phylum Firmicutes (including species such as *Lactobacillus, Clostridium, Enterococcus,* and *Ruminococcus*) and gram-negative bacteria knowns as Bacteroidetes (with species such as *Bacteroides* and *Prevotella*), but there are many others such as the common (and beneficial) species *Bifidobacterium* (of the phyla Actinobacteria). Individual bacteria may be considered commensal (good), while others are problematic. They need to be present in balanced amounts for a healthy microbiome. Microbiome stool tests can classify if you have a deficiency of good bacteria, as well as an overabundance of opportunistic (potentially bad) vs. pathogenic (ugly) bacteria.

- **Probiotic bacteria** (sometimes called commensal species): These are generally helpful to us as their hosts. They help with digestion, producing SCFAs and keeping the peace in the gut. Some species include *Bacteroides, Bifidobacteria, Clostridia* (butyrate-producing strains), *Enterococcus, Escherichia* (certain strains), *Lactobacillus, Enterobacter, Akkermansia, Faecalibacterium,* and *Roseburia.*

- **Opportunistic bacteria** usually behave when conditions are balanced but can become harmful in large numbers or during host stress: *Bacillus, Eschericha* (some strains), *Enterococcus, Morganella, Pseudomonas, Staphylococcus,* and *Streptococcus.*

- **Pathogenic bacteria:** The presence of the ugly (pathogenic and inflammatory/autoimmune-related) bacteria can lead to severe digestive distress and various diseases, including autoimmune disease. These include *Campylobacter, Citrobacter, Clostridium difficile,* enterohemorrhagic *E. coli, Klebsiella, M. avium* ssp. paratuberculosis, and *Proteus.*

The Role of Beneficial Bacteria

Beneficial bacteria in the gut play a powerful role in maintaining overall health, acting like tiny hardworking multitaskers. They help break down food, aiding digestion and allowing us to absorb vital micronutrients. For example, *Lactobacillus* and *Bifidobacterium* can support nutrient extraction. These beneficial microbes are also the guardians of the gut lining, ensuring its integrity and making sure harmful pathogens don't slip through and cause trouble. The gut is home to over 70 percent of the body's immune system, and beneficial bacteria help regulate this complex system, ensuring it responds appropriately without becoming overactive. For example *Lactobacillus acidophilus, L. casei, Bifidobacterium lactis,* and the beneficial yeast *Saccharomyces boulardii* have been shown to increase the number of intestinal-defending IgA-producing cells.

These good probiotic bacteria also have a hand in balancing our hormone levels, including estrogen and thyroid hormones, which have far-reaching effects on everything from energy to mood. They can enhance carbohydrate metabolism supporting blood sugar balance and even produce essential nutrients like vitamin K and folate. Perhaps even more fascinating, beneficial gut bacteria synthesize neurotransmitters such as serotonin, impacting not only our gut but also our brain and mood—affecting anxiety and depression.

They can also support our metabolism. And their role doesn't stop there! These bacteria break down dietary fiber, creating short-chain fatty acids (SCFAs) like butyrate, which are essential for reducing inflammation, improving gut barrier function, and modulating gut pH. This helps prevent the growth of pathogenic bacteria, ensuring that our gut stays balanced and healthy. Without these beneficial bacteria, our bodies simply don't function as smoothly!

When the number of beneficial bacteria in the gut is low or they are outnumbered, the entire balance of the microbiome can shift in favor of opportunistic and pathogenic bacteria. When beneficial bacteria are depleted, opportunistic bacteria seize the opportunity to multiply. These opportunistic bacteria, which usually exist in the gut in small numbers and act like "good citizens" when enough probiotic bacteria are present, can cause problems when left unchecked, especially if we are under stress. Interestingly, these bacteria have adrenaline sensors and increase their virulence in response to our fight-or-flight hormone, adrenaline. They can produce excess gas, trigger low-grade inflammation, and contribute to symptoms like bloating, constipation, and diarrhea.

As the balance tips further, pathogenic bacteria, which are more harmful, can begin to dominate. Pathogens such as *E. coli*, *Clostridium difficile*, and *Salmonella* can cause infections, damage the gut lining, and release toxins that lead to more serious issues such as intestinal permeability, chronic inflammation, and even systemic infections. This imbalance, known as dysbiosis, can set off a cascade of digestive and immune-related symptoms, often worsening conditions such as IBS, SIBO, and autoimmune diseases.

Bacterial By-Products: Made by the Microbiome

The bacteria living in your gut can make various by-products that will either benefit or harm the body.

Beneficial By-Products: Short-Chain Fatty Acids (SCFAs)

SCFAs, produced when beneficial gut bacteria ferment fiber, are key for gut health and energy for the cells lining the colon. They also support metabolism, may protect against digestive disorders and colon cancer, and help with weight management. There are a few main types of SCFAs.

Butyrate
Critical for regulating tight junctions, promoting mucus production, and repairing intestinal cells. Low butyrate can cause IBS-like symptoms such as diarrhea and abdominal pain. Butyrate is made by anaerobic bacteria in the gut, with Firmicutes being key players, through fermenting dietary fiber such as resistant starch.

Propionate
Propionate, produced by *Bacteroides* and *Akkermansia* bacteria by fermenting beta-glucan (a prebiotic fiber found in oats and barley), helps regulate blood sugar, appetite, and intestinal inflammation. Low propionate is linked to IBS.

Acetate
Beneficial bacteria such as *Bacteroides*, *Bifidobacteria*, and *Akkermansia* ferment inulin (found in chicory root, garlic, onions, leeks, and asparagus) to make acetate, the most abundant SCFA, which supports gut barrier function, modulates inflammation, and may protect against colitis.

Potentially Problematic By-Products
Acetaldehyde
A toxic by-product of alcohol metabolism, acetaldehyde can also be produced by *Lactobacillus, Enterococcus faecalis, Streptococcus, Klebsiella pneumoniae, Clostridium,* and *Candida,* and can cause brain fog, headaches, fatigue, and nausea.

Ammonia
Ammonia is a neurotoxic waste product of protein digestion that accumulates with constipation and poor stomach acid. It is also produced

by certain gut bacteria, including *Proteus, Klebsiella pneumoniae, Enterobacter, Pseudomonas,* and *Clostridium perfringens,* and may cause confusion and fatigue.

Histamine
Histamine released during allergic reactions and produced by bacteria such as *Lactobacillus* spp., *Morganella* spp., *Pseudomonas aeruginosa, Citrobacter freundii, Klebsiella pneumoniae, Proteus mirabilis, Enterobacter* spp., *Escherichia* spp., *Fusobacterium* spp., and *Clostridium perfringens.* Histamine intolerance can cause symptoms such as headaches, hives, and gut issues when the body struggles to break it down. Gut pathogens such as *H. pylori,* mold, *Blastocystis hominis,* and *Dientamoeba fragilis* can also trigger excessive histamine release.

Hydrogen Gas
Hydrogen gas is the result of carbohydrate fermentation in the gut and *Firmicutes* and *Bacteroides* are the two main producers. Hydrogen gas can support the production of butyrate, which can have beneficial effects on health. However, extremely high levels of hydrogen may indicate gut issues such as SIBO, enzyme deficiencies, or altered transit time.

Methane
High methane levels produced predominantly by *Methanobrevibacter smithii* slow intestinal transit time, may lead to weight gain by increasing the amount of calories absorbed by the host, and are associated with IBS-C, SIBO, and intestinal methanogen overgrowth (IMO).

Lipopolysaccharide (LPS)
LPS, often referred to as an "endotoxin," is a molecule found on gram-negative bacteria that, when released, causes increased intestinal permeability, inflammation, and activation of immune cells. LPS has been linked to IBD, metabolic issues, obesity, autoimmunity, and yes, IBS.

Beta-Glucuronidase

Beta-glucuronidase is an enzyme that disrupts the glucuronidation process, which normally packages compounds such as estrogen, testosterone, xenobiotics, mold mycotoxins, and pharmaceuticals for removal. Instead of allowing them to leave, beta-glucuronidase can "cut open" these packages, allowing the substances to reenter circulation. Excess beta-glucuronidase can lead to hormonal imbalances, such as estrogen excess (which is linked to constipation), increased medication side effects, and poor toxin clearance. Furthermore, it can lead to a deconjugation of bile acids, potentially impacting fat digestion. High levels are associated with cancers, autoimmune conditions, and inflammatory conditions. Bacteria that produce beta-glucuronidase include *E. coli*, *Clostridium*, *Bacteroides fragilis*, *Staphylococcus*, *Ruminococcus*, *Eubacterium*, and *Peptostreptococcus*.

What Causes Dysbiosis?

Numerous factors affect the composition of the microbiota, including:

- Antibiotics: While antibiotics are great at wiping out bad bacteria, they often take down the good ones, too. Broad-spectrum antibiotics, like amoxicillin and ciprofloxacin, are especially guilty of reducing microbial diversity and allowing opportunistic and pathogenic bacteria, including the life-threatening, colitis-causing *Clostridium difficile* bacteria, to flourish. (Fortunately, the yeast-based probiotic *Saccharomyces boulardii* can help restore balance and even prevent or combat *C. diff.*)

- Pesticides and herbicides: Glyphosate, the active ingredient in the herbicide Roundup, tends to harm beneficial bacteria while allowing potentially harmful bacteria to thrive. Animal studies show that glyphosate reduces beneficial species such as *Lactobacillus* and *Butyricicoccus,* which produce the protective short-chain fatty acid butyrate. Glyphosate exposure can also lead to an overgrowth of *Clostridia* and can cause other bacterial imbalances and SIBO.

- Mold: Did you know that penicillin was derived from *Penicillium notatum* mold? Just like taking too many antibiotics, mold exposure can shift the microbiome, killing our good bacteria.

- Infections: Various infections can shift the microbiome by displacing healthy bacteria. For example, a school of thought believes that *Blastocystis hominis* parasites result in dysbiosis because they "eat" beneficial *Lactobacillus* bacteria, while *H. pylori* infection (as well as the antibiotics used to treat it) results in a reduction in bacteria diversity.

- Stress: Stress can weaken the immune system, making it harder for the body to fight off harmful bacteria and promoting dysbiosis. For instance, social stress can reduce anti-inflammatory microbes and increase inflammation, leaving us more vulnerable to illness. Research also shows that stress hormones such as epinephrine (adrenaline) can boost bacterial adhesion and biofilm formation, increasing their virulence.

- Lifestyle factors: Exercise, sleep, alcohol, and nicotine all affect gut health. While regular exercise promotes diversity in the microbiome, alcohol and nicotine can create an environment in which bad bacteria take over. So, while we all have our vices, it's worth considering how they might be nudging our microbiome in the wrong direction.

- Thyroid hormone imbalance: Thyroid hormones are closely linked to gut health. Hypothyroidism interrupts bile function, affecting digestion and nutrient absorption, which can result in a reduction of bacterial diversity and abundance.

- Digestive enzyme deficiency: When food isn't digested properly, it can become a feast for pathogenic and opportunistic bacteria, supercharging their ability to proliferate. Supporting healthy enzyme function is essential for preventing dysbiosis.

- Diet: We are what we eat! A fiber-rich diet helps support beneficial bacteria, while eating one high in saturated fats, processed foods, additives, and refined sugars (the all-too-common standard American diet) feeds the bad ones. As a caveat, I want to be clear that certain types of triggers, such as an infection or overgrowth of opportunistic bacteria (SIBO) or yeast (SIFO), may lead to symptoms worsening by adding extra fiber. Clearing the infection and/or bacterial overgrowth would be the first priority.

Root Cause Research Corner: The Mighty Microbiome and Celiac Disease

A deficiency of beneficial bacteria along with a genetic predisposition and environmental triggers has been shown to play a role in the development of many diseases.

One example that is very relevant to IBS is celiac disease.

While we know that the likelihood of developing celiac disease is associated with a genetic predisposition and the amount of gluten consumption, emerging studies are showing that the microbiome could be the environmental trigger that actually leads to the autoimmune response to gluten in those who are genetically susceptible.

Researchers hypothesize a microbiome low in beneficial bacteria (potentially due to antibiotic use) could lead to gluten reactions,

> as beneficial bacteria species such as *Bifidobacterium* and *Lactobacillus* are excellent at digesting gluten. Interestingly, researchers believe this dysbiosis pattern may be more relevant than genes!

So How Do You Know You Have Dysbiosis?

Many people aren't fully aware that they have gut dysbiosis, since not everyone experiences digestive symptoms. But signs like gas, bloating, constipation, diarrhea, or cramping can be a giveaway. That said, not all dysbiosis leads to obvious gut issues—sometimes it shows up in more subtle ways.

You can officially test for dysbiosis with a functional stool test, but if you have IBS or related symptoms, chances are your gut needs support regardless! Probiotics and gut-healing protocols can often help without the need for testing, though testing may offer some more specific guidance.

Testing

- Various comprehensive stool analysis (CSA) tests on the market can identify a lack of beneficial bacteria, an overgrowth of opportunistic bacteria, potentially pathogenic bacteria, excess levels of beta-glucuronidase, digestive enzyme deficiencies, poor bacterial diversity, low butyrate levels, and low levels of secretory IgA, a marker of gut immunity. The Vibrant Wellness Gut Zoomer 3.0 test offers the most helpful guidance for choosing probiotics and prebiotics based on results. Most of the other CSA tests on the market don't offer much guidance for rebalancing the microbiome.

- I have become very interested in using targeted microbiome tests including Enbiosis and Viome Gut Intelligence Test to restore microbial balance. While they don't test for the digestive markers and infections that comprehensive stool analysis (CSA) tests can find, they analyze the microbiome and provide personalized recommendations for foods, prebiotics, and probiotics.

- Enbiosis employs microbiome testing and uses artificial intelligence–based technologies to interpret the results and offer targeted solutions. It focuses on identifying imbalances, particularly in bacterial diversity, and suggests personalized food and supplement recommendations. A multicenter randomized trial showed that the AI-driven recommendations have helped 78 percent of people with IBS.
- Viome Gut Intelligence Test uses advanced RNA sequencing to analyze the activity of microbes in your gut, offering a snapshot of how well your gut microbiome is functioning. It then provides personalized food and supplement recommendations to improve your gut health, digestion, and even mental well-being.

Treatment Options

Generally, the treatment for dysbiosis is focused on increasing the number of beneficial bacteria through probiotic supplements, though using prebiotics and diet can also create big shifts in the microbiome. In some cases, clinicians may also utilize protocols to clear out pathogenic microbes.

While a comprehensive stool analysis may help with knowing which bacteria are deficient, and the Gut Zoomer and targeted microbiome tests can help determine which probiotics, foods, and prebiotics may be the most helpful to rebalance your microbiome, many people with IBS can also benefit from trialing probiotics without testing.

Probiotics

Probiotics are beneficial bacteria that support our gut health and overall well-being. Found in the gut, in fermented foods and probiotic supplements, they aid in digestion, boost immunity, reduce inflammation, and even impact our mood. Probiotics can help ameliorate the symptoms of IBS through improving the gut's microbial balance, boosting the gut's immune response, and making the gut less susceptible to infections through producing beneficial by-products such as butyrate. Butyrate can block pathogen adhesion, which makes infections less likely to take hold; can reduce gut inflammation; and can stimulate the production of secretory IgA, our gut's first line of immune defense. Probiotics can enhance gut barrier function by helping to downregulate mucosal immune activation while increasing the mucus layer in the gut. They can also reduce visceral hypersensitivity.

Most Helpful Strains in IBS

Emerging research continues to highlight the therapeutic potential of specific probiotic strains for managing IBS symptoms. Different strains may have different beneficial effects on certain IBS symptoms. While individual results can vary, here are the probiotic types that have shown the most promise.

Lactobacillus-Based Probiotics

Lactobacillus-based probiotics are the most widely researched and commonly used and can be very helpful in rebalancing gut dysbiosis, relieving IBS symptoms, and assisting with fiber digestion, especially if testing has indicated low levels. There are various strains that have been studied to show benefits for IBS, with *Lactiplantibacillus plantarum* the most likely to reduce the formation of gas and significantly improve the quality of life in people with IBS after four weeks of use. People who received *Lactobacillus acidophilus* had the lowest incidence of adverse events.

Some of the microbes present in up to 75 percent of cases of SIBO are actually *Lactobacillus* bacteria (good bacteria in the wrong part of the body), which means taking *Lactobacillus* probiotics (and the prebiotics that feed them) can actually worsen symptoms! (See chapter 9 for more on SIBO and the full SIBO protocol.)

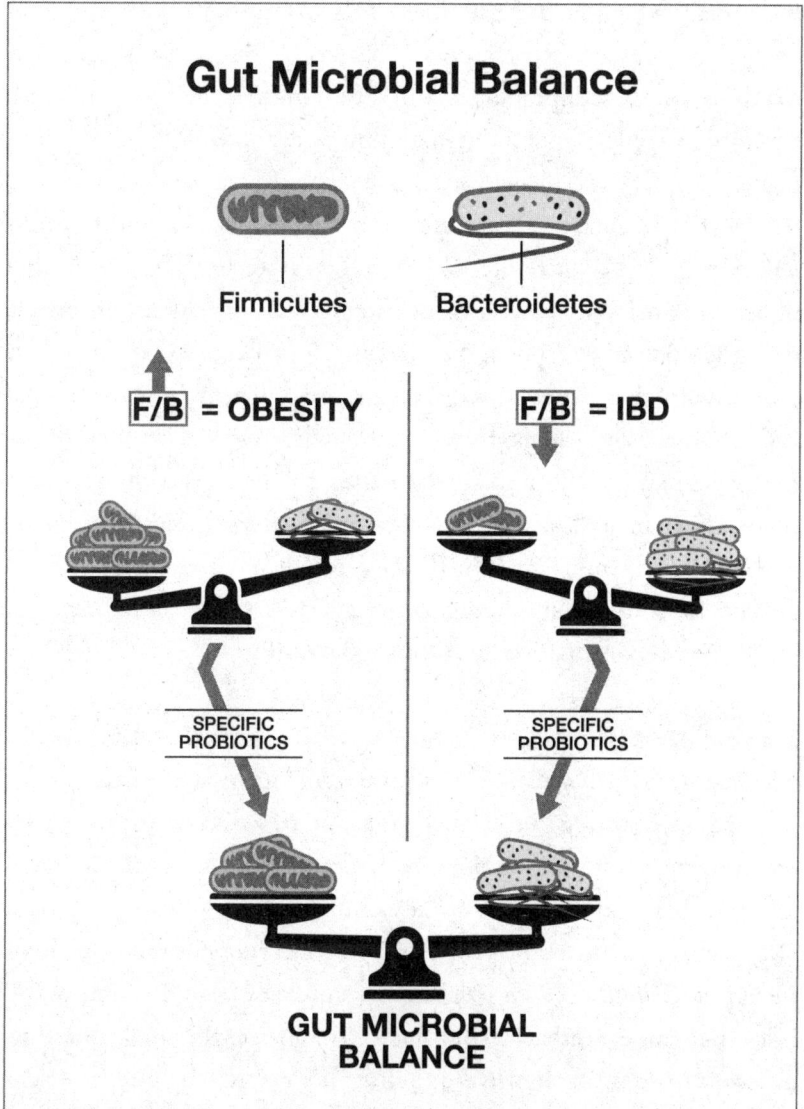

Bifidobacteria-Based Probiotics

Because people with IBS often have lower amounts of the beneficial *Bifidobacterium sp.*, supplementing often helps IBS symptoms, especially in those with constipation. Boosting *Bifidobacteria* may help relieve constipation by increasing the amount of the beneficial SCFA acetic acid, which helps break down fats and carbohydrates while reducing potentially pathogenic bacteria. Supplementing with *Bifidobacteria*-based probiotics can also improve bloating, cramps, straining, urgency, and abdominal pain and reduce inflammation in people with IBS and ulcerative colitis.

The FUT2 gene has been associated with lowered amounts of *Bifidobacteria*, which contributes to IBS and is linked to IBD, with studies indicating an increased risk of developing Crohn's disease in people with the non-secretor phenotype (about 20 percent of Caucasians). A person with that genetic predisposition may benefit from additional *Bifidobacteria* supplementation. Additionally, people with fiber digestive issues may benefit from *Bifidobacteria*, as they're known to support proper fiber breakdown. *Bifidobacterium longum* is one of the most widely studied strains for IBS. *Bifidobacterium lactis* has demonstrated benefits for constipation-predominant IBS (IBS-C). It can improve gut motility, ease constipation, and reduce discomfort.

Saccharomyces boulardii

Saccharomyces boulardii is a powerful probiotic yeast, often recommended for restoring gut balance. *S. boulardii* works by increasing secretory IgA, a gut-protective antibody that helps neutralize pathogens and stop harmful bacteria from attaching to the gut wall. This yeast also helps to improve gut permeability by clearing out gut infections, including *Candida, Blastocystis hominis,* and SIBO. Unlike some probiotics that can exacerbate SIBO due to colonizing the small intestine, *S. boulardii* doesn't colonize the gut but rather sweeps up gut pathogens on its way through the entire digestive tract. Because it is a yeast and not a bacterium, like most probiotics, it can't be killed by bacteria-targeting antibiotics, making it a go-to for preventing antibiotic-related dysbiosis and helping combat antibiotic-induced *Clostridium difficile* infections. *S. boulardii* may be particularly useful for diarrhea, including acute and postinfectious diarrhea. If you have Crohn's disease, *S. boulardii* may not be right for you. While there are no studies of it being harmful, in theory *S. boulardii* may cross-react with the anti-*Saccharomyces cerevisiae* (another type of yeast) antibodies commonly present in Crohn's disease.

Quality options include Rootcology *S. Boulardii*, Designs for Health FloraMyces, and Pure Encapsulations *Saccharomyces boulardii*. Therapeutic doses range from 5 billion to 15 billion CFUs, taken 2 to 4 times daily.

Spore-Based Probiotics

Naturally occurring in soil, these probiotics promote the growth of beneficial bacteria and increase microbial diversity. Unlike most traditional probiotics, they have a protective shell that helps them remain stable and resistant to stomach acid's low pH, resulting in the delivery of more usable probiotics to the intestines. Spore-based probiotics have the ability to boost *Lactobacillus* colonies indirectly, so they can be used concurrently with *Lactobacillus* probiotics, as well as in place of them. Unlike *Lactobacillus* probiotics, spore-based probiotics can reduce SIBO and increase gut diversity by boosting the growth of other beneficial flora.

Some names for spore-based probiotics include *Bacillus coagulans*, *Bacillus clausii*, and *Bacillus subtilis*. *B. coagulans* seems to be especially helpful, as it had the highest probability of improving IBS symptoms like abdominal pain, bloating, and straining, as well as being helpful for both constipation and diarrhea.

Brands to consider include Rootcology Spore Flora, Microbiome Labs MegaSporeBiotic, and Designs for Health ProbioSpore. The starting dose for the above-mentioned probiotics is generally ½ capsule per day, while the therapeutic dose is 2 capsules per day.

Best Practices in Using Probiotics

Consider Multiple Strains vs. Individual *Lactobacillus* and *Bifidobacteria* Strains

Many strains of probiotics have been shown to be beneficial for those with IBS. While you can supplement with individual strains of probiotics, you may be more likely to experience synergistic benefits by incorporating multiple strains. Remember that probiotic diversity is associated with greater health and improved gut function.

Multistrain blends include:

- Low Dose: SFI Health Ther-Biotic Pro IBS Relief: A clinically studied blend of *Lactiplantibacillus plantarum, Lactobacillus acidophilus,* and *Bifidobacterium lactis* probiotics, it has been shown to significantly relieve IBS symptoms with a 79 percent reduction in constipation and a 70 percent reduction in diarrhea within twelve weeks. It is a medical-grade food that contains over 21 billion CFU of targeted probiotics per serving, along with a low FODMAP prebiotic to synergistically support the probiotics.

- Mid-Range: Various high-quality companies have formulated therapeutic doses of a mix of diverse *Lactobacillus, Bifidobacteria,* and beneficial strep strains within the 50 billion CFUs range. Rootcology ProB 50, Pure Encapsulations Probiotic 50B, Xymogen ProbioMax Complete DF, and Ortho Molecular Ortho Biotic are some quality options.

- Ultra-High Dose: Visbiome/VSL#3: Visbiome/VSL#3 is a high-potency probiotic formulation that includes eight different strains of beneficial bacteria (*Lactobacillus* and *Bifidobacterium* species) with a lot of research—and some controversy—behind it. VSL#3 is the strain that is often cited in studies. However, the patent holder for the formulation, Claudio De Simone, left the manufacturer of VSL#3, and the probiotic formulation went with him to a new company that now uses this formulation in Visbiome probiotics. This formulation has been studied in several clinical trials for IBS and has shown effectiveness in reducing bloating, improving stool consistency, and alleviating abdominal discomfort.

Consider Therapeutic Dosing for Probiotics

Most grocery stores and health food stores sell *Lactobacillus*-based probiotics that contain 5–10 billion colony-forming units (CFUs) of one probiotic strain. While this seems like a really big number, in reality, we have 1 trillion bacteria in our gut, and that small amount is not likely to make a difference. In fact, most probiotic supplements contain only enough probiotics to *maintain* an already healthy gut, not to restore gut microbe balance. I've often found the doses of *Lactobacillus*- and *Bifidobacterium*-based probiotics required to make a shift are in the range of 50–500 billion CFUs. A reminder that if you've never taken probiotics before, you will want to start low and go slow (see page 218).

Consider Multiple Species of Probiotics

Different species of probiotics often work synergistically, and I sometimes suggest the beneficial yeast *Saccharomyces boulardii*, a spore-based probiotic, and a *Lactobacillus*-based probiotic for people with digestive issues. This is an approach I have personally used to induce and maintain remission from autoimmune disease and digestive issues. It's also the method of choice for Dr. Michael Ruscio, a clinical researcher, author, and adjunct professor. He calls it the "triple therapy probiotic regimen." He found that patients whose symptoms were not improving with the use of a single probiotic would see improvement with the addition of a probiotic from a different category. Symptoms would improve even more by adding the third category of probiotics to their regimen.

Start Low and Go Slow with Dosing Probiotics

It's important to start at a low dose with probiotics and work your way up to a full dose to avoid gas, bloating, diarrhea, or constipation that can result from significant changes in the balance of the microbiome. As gram-negative bacteria and pathogens in the digestive system die or are displaced, they may release lipopolysaccharides (LPS) and other toxic by-products as they are cleared. These by-products may cause symptoms, including headaches, fatigue, intestinal distress, muscle soreness, or flu-like symptoms. This is known as a "die-off reaction" and can occur with high doses of probiotics and rapid shifts in the microbiome, and can generally last three to seven days. I recommend incorporating one probiotic at a time, until you reach the full dose of that probiotic with no gastrointestinal issues.

In functional medicine training, there's a popular saying: "Start low and go slow . . . but go." It's such a perfect way to think about probiotic dosing. You ease in gently, but you don't stay stuck—progress is the goal! I love how this approach respects our body's need for a gradual adjustment, while still keeping the focus on moving forward with healing.

Tailoring to Symptoms

Considerations for IBS-D

Saccharomyces boulardii, Bifidobacterium infantis, and *Lactiplantibacillus plantarum* have been particularly effective in resolving diarrhea and reducing inflammation.

Considerations for IBS-C

Bifidobacterium lactis and *Lactiplantibacillus plantarum* are often recommended to help regulate bowel movements and reduce bloating.

B. lactis has demonstrated benefits for constipation-predominant IBS. It can improve gut motility, ease constipation, and reduce discomfort.

Considerations for SIBO

If you suspect you have SIBO, consider avoiding *Lactobacillus*-based probiotics and using SIBO-safe probiotics, such as *Saccharomyces boulardii*, spore-based probiotics, as well as *Bifidobacteria*-containing probiotics until SIBO is properly treated. Avoid using prebiotics such as inulin, fructooligosaccharides (FOS), galactooligosaccharides (GOS), and resistant starch until you have ruled out and treated SIBO and/or *Klebsiella*.

> ### The Power of Poop to Rebalance the Microbiome
>
> Fecal transplants, also known as fecal microbiota transplantation (FMT), have been used to treat recurrent *Clostridium difficile* infections, with about a 90 percent success rate. By restoring microbial diversity with screened donor bacteria, FMT helps rebuild the microbiome and reduces the risk of future *C. diff* infections, which commonly recur after antibiotic treatment.
>
> There's also growing interest in using FMT for conditions like Crohn's disease and ulcerative colitis, where it has shown promise in achieving and maintaining remission. However, results in IBS are less consistent, benefits often fade, and repeated treatments have limited success.
>
> There are also risks to FMT. The microbiome is highly personalized, and transferring bacteria from one person to another can lead to unintended consequences. For example, studies in mice have demonstrated that transferring microbiota from mice with lupus can induce autoimmunity in genetically susceptible mice. Human cases have also reported adverse effects, such as systemic

> inflammatory response when "heathy" recipients received fecal transplants from "healthy donors." Although measures are taken to use healthy donors whenever possible, sometimes a person may be healthy for all intents and purposes, yet their microbiome can trigger autoimmunity in someone who has different genes and thus is genetically susceptible, as when we mix different genes with different germs, we get different results. A small case report study I reviewed about ten years ago found two cases of new-onset autoimmunity in fecal microbiota recipients.
>
> Given the complexities of altering the microbiome, I would encourage exploring less extreme measures for IBS before using poop as medicine.

What About Fiber and Prebiotics?

A common recommendation for IBS is to eat more fiber and to take prebiotics, to feed the microbiome. These are both controversial, especially when looking at health through the lens of a root cause approach, bio-individuality, and clinical research.

While prebiotics are promoted as "food for our beneficial bacteria," they don't work the same way for everyone, especially for those of us with sensitive digestive systems.

One big issue is that prebiotics, which are essentially fibers that feed the bacteria in our gut, can sometimes end up feeding the wrong kind of bacteria (or the bacteria that are in the wrong places)!

For someone with IBS caused by SIBO, this can lead to worsening symptoms such as gas, bloating, and discomfort. It's not uncommon for people to try fiber/prebiotics, only to find they're suddenly dealing with more digestive upset, not less!

Despite the marketing hype of using prebiotics to boost beneficial bacteria, the research studies on common prebiotics in IBS have not been impressive, either! A 2019 meta-analysis of prebiotics including inulin, FOS, pectin, oligofructose, partially hydrolyzed guar gum, and beta-galactooligosaccharide concluded that "[p]rebiotics do not improve gastrointestinal symptoms or quality of life in patients with IBS or other functional bowel disorders, but they do increase *Bifidobacteria*," making the case for recommending prebiotics somewhat weak. While increasing *bifidobacteria* might sound beneficial, it doesn't necessarily translate to symptom relief for IBS. In fact, some people with IBS, especially those with SIBO or fermentable carbohydrate sensitivities, may find that prebiotics worsen bloating, gas, and discomfort. This reinforces the importance of a personalized approach. Rather than assuming prebiotics are universally helpful, it's essential to assess individual tolerance and needs.

Remember that you can tailor your fiber intake according to the kind of IBS you're experiencing. For more, see chapter 4.

Help for Hemorrhoids

Hemorrhoids are common in people with IBS, affecting about 33 percent of cases—especially those with IBS-C, where straining from constipation increases risk. Diarrhea can also irritate and worsen hemorrhoids.

Gut dysbiosis may contribute by triggering inflammation and constipation. While high-fiber diets are often recommended, some people with IBS struggle to digest fiber, which can worsen symptoms. In these cases, digestive enzymes, such as Rootcology Broad Spectrum Enzymes, may help support fiber breakdown and promote well-formed stools.

Stool softeners may ease straining short term but aren't a long-term fix. (See Chapter 16 for deeper constipation solutions.)

For relief:

- Sitz baths can soothe pain and inflammation.

- Venous-support supplements may reduce swelling:
  » Butcher's broom helps veins contract and reduce pain.
  » Vitamin C supports vein integrity via collagen production.
  » Diosmin + hesperidin reduce inflammation and restore vein function.

- Horse chestnut is anti-inflammatory but should be used for no more than four weeks due to potential liver toxicity.

- Some people also find relief from homeopathic remedies like Boiron Hemcalm (ointments or suppositories), which include Aesculus, Hamamelis, and Nux vomica.

- Topical treatments can ease discomfort:
  » Phenylephrine reduces swelling.
  » Lidocaine, benzocaine, and dibucaine offer temporary numbing relief.
  » Steroid creams reduce inflammation but should be used for no more than a week and only under medical supervision.

Tailoring Prebiotic Recommendations to IBS

Common prebiotics include resistant starch, inulin, FOS, GOS, partially hydrolyzed guar gum (PHGG), psyllium husk, and beta-glucan. Each has a unique profile and may be appropriate or inappropriate depending on the circumstances.

Inulin, FOS, and GOS

These are considered FODMAPs and generally not as well tolerated by people with IBS-D and SIBO, but may be helpful for IBS-C.

- FOS is especially poorly tolerated and has been shown to increase visceral hypersensitivity and inflammation in IBS. It is commonly added to probiotic formulations.
- Inulin can be a helpful prebiotic for constipation, especially when used in doses under 10 grams a day, as higher doses worsened symptoms of flatulence and bloating.
- Common dietary sources of inulin and FOS include chicory root, garlic, onions, asparagus, and Jerusalem artichokes, while sources of GOS include legumes such as lentils and chickpeas.

Resistant Starch

Resistant starch is able to pass through the stomach and small intestine without being digested until it reaches the colon, where it feeds friendly bacteria and is fermented by them into beneficial SCFAs, including butyrate which strengthens the integrity of the cells lining the gut. While there are no specific studies I could find for using resistant starch for IBS, it has shown to increase butyrate-producing bacteria and has shown benefits in both diarrhea and constipation. It can also help with balancing blood sugar. Although it's not a FODMAP, it can feed *Klebsiella*, a pathogenic microbe that sometimes causes SIBO.

In addition to dietary sources of resistant starch (see page 224), it is also available as a powder supplement. Although prebiotics can generally be taken along with probiotics, when it comes to resistant starch, I recommend taking it blended in a beverage or mixed with food, at bedtime. This way, it will help stabilize blood sugar levels and improve sleep quality. Designs for Health PaleoFiber RS blends two forms of resistant starch, organic green banana flour and organic potato starch, to fuel beneficial microbes.

> ### Dietary Sources of Resistant Starch
>
> The best dietary food sources for resistant starch include green banana, raw potato starch, raw plantains, legumes, and oats. Rice and potatoes that have been cooked, *then* cooled, are also excellent sources, as cooking and cooling actually increase the levels of resistant starch. And yes, you can reheat them after cooling with no changes to the resistant starch level. Cooked beans and pasta can be cooled and reheated as well. Please note that some resistant starches such as green bananas, oats, and plantains lose some of their resistant starch when cooked.

Partially Hydrolyzed Guar Gum (PHGG)

PHGG is a water-soluble fiber that has shown great promise for people with IBS because it tends to be well-tolerated across the board and may help regulate bowel movements, making it useful for both constipation (IBS-C) and diarrhea (IBS-D). It also promotes the growth of beneficial bacteria without causing excessive bloating or gas. Sources include guar gum supplements (often labeled as Sunfiber).

Psyllium Husk

Psyllium is a soluble fiber that can help normalize bowel movements, whether you're dealing with constipation or diarrhea. Psyllium has shown effectiveness in regulating IBS symptoms by bulking stool and reducing abdominal pain. It's especially beneficial for IBS-M (mixed bowel habits). Sources include psyllium husk supplements such as Metamucil.

Beta-Glucan

Beta-glucan is another soluble fiber known to improve digestion and immune response. It can help modulate gut bacteria and reduce inflammation, which can benefit IBS patients. Common sources include oats, barley, and certain mushrooms.

Prebiotic and Fiber Blend

For prebiotics plus a blend of fibers, consider Pure Encapsulations PureLean Fiber. It contains ingredients such as PHGG and flaxseed fiber.

Best Practices for Prebiotics

SIBO testing, CSA, and microbiome mapping can be incredibly helpful for tailoring prebiotic recommendation. Even if you don't use them, here are some considerations:

- Because SIBO is present in at least 30 percent of people with IBS, my general approach is to avoid using FOS, GOS, and inulin in people with IBS-D until SIBO has been ruled out and treated.

- Additionally, for people who may present with arthritis or ankylosing spondylitis (AS), I would insist on getting a CSA and would avoid resistant starch until a *Klebsiella* overgrowth was ruled out. *Klebsiella* is a common trigger of SIBO, arthritis, and AS and can be fed by resistant starch.

- If I were to make a recommendation for someone without seeing their CSA or targeted microbiome test, I would recommend taking probiotics for at least two weeks before introducing prebiotics.

- For both diarrhea and constipation, I would consider PHGG, beta-glucan, or psyllium. I would avoid inulin in diarrhea, but consider it in constipation.

Additionally, in some cases, rather than taking prebiotics, I may instead recommend taking an aloe or butyrate supplement.

Non-Prebiotic Ways to Support Probiotic Growth
Aloe vera
Aloe vera is not traditionally considered a prebiotic, but it does have prebiotic properties and can help improve the growth of different *Lactobacilli* species such as *L. acidophilus, Lactiplantibacillus plantarum,* and *L. casei*. It's also very helpful for constipation! Aloe can be taken as a liquid or capsule. Nature's Way Organic Aloe Vera Whole Leaf Juice is a liquid option, and capsule options include Rootcology Aloe (1 capsule at breakfast) and Designs for Health Aloe/200x.

Butyrate
Probably the most gut-supportive compound produced by beneficial colonic bacteria, this supplement offers butyrate directly, in a bit of "if you build it, they will come" fashion. As butyrate is both made by good bacteria and feeds the good bacteria, one way to ensure a healthy bacterial balance is to ensure you maintain adequate levels of this important nutrient to modulate gut flora and support gut barrier integrity. Butyrate has been found to be helpful in both constipation and diarrhea at doses of 150–300 mg per day. Rootcology Butyrate Balance is a high-quality option, as is Designs for Health Tri-Butyrin Supreme, Pure Encapsulations Butyrate, and Healthy Gut Company TriButyrin-X.

General Treatment Options for Dysbiosis
Probiotic-Rich Fermented Foods and Vegetables
Fermented foods like sauerkraut and other fermented vegetables (that are kept in the refrigerator section of the grocery store or are homemade and refrigerated) have an abundance of beneficial bacteria, such as *Lactobacillus* and *Bifidobacterium,* and can be very helpful in rebalancing the gut flora.

Kefir and yogurt are also filled with good bacteria, but if you're sensitive to dairy, consider fermented coconut water or fermented coconut yogurt.

Reseeding your gut with fermented foods and probiotics too quickly can cause temporary digestive discomfort, changes in bowel movements, muscle aches, headaches, and skin sensitivity as your body adjusts to the change. In order to minimize these potential side effects from changing your gut flora too rapidly, I always recommend slowly introducing probiotic-rich foods. Please note that fermented foods can exacerbate SIBO (chapter 9) or histamine intolerance (chapter 4). Those with an adverse reaction to fermented foods may need to test and treat SIBO and/or address histamine-producing microbes such as *H. pylori* bacteria or protozoa (chapter 14) to get full relief from IBS.

Tailoring Your Protocol Based on Microbiome Testing Results

While broad-spectrum probiotics can benefit most people, there are times when microbiome testing helps tailor your protocol more precisely. Here's how certain patterns in microbiome testing might guide your treatment plan:

Low *Akkermansia*

Akkermansia helps to maintain gut lining and metabolism. When levels are low, you might experience weight gain, metabolic imbalances, or inflammation. To boost *Akkermansia*, consider supplementing with Pendulum Akkermansia and Designs for Health PhytoBiome, which contains prebiotic polyphenols that promote the growth of *Akkermansia*. Additionally, incorporating polyphenol-rich foods such as pomegranate, cranberries, and green tea can support *Akkermansia* levels.

Overgrowth of Pathogenic *Streptococcus* Bacteria

While certain Streptococcus strains are beneficial, like *Streptococcus thermophilus*, which aids digestion, an overgrowth of pathogenic *Streptococcus* can lead to gut dysbiosis, increased inflammation, digestive discomfort, and even obsessive thoughts. Taking the beneficial *Streptococcus thermophilus* can displace pathogenic strep, while herbs such as berberine or St. John's-wort can reduce pathogenic overgrowth and restore balance.

Overgrowth of Pathogenic *Clostridia*

Certain *Clostridia* species, particularly *Clostridium difficile*, can wreak havoc on the gut, leading to severe diarrhea, inflammation, and even more serious complications. Addressing *Clostridia* overgrowth is crucial, and *Saccharomyces boulardii*—a beneficial yeast—can help displace *Clostridia*. Biocidin Botanicals Biocidin Liquid, the broad-spectrum herbal antimicrobial, can also work against *Clostridia*.

Opportunistic *E. coli* Overgrowth

Opportunistic strains of *E. coli* can disrupt gut health, leading to symptoms like bloating, constipation, or diarrhea. To target these strains, *E. coli*–eating benevolent viruses, known as bacteriophages or phages, selectively infect and destroy *E. coli*. *E. coli*–eating phages include LH01-Myoviridae, LL5-Siphoviridae, T4D-Myoviridae, and LL12-Myoviridae and can be taken as stand-alone products or in combination with probiotics. High-quality options include Designs for Health Probiophage DF, Life Extension-FLORASSIST® GI with Phage Technology, and Body Ecology EcoPhage. They contain four different types of phages and target *E. coli*, a common overgrowth associated with SIBO and IBS.

Low Levels of Beneficial *E. Coli* (*E. Coli* Nissle)

Not all strains of *E. coli* are harmful! This particular strain of *E. coli* was isolated by Alfred Nissle in 1917 and is considered to be beneficial. It has been shown to be as effective in maintaining remission of ulcerative colitis as mesalazine, a first-line anti-inflammatory prescription drug used to treat IBD. It's also been shown to restore gut barrier function in those with IBS. If your microbiome test shows low levels of this strain, you may benefit from *Mutaflor*, a probiotic supplement containing *E. coli Nissle*. Although it's primarily available in Germany, some importers ship it to the U.S.

Autoimmune Triggers Including *Klebsiella*

Klebsiella species, often linked to autoimmune conditions like ankylosing spondylitis and reactive arthritis, can trigger inflammation and immune dysregulation. Reducing *Klebsiella* levels with antimicrobial herbs such as berberine and oil of oregano can help manage this overgrowth and reduce autoimmune risks.

Firmicutes: Bacteroides Ratio

Some cases of IBS show a high *Firmicutes: Bacteroidetes* ratio, which appears to correlate with higher weight and psychological symptoms including depression and anxiety, while other cases of IBS and IBD may have a low *Firmicutes: Bacteroidetes* ratio. *Bacillus* probiotics can increase firmicute bacteria, while *Bifidobacteria* probiotics and *S. boulardii* can increase *bacteroidetes*.

Chapter Summary

- Dysbiosis in the microbiome occurs when we have an imbalance among beneficial bacteria (that help us digest foods and extract nutrients and keep the peace in the gut), opportunistic bacteria (that can become problematic when stressed), and pathogenic microbes (that can cause *a lot* of trouble).

- Restoring balance by promoting beneficial bacteria (probiotics) can significantly help to resolve diarrhea, constipation, and other IBS-associated symptoms, and may also improve and/or prevent many autoimmune issues, hormonal imbalances, health conditions, and even help us reach a healthier weight.

- Common causes of dysbiosis include antibiotics, environmental toxins (glyphosate, mold), infections, stress, the Standard American Diet, poor sleep, alcohol, nicotine, thyroid hormone imbalance, and digestive enzyme deficiency.

- A comprehensive stool analysis test can identify dysbiosis if you have IBS-related symptoms, but there's a good chance you do not need to test to benefit from probiotics.

- Ways to add probiotics include eating fermented foods and vegetables and supplementing with *S. boulardii,* a beneficial yeast, spore-based probiotics, individual strain probiotics, and multiple strain probiotics.

- Once the gut has been repopulated with probiotics, prebiotics may help some people.

- If you find some probiotics/prebiotics make you feel worse, you may wish to consider testing for SIBO and potentially pathogenic bacteria.

Visit https://ibsrootcause.com/bonus for notes on this chapter.

CHAPTER 8

Intestinal Permeability

When healthy, our intestines serve dual roles—they're both a barrier and a filter. Picture the lining of the gut as a meticulously woven cloth, composed of cells tightly linked by structures akin to thread fibers. These intercellular tight junctions open selectively to absorb essential nutrients from the food we eat and close to block harmful substances like partially digested food, pollen, feces, dead cells, and bacteria from entering our bloodstream. This selective permeability is crucial for maintaining overall health and preventing unwanted materials from circulating throughout our bodies.

If those intestinal tight junctions become damaged and/or loose, we develop what's known as intestinal permeability (IP), commonly referred to as "leaky gut." Intestinal permeability allows toxic substances to pass into the bloodstream, triggering inflammation and several IBS-related symptoms such as gas, bloating, abdominal pain, and indigestion. IP may be the true cause behind the heightened perception of pain seen in IBS known as "visceral hypersensitivity."

Root Cause Research Corner: Visceral Hypersensitivity and Intestinal Permeability

Intestinal permeability (leaky gut) is a key contributor to visceral hypersensitivity, a heightened pain response in internal organs that affects 30 to 40 percent of people with IBS. When the gut barrier is compromised, toxins can leak into the bloodstream, triggering pain pathways and amplifying discomfort from otherwise mild stimuli.

Research shows increased intestinal permeability is more common in IBS, affecting 37 to 62 percent of those with IBS-D, 17 to 50 percent with post-infectious IBS, and 4 to 25 percent with IBS-C. It's also frequently seen in children with functional GI issues and food allergies.

Beyond digestive symptoms, intestinal permeability can lead to immune dysfunction and autoimmunity. Dr. Alessio Fasano's "three-legged stool" model proposes that genetic predisposition, environmental triggers, and intestinal permeability are all required for autoimmune diseases to develop. Studies have linked leaky gut to nearly every autoimmune condition, from Hashimoto's to vitiligo.

When I was dealing with both IBS and Hashimoto's, healing my gut made a profound difference. In my experience, and in helping thousands of others, addressing intestinal permeability is one of the most powerful steps for long-term healing, often leading to symptom relief and autoimmune remission.

What Causes Intestinal Permeability?

Intestinal permeability may occur for a variety of reasons. For example, an imbalance of gut bacteria can disrupt the integrity of the gut's protective mucus barrier. This imbalance reduces the production of butyrate and other protective short-chain fatty acids (SCFAs), while in-

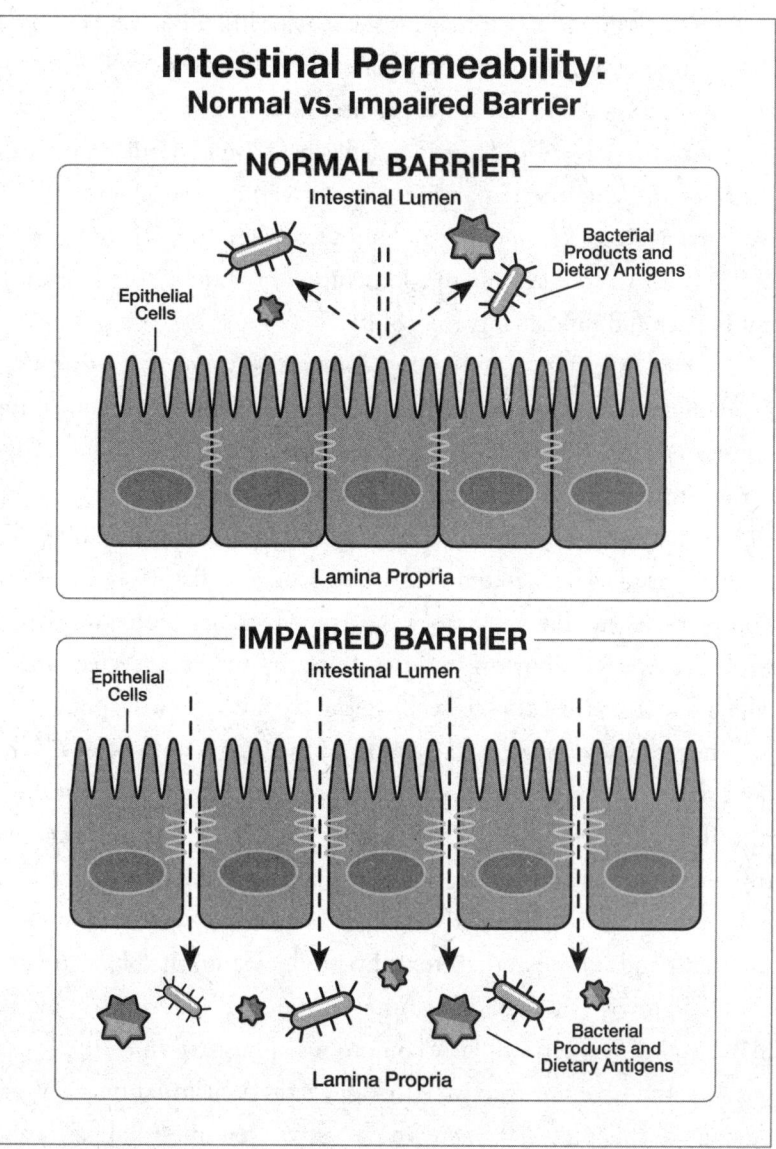

Normal barrier function allows for proper filtering of nutrients and toxins, while impaired barrier function allows for problematic substances to cross into our circulation.

Image by Dave Kinzel, adapted from Takuya Suzuki and Hiroshi Hara, "Role of Flavonoids in Intestinal Tight Junction Regulation," *The Journal of Nutritional Biochemistry* 22, no. 5 (2011), figure 1.

creasing inflammation-promoting substances like LPS, which loosens the tight junctions between intestinal cells. A deficiency of *Bifidobacteria* has been linked to intestinal permeability.

Digestive enzyme and nutrient deficiencies (in particular pancreatic enzymes and zinc and glutamine, respectively) can weaken the intestinal barrier. Research suggests glutamine synthesis may be impaired in people with IBS-D, leading to a loosening of the tight junctions of the gut barrier and intestinal permeability.

Various infections—from parasites such as *Blastocystis hominis* and *Dientamoeba fragilis* to bacteria such as *H. pylori* and viruses, including norovirus—can also lead to increased intestinal permeability. These pathogens may disrupt the barrier function by damaging the gut's protective mechanisms or by directly attacking the intestinal lining. For example, studies have found *B. hominis* protozoa disturb barrier function by breaking down secretory IgA, the GI tract's protective barrier, while *H. pylori* can burrow into the stomach lining and secrete urease, which damages the epithelial cells lining the surface of the gut.

The pathogenic yeast (and member of the fungi family) *Candida* has been shown to contribute to the development of intestinal permeability by using its branching form (known as hyphae) to weaken and penetrate the intestinal barrier, leaving holes in the intestinal wall. Once these holes are created, this fungal pathogen is able to release several endo- (internal) and exo- (external) toxic by-products into the bloodstream.

Overgrowths of bacteria or fungi in the small intestine, known as SIBO and SIFO, can similarly compromise intestinal integrity.

Any food we are reactive to causes irritation, inflammation, and damage to the intestinal tract, which can worsen intestinal permeability. There are also some foods that induce intestinal permeability in everyone who consumes them, though notably with varying degrees.

Gluten (specifically, the gliadin proteins that make up gluten) can alter the properties of the cells that make up the intestinal barrier and thus weaken the structure of the barrier. Studies suggest that the impact of gluten consumption can induce gut permeability for minutes to months at a time, depending on the individual (as you may have guessed, those with celiac disease are on the higher end of this).

Capsaicin, a component found in spicy peppers (including chili peppers and cayenne peppers (but not bell peppers), is also an inducer of intestinal permeability, through causing structural damage to the gut lining. Researchers (and many people with IBS), have found that spicy foods are a common IBS trigger, and perhaps this is why.

Moreover, stress, both chronic and acute, and the use of certain medications—such as proton pump inhibitors, NSAIDs, antibiotics, steroids, and hormonal therapies—have been linked to increased gut permeability. These substances and conditions disrupt the gut flora and mucosal lining, leading to inflammation and a breakdown of the gut barrier. Studies have found that NSAIDs increase intestinal permeability within twelve to twenty-four hours of intake. This is a big issue for people who take them long term.

Additionally, environmental toxins such as mold and glyphosate further exacerbate this condition.

Finally, alcohol consumption can directly damage the tight junctions between epithelial cells, increasing intestinal permeability while also disturbing the microbial balance within the gut. One study found a moderate amount of alcohol (about 1 drink per day) could significantly increase the risk for SIBO.

Factors That Increase Intestinal Permeability

- Advanced age: As we age, the regeneration of gut cells slows down.
- AGES (advanced glycosylation end products): Formed when protein or fat combine with sugar in the bloodstream; can increase oxidative stress and inflammation, damaging gut lining.

- **Alcohol:** Excessive alcohol consumption can directly damage the cells lining the intestine.
- **Antibiotics:** While fighting infections, antibiotics can also kill beneficial gut bacteria, disrupting the microbiome balance.
- **Capsaicin:** Found in hot peppers, capsaicin can irritate the gastrointestinal lining.
- **Digestive enzyme deficiencies:** Without sufficient digestive enzymes, food isn't properly broken down, leading to gut irritation.
- **Female hormones:** Hormonal fluctuations can affect gut barrier function.
- **Food allergies:** Inflammatory responses to food allergens can damage intestinal tissues.
- **Gliadin (Gluten):** Gliadin, a component of gluten, can trigger the release of zonulin, a protein that regulates gut permeability, especially in those with gluten sensitivity or celiac disease.
- **IBD (inflammatory bowel disease):** Conditions such as Crohn's disease and ulcerative colitis involve chronic inflammation of the gut, which can damage the mucosal lining.
- **Intestinal infections:** Infections from parasites or bacteria can damage the gut lining and disrupt tight junctions.
- **L-alanine:** This amino acid can influence gut barrier function, but its exact role in intestinal permeability needs further research.
- **Large amounts of tryptophan:** High levels of tryptophan may affect serotonin production and gut function, potentially impacting permeability.
- **Linoleic acid:** An omega-6 fatty acid that, in excessive amounts, can promote inflammation in the gut.

- Nutrient depletions: Deficiencies in nutrients such as zinc and glutamine can impair the repair and maintenance of the gut lining.
- NSAIDs (nonsteroidal anti-inflammatory drugs): Can damage the gut lining and decrease mucus production.
- Overgrowth of bacteria in the small intestine: Known as SIBO, this condition can lead to the production of bacterial toxins that damage the gut lining.
- Pathogenic bacteria: Harmful bacteria can cause infections and inflammation, disrupting gut integrity.
- PPIs (proton pump inhibitors): These drugs reduce stomach acid, which can lead to bacterial overgrowth and nutrient malabsorption.
- Psychological stress (anger, fear): Stress can trigger changes in gut physiology that reduces barrier function.
- Reactive/triggering foods: Reactive foods can cause an immune response or irritation in the gut.
- Steroids: While reducing inflammation, steroids can also weaken immune function and thin mucosal barriers.
- Strenuous exercise: Intense physical activity can stress the body and temporarily weaken gut barriers.
- Surgery/Trauma: Physical damage to the body, including to the gut itself, can disrupt the intestinal lining.
- Toxins: Environmental toxins, like pesticides and heavy metals, can damage the gut lining.
- Unsaturated fats: While generally healthy, excessive intake of certain unsaturated fats without balance can promote inflammation in the gut.

How Do You Know You Have Intestinal Permeability?

Generally speaking, intestinal permeability in itself is not symptomatic, but research suggests that IP is a common feature in people with autoimmunity, IBD, and IBS-D. Intestinal permeability can be measured via testing.

Zonulin is a protein that acts as a gatekeeper, helping to maintain the integrity of the gut barrier by modulating the tight junctions between cells in the gut lining. When zonulin levels increase, this signals the tight junctions to relax, allowing larger molecules and potentially harmful substances to pass through the intestinal barrier into the bloodstream. This can be a stand-alone test, and is also offered as part of various comprehensive stool analysis tests on the market. I prefer the comprehensive tests, because they can also uncover some of the causes behind intestinal permeability, such as a lack of beneficial bacteria, an overgrowth of opportunistic bacteria, potentially pathogenic bacteria, digestive enzyme deficiencies, potential pathogens, markers of gut inflammation such as calprotectin, poor bacterial diversity, and low butyrate levels.

The mannitol-lactulose intestinal permeability test measures how well your intestinal barrier is functioning by analyzing the ratio of two sugars, lactulose and mannitol. Normally, mannitol, a monosaccharide, is easily absorbed, while lactulose, a disaccharide, isn't—unless the intestinal lining is compromised. After drinking a premeasured amount of these sugars, you collect a urine sample over six hours. If your lactulose-to-mannitol ratio is high, it suggests increased intestinal permeability.

Healing Intestinal Permeability with Repairing Protocols

If you were to tell your conventionally trained doctor you have "leaky gut" there's a chance you might notice a subtle eye roll from the doctor. In conventional medicine circles, the term "leaky gut" is often dismissed as a made-up condition with no scientific validity, however, funny enough there are over 25,000 research articles on PubMed on intestinal permeability, the medically accepted term that means the same thing!

However, addressing intestinal permeability is a key feature of integrative functional medicine. The 5R framework is often used in functional medicine practitioners to heal and support intestinal permeability, and is focused on removing reactive foods and infections, replacing digestive enzymes, reinoculating the gut flora with beneficial microbes, rebalancing the lifestyle, and using repairing protocols to help with healing and sealing the intestinal lining. This book incorporates all of the 5 Rs, and this chapter will specifically focus on repairing protocols.

A healthy gut is essential for overall well-being, and by focusing on reducing inflammation, adding in gut-healing foods, and incorporating targeted supplements, we can support a strong, resilient gut lining. Please note that these interventions work best in conjunction with the other 4 Rs.

The 5R Framework for Gut Health

1. Remove: In this step, any foods causing a reaction or that someone is sensitive to are eliminated. If there are known infections, including bacterial, fungal, and parasitic infections, they may be eradicated in this step. For help removing:

    • Reactive foods and dietary triggers, see chapter 4.

- Infections, see chapter 10.
- Toxins, see chapter 14.

2. **Replace:** Next, key digestive enzymes, hydrochloric acid, and bile are added, to support optimal digestion and nutrient absorption. For help replacing:
   - Digestive enzymes and optimizing digestion, see chapter 5.
   - Gut-supporting nutrient depletions, see chapter 6.

3. **Reinoculate:** Start rebuilding the beneficial gut flora through the use of probiotics and fermented foods to help the gut thrive. For help reinoculating:
   - The microbiome, see chapter 7.

4. **Repair:** Key nutrients, such as glutamine, and anti-inflammatory foods, such as bone broth, are used to support the repair of the gut lining. The treatment recommendations in this chapter will focus on repair.

5. **Rebalance:** This step is related to lifestyle modifications to support the gut including reducing stress, getting enough sleep, and regular exercise. You may also need to incorporate liver and adrenal support. For help rebalancing:
   - Stress hormones, see chapter 11.

Food as Medicine

Eliminating inflammatory foods is a significant step toward repairing intestinal permeability. Following a gluten-free diet may be helpful, as gluten has been found to activate zonulin release in people with and without celiac disease, though levels were much higher in people with celiac disease.

Additionally, incorporating a diet rich in omega-3 fats and low in omega-6 fats can further aid in healing the gut. For example, a study involving 68 women compared the effects of a Mediterranean diet to a standard diet over three months. Those following the Mediterranean diet, which is naturally higher in omega-3 fats, experienced reduced zonulin levels and enhanced intestinal barrier integrity. This suggests that adjusting your dietary fats can play a crucial role in maintaining gut health.

Focusing on omega-3 fatty acids is crucial for managing intestinal permeability, as they help strengthen the gut lining and reduce inflammation. Omega-3s such as EPA (eicosapentaenoic acid) and DHA (docosahexaenoic acid), found abundantly in fish such as salmon, mackerel, and sardines, are integral for maintaining the integrity of the intestinal barrier. They also counteract inflammation, which is pivotal in preventing and managing issues related to intestinal permeability.

In addition to omega-3s, other beneficial fats play important roles in gut health. Short-chain fatty acids (SCFAs) like butyrate, propionate, and acetate, which are produced when fiber (especially from oats) is fermented by gut bacteria, nourish colon cells and help maintain a healthy gut barrier. Butyrate is found in dairy products like butter and ghee, and if tolerated, these foods can support the cells lining the gut.

Medium-chain triglycerides (MCTs), found in coconut oil and palm kernel oil, are also beneficial for the gut. They not only help improve the gut barrier function but also possess antimicrobial properties that protect against harmful pathogens. Lauric acid, a type of MCT, is notably effective in this regard.

Conversely, it's wise to limit omega-6 fatty acids, commonly found in processed foods and certain vegetable oils like corn and sunflower oil. While necessary in moderation, an excess of omega-6 fatty acids can promote inflammation, potentially worsening intestinal permeability if not balanced with adequate omega-3 intake.

Incorporating these beneficial fats while managing the intake of less helpful ones can significantly support the health of your gut barrier and reduce the risk of intestinal permeability.

Adding foods with antioxidant and anti-inflammatory properties can also support the intestinal linking. The MaPLE randomized controlled trial focused on the role of dietary polyphenols, a class of compounds naturally found in plant foods, in improving intestinal health, and revealed that a diet rich in polyphenols could reduce serum zonulin levels and improve gut microbiome composition by increasing populations of fiber-fermenting and butyrate-producing bacteria in the gut. Foods high in polyphenols include berries, nuts, dark green vegetables, and dark chocolate, as well as beverages like tea and coffee. Regularly including these foods in your diet can help strengthen the gut barrier.

Polyphenol Rich Foods

- Berries: Blueberries, blackberries, raspberries, strawberries, and cranberries are particularly high in anthocyanins, a type of polyphenol that has antioxidant and anti-inflammatory effects.
- Dark chocolate/cocoa: Rich in flavonoids, particularly epicatechin, which supports cardiovascular health and has antioxidant properties.
- Olives and olive oil: Contain hydroxytyrosol and oleuropein, which have anti-inflammatory and antioxidant effects.
- Nuts: Pecans, hazelnuts, and walnuts are high in polyphenols, contributing to their heart-healthy benefits.
- Herbs and spices: Oregano, rosemary, thyme, sage, cloves, cinnamon, turmeric, and ginger are packed with polyphenols and have antimicrobial and anti-inflammatory effects.

- Tea: Both green and black tea are rich in catechins and flavonoids, which promote heart health and offer antioxidant benefits.
- Red wine: Rich in resveratrol, which is associated with cardiovascular benefits and antiaging properties (in moderation).
- Fruits: Grapes, apples, cherries, pomegranates, and plums are high in various polyphenols like anthocyanins, flavonoids, and resveratrol.
- Vegetables: Artichokes, spinach, red onions, purple cabbage, and shallots contain quercetin and other flavonoids.
- Legumes: Black beans, kidney beans, and lentils have high polyphenol content and offer gut health benefits.
- Coffee: Coffee is rich in chlorogenic acid, a powerful antioxidant that supports metabolism and overall health.
- Whole grains: Oats, quinoa, and buckwheat are rich in phenolic acids, supporting heart health and digestion.
- Seeds: Flaxseeds and chia seeds contain polyphenols that help reduce inflammation and support digestion.

Gelatinous foods, like bone broth and gelatin, are powerful allies when it comes to healing intestinal permeability. These foods are rich in collagen and amino acids like glycine and glutamine, which work together to repair and strengthen the gut lining. Glycine stimulates the production of stomach acid, which is essential for digestion, while glutamine supports the maintenance of a healthy mucosal layer in the gut. This protective layer acts as a barrier, preventing harmful substances from leaking through the gut wall. Gelatin in the gut will also draw fluid into the intestine, improving gut motility and supporting healthy bowel movements

By incorporating gelatinous foods into your diet, you're providing your gut with the tools it needs to restore its integrity and reduce inflammation, ultimately helping to seal those "leaks" and promote overall digestive health.

I love recommending bone broth and homemade polyphenol-rich jello to support intestinal repair.

Bone broth has surged in popularity as a Paleo diet staple, though it has been a healing tradition worldwide for millennia. Bone broth is packed with nutrients from simmered bones, including collagen and gelatin, and contains key amino acids like glycine, proline, and glutamine, essential for intestinal and immune cell energy. Additionally, bone broth provides glucosamine and chondroitin sulfate for joint health, and minerals like calcium, magnesium, and zinc. Easily made at home in a slow cooker, bone broth is both a nourishing and a simple addition to a healthy diet. Here's how I make it:

Simple Bone Broth Recipe

4 to 5 organic chicken legs

1 tablespoon apple cider vinegar

2 stalks celery

1 onion

6 to 8 large carrots

Purified water

Sea salt to taste

Black pepper to taste

1. Place the chicken, vinegar, and vegetables in a slow cooker.
2. Fill with water to 1 inch below the top of the slow cooker, cover, and cook on high for 8 to 12 hours.
3. Season with salt and pepper to taste.
4. Strain, pour into jars, and refrigerate (or freeze).

> ### What if I Can't Tolerate Bone Broth?
>
> Some people can't tolerate bone broth or glutamine due to histamine intolerance or the over-conversion of glutamate to glutamine. I've found supplementing with P5P (the active version of B_6) can help significantly with these kinds of reactions. To learn more, see the box in chapter 6 (page 179). You may also want to avoid bone broth until the histamine intolerance has been addressed (see chapter 4). Consider using meat broth, which is low in histamine, as a stepping-stone before eventually introducing bone broth.

Gelatin is a flavorless, colorless, jellylike substance made by processing animal bones, cartilage, and skin. It's used in many foods like marshmallows, gummy candies, soups, broths, and sauces and has been consumed as a food and used therapeutically throughout history. The most abundant amino acid in gelatin is glycine, and it also contains glutamic acid, which is converted into glutamine in the body and can help maintain a healthy mucosal lining and support digestion.

Of course, we don't want to eat gelatin in just any form (gummy bears, especially ones made with maltitol, probably won't make your stomach feel great). I recommend avoiding the more processed foods that contain gelatin, as they will likely include other additives like artificial colors, thickeners, sweeteners, and preservatives that may actually be detrimental to the gut. Using gelatin at home in recipes is the best way to reap all of its benefits. Here's my homemade Polyphenol Anti-Inflammatory Jello recipe.

Polyphenol Anti-Inflammatory Jello

Serves: 4

Prep time: 2 minutes

Cook time: 5 minutes, plus 2 to 4 hours to cool

2 cups organic concord grape juice

2 cups tart cherry juice

4 tablespoons gelatin

1 cup blueberries (if tolerated)

1. Pour 2 cups of cold juice into a glass container.
2. Add the gelatin to the cold juice, mix, and let sit for one minute.
3. In a small pan on medium low, heat the two remaining cups of juice for 5 minutes.
4. Slowly pour the hot juice into the gelatin mixture while whisking until fully incorporated.
5. Add the blueberries.
6. Pour the mixture into a 8×8 baking dish and refrigerate for 2 to 4 hours.
7. Cut into desired shapes and serve.

Polyphenol Supplements for Gut Health

Polyphenol supplements are derived from plant sources rich in polyphenols and can help support gut barrier integrity.

Common Polyphenol Supplements

- **Resveratrol:** Found in red wine, grapes, and berries, resveratrol is known for its antiaging and anti-inflammatory benefits, and has been shown to decrease pro-inflammatory cytokines in the gut and decrease gut vascular permeability.
- **Quercetin:** A flavonoid present in apples, onions, and green tea, which can enhance intestinal barrier function and help modulate the composition of gut microbiota, and plays a protective role

for the gut and intestinal immune tolerance. High-quality resveratrol and quercetin supplements are available from various companies.

- Curcumin: Curcumin is the active component of turmeric and is revered for its anti-inflammatory benefits. It has also been shown to regulate intestinal barrier function. Research has found curcumin helps to modulate all four layers of the intestinal barrier and helps protect the intestines from damage. Incorporating turmeric into your diet is one way to get curcumin, and a supplement like Rootcology Curcumin Absorb or Thorne Curcumin Phytosome may be helpful for achieving a therapeutic dose, which is usually between 500 and 2,000 mg per day.
- Green tea extract (EGCG): A powerful polyphenol found in green tea, known for its antioxidant properties and its potential to support metabolism and gut health.
- Grape seed extract: Rich in proanthocyanidins, grape seed extract supports cardiovascular health and has strong antioxidant properties.
- Olive leaf extract: Contains polyphenols such as oleuropein, which supports heart health and has anti-inflammatory benefits.
- Pomegranate extract: High in ellagitannins and punicalagins, pomegranate extract supports gut health and reduces oxidative stress.
- Blueberry extract: Contains anthocyanins, a type of polyphenol known for its cognitive and heart health benefits.

Supplements for Repairing the Gut Lining

Because intestinal permeability is caused by multiple factors, we take a multifactor approach that involves strengthening the gut lining, supporting the production of mucus, reducing inflammation, and restoring the balance of beneficial bacteria.

Key strategies include tightening the tight junctions between gut cells, promoting the production of gut-protective mucus, and addressing inflammation with specific supplements, herbs, and nutrients. We've already discussed many interventions that are important for intestinal permeability, such as glutamine, zinc, probiotics, and butyrate in previous chapters and, I will list them briefly here as well.

Glutamine

Glutamine is the most widely studied substance for healing intestinal permeability. Studies have found supplementation of this important amino acid in people with IBS-D significantly reduced intestinal permeability and improved IBS-related symptoms, especially diarrhea and abdominal pain.

Zinc

A deficiency has been associated with increased intestinal permeability, susceptibility to infections, and reduced detoxification of bacterial toxins. Replenishing zinc has been shown to repair intestinal permeability, lower gut inflammation, and promote a balanced gut microbiome. Zinc carnosine (zinc chelated with the amino acid L-carnosine) is the preferred form of zinc for gut health because it remains intact in the presence of stomach acid and adheres to gut wounds more effectively.

Probiotics

An abundance of beneficial bacteria, including spore-based probiotics and the beneficial yeast-based probiotic *S. boulardii,* can support gut integrity and healthy levels of zonulin by helping restore a balanced microbiome and protecting the gut mucosa from injury as a result of toxins, allergens, and pathogens.

Butyrate

The important SCFA butyrate supports the integrity of the intestinal lining by regulating the tight junctions and supporting intestinal mucus production.

Substances That Help "Tighten" the Tight Junctions
Berberine

This compound, found in a variety of plants, has a number of beneficial effects on the gut. By modulating certain pathways, berberine has been found to reduce intestinal permeability and increase the thickness of the mucus layer in the gut. In a study on diabetic rats, high doses of berberine were found to decrease intestinal permeability by 27.5 percent. Please note that berberine is very helpful for many people with IBS but may not be appropriate for people with extreme diarrhea and IBD (see chapter 15). High-quality options include Rootcology Berberine, NOW Foods Berberine, Candibactin-BR (an herbal formulation containing berberine), Integrative Therapeutics Berberine, Designs for Health Berb-Evail, and Pure Encapsulations Berberine UltraSorb.

Immunoglobulins

Immunoglobulins, or antibodies, are a key part of our immune system, helping to protect against harmful bacteria, viruses, and fungi. In the gut, they bind to microbes and neutralize them before they can cause harm. Supplementing with immunoglobulin G (IgG) has been shown to reduce inflammation by lowering pro-inflammatory cytokines and binding to harmful bacteria, ultimately improving gut barrier function. This approach has been beneficial for conditions like IBS and IBD.

Colostrum is the first form of milk produced after birth and is rich in IgG antibodies that support gut and immune health. Cow's colostrum, which is similar to human colostrum, has shown benefits for digestive disorders, including IBD, as early as the 1950s. However, since it's dairy-derived, it may not be suitable for those with lactose intolerance. ARMRA Colostrum is a popular high-quality option, and some people with lactose intolerance have reported they can tolerate it.

For those sensitive to cow's dairy, camel colostrum is an alternative. Studies show around 80 percent of people who are sensitive to cow's milk can tolerate camel milk, which is also rich in immunoglobulins and supports gut health. Desert Farms is a trusted brand for camel colostrum.

Serum-derived bovine immunoglobulin (SBI) is a dairy-free immunoglobulin option, typically used in conditions like IBD, IBS-D, and chronic diarrhea. One study found that 76 percent of IBD patients experienced symptom improvement after twelve weeks of taking 5 grams of SBI daily (improvements were seen in about 49 percent of people in just one week). SBI is available through prescription products like EnteraGam and OTC brands such as Ortho Molecular Products and Microbiome Labs.

For another dairy-free option, hyperimmune egg powder is made by vaccinating chickens to produce antibodies against common human pathogens, including *E. coli, Salmonella, Klebsiella, Staphylococcus,* and *Streptococcus.* Antibodies to the pathogens (IgY immunoglobulins) are then found in the eggs of the chickens and transformed into a powdered supplement. Hyperimmune egg powder has been found to inhibit bacterial growth, adhesion to the gut lining, and toxin production. It may help support the immune function of the gut and modulate cytokine production. Case studies on two patients with IBS found hyperimmune egg powder improved stool consistency and frequency. XYMOGEN: Ig 26 DF and IgY Nutrition IgY Max are high-quality hyperimmune egg supplement options.

Larazotide is a promising zonulin inhibitor that helps protect the integrity of the gut lining by blocking zonulin, keeping tight junctions closed. Originally larazotide was available only as an investigative medication though clinical trials as an adjunct to the gluten-free diet for celiac disease. However, it recently became available as a prescription via compounding pharmacies and through some supplement companies and may offer broader benefits for other gut-related issues.

Substances That Support the Intestinal Mucous Membrane

Seacure

A whole-food-based supplement made from deep-ocean whitefish, this contains naturally occurring nutrients from the fish, including omega-3 fatty acids. I have personally used this supplement in people with IBS with good results, and many other practitioners report Seacure reduces symptoms and restores gut integrity in their patients with Crohn's disease and IBS. Seacure has been studied and found to reduce gastric injury by 59 percent and increase cell proliferation. Seacure also contains high concentrations of glutamine and glutamine-containing peptides, which are also likely responsible for the gut benefit of the supplement.

N-Acetyl Glucosamine (NAG) and Glucosamine

NAG, at daily doses of 6 grams, has also been shown to help restore intestinal permeability by acting as a cytoprotective agent and supporting normal functioning of the mucous membrane in the gut. Glucosamine, a related compound best known for joint health, also supports gut health by strengthening the intestinal lining and reducing inflammation, which helps to prevent intestinal permeability and soothe digestive discomfort. Consider Jarrow Formulas N-A-G at a dose of 700 to 6,000 mg per day.

Mucilaginous Herbs

These botanicals, which include DGL (deglycyrrhizinated licorice), slippery elm, marshmallow, chamomile, okra extract, and cat's claw, can provide support for healthy intestinal function by coating and soothing the intestinal lining, promoting the healing of ulcers and inflamed tissue, and reducing cramping by relaxing the intestines. Consider these high-quality blends: Rootcology Gut R&R, Biosense Clinic MucosaHeal, Designs for Health GI Revive, XYMOGEN GI Balance Powder, DaVinci Laboratories G.I. Benefits, Pure Encapsulations G.I. Fortify, and ReLeaf MucosaCalm.

N-acetylcysteine (NAC)

NAC is a precursor to glutathione (our master antioxidant) and promotes intestinal health by helping to detoxify intestinal bacteria and by breaking down biofilms that house gut pathogens. NAC offers significant gastro-protective effects, potentially by increasing the viscosity of the mucus that protects the gut lining. Consider taking 1,800 mg daily with food of Rootcology Pure N Acetyl Cysteine, Pure Encapsulations NAC, or Designs for Health N Acetyl-Cysteine.

> ## Intestinal Permeability Support Blends
>
> Oftentimes, using a few of the intestinal linking supportive ingredients mentioned in this section produces synergistic results on the gut. A few companies offer a mix of ingredients, such as L-glutamine, zinc, quercetin, glucosamine, and mucilaginous herbs in one convenient, easy-to-use product. I prefer using the powders due to their ease of use (and fewer pills to swallow), but you may prefer to purchase stand-alone products if you have a sensitivity to one of the ingredients. My favorite options include Rootcology Gut R&R, Pure Encapsulations G.I. Fortify, DaVinci Laboratories G.I. Benefits, XYMOGEN GI Balance Powder, Designs for Health GI Revive, Biosense Clinic MucosaHeal, ReLeaf MucosaCalm

Chapter Summary

- Intestinal permeability is present in most people with IBS-D and some people with IBD-C.

- Intestinal permeability can be a driver of gas, bloating, abdominal pain, indigestion, and visceral hypersensitivity.

- Intestinal permeability has various causes, including gut infections, bacterial and/or fungal overgrowths, and nutrient depletions.

- The 5 Rs can help resolve intestinal permeability:
    - Remove reactive foods, toxins, and infections.
    - Replace digestive enzymes and nutrients.
    - Reinoculate the microbiome with probiotics.
    - Repair the gut lining with gelatinous foods and nutrients.
    - Rebalance stress.

- Omega-3 fatty acids, MCTs, vitamins A and D, gelatinous foods, polyphenols, glutamine, zinc, probiotics, butyrate, berberine, immunoglobulins, N-acetyl glucosamine (NAG), mucilaginous herbs, and NAC can help with intestinal permeability.

Visit https://ibsrootcause.com/bonus for notes on this chapter.

CHAPTER 9

Intestinal Overgrowth

Have you ever felt bloated and constipated after eating or noticed your IBS symptoms getting worse over time? If so, you might be dealing with SIBO (small intestinal bacterial overgrowth), a common root cause of IBS. But here's what many don't realize—there's more than one type of microbial overgrowth that can lead to these uncomfortable symptoms.

This chapter will dive deep into SIBO, including a form called methane-dominant SIBO, or intestinal methanogen overgrowth (IMO), where the issue isn't caused by bacteria, but by archaea—most notably, *Methanobrevibacter smithii* (*M. smithii*).

We will also cover the overgrowths caused by the opportunistic yeast *Candida* in both the small intestine, often called small intestinal fungal overgrowth (SIFO), and the large intestine (sometimes called intestinal candidiasis).

Thanks to the pioneering research of Dr. Mark Pimental, the connection between SIBO and IBS is more widely recognized by practitioners. However, many treatments fall short. Some practitioners recommend long-term low FODMAP diets to "starve out" the bacteria, but this only addresses symptoms temporarily and doesn't tackle the root cause—plus, it can reduce gut diversity in the long run, which leads to more issues down the road.

Others take a more aggressive approach, using antibiotics, antimicrobial herbs, or even the elemental diet to clear the overgrowth. While people report these methods do provide relief, SIBO often returns if the protocols are too short, are used incorrectly, or are incomplete. In my experience, the key is not just to address the overgrowth but to uncover and treat the underlying causes that allowed it to develop in the first place. This often includes supporting digestive enzymes, improving gut motility, and clearing out other gut infections that have created an environment for overgrowth.

We'll explore how to do just that in this chapter and take a key step toward restoring gut health by addressing both SIBO and Candida overgrowths. For the infections that can contribute to these issues, stay tuned for chapter 13!

Small Intestinal Bacterial Overgrowth (SIBO)

Our small intestine is meant to be relatively clear of bacteria, while the large intestine houses most of our bacterial friends and foes. Small intestinal bacterial overgrowth, or SIBO, is what happens when bacteria from the large intestine (good or bad) make their way into the small intestine and grow in large numbers. Many studies have linked IBS and SIBO, with one 2018 meta-analysis of over fifty studies finding that one third of IBS patients tested positive for SIBO.

The symptoms of SIBO and IBS overlap (belching, bloating, constipation, diarrhea), and studies have generally found people with IBS are more likely to have SIBO (ranging from 19 percent to 37 percent) compared to healthy controls (0 percent to 12 percent). SIBO often presents with bloating after eating and is connected with the annoying "I woke up with a flat stomach and now I look pregnant" syndrome. This is caused by all of those bacteria in the small intestine fermenting food there and generating too much gas as a by-product.

SIBO contributes to other digestive symptoms because it can result in intestinal permeability as the body tries to get rid of the excess bacteria in the small intestine (and contributes to the holes being created in the intestinal wall) and reduce levels of key digestive enzymes, making it harder to break down foods.

How Do You Know You Have SIBO?

Testing is generally required for a diagnosis of SIBO, but symptoms can point you in the direction of whether you should pursue SIBO testing (or another type of gut test).

If you've noticed fibrous foods, fermented foods, histamine-containing foods, prebiotics, cruciferous veggies, and/or the use of probiotics seem to cause a flare-up in your digestive symptoms, there's a good chance you have an overgrowth in your small intestines.

That is because these foods feed the bacteria in your intestines and cause them to multiply, contributing to the overgrowth.

Also, if taking antibiotics or antimicrobials (even for an unrelated cause) lessens your digestive symptoms, this is another indication SIBO may be at play.

Additionally, consider the following risk factors and symptoms.

Risk Factors

Two or more of the following risk factors may indicate a moderate risk. More than four suggests a severe risk.

- History of food poisoning (gastritis)
- History of taking PPIs or acid-suppressing medications
- Gastric surgery for obesity or ulcers
- A structural defect in the small intestine
- An injury to the small intestine
- An abnormal passageway (fistula) between two segments of the bowels

- Crohn's disease, intestinal lymphoma, or scleroderma involving the small intestine
- History of radiation therapy to the abdomen
- Diabetes
- Diverticulosis of the small intestine
- Adhesions caused by previous abdominal surgery
- Hypothyroidism
- *H. pylori*
- Immunodeficiency
- Age, as gastrointestinal motility decreases with age
- Celiac disease
- History of using bowel-function-slowing narcotic drugs, including prescription opioids such as codeine, hydrocodone (Vicodin), and oxycodone (OxyContin, Percocet)

Symptoms

Three or more of the following symptoms may indicate a moderate risk. More than ten suggests a severe risk.

- Alternating constipation and diarrhea
- Chronic diarrhea
- Chronic constipation
- Restless legs at night
- Burping after meals
- Bloating within one hour after meals (you feel better when fasting and skipping meals)
- Worsening of gut symptoms when using fiber products
- Digestion symptoms improve while on antibiotics (even for unrelated issues)
- Prebiotics (i.e., fructooligosaccharides [FOS] and inulin) in probiotic formulas make symptoms worse

- Lactose intolerance
- Fructose intolerance
- Fibromyalgia symptoms
- Interstitial cystitis (chronic bladder pain)
- Have had gut problems since a bout of food poisoning
- Chronic B$_{12}$ deficiency
- Foul-smelling gas/wind
- Diabetes
- Multiple food sensitivities
- Gluten intolerance
- Diagnosed celiac disease and off gluten but still have gut symptoms
- Chronic low iron or low ferritin levels with no apparent cause

Types of SIBO

There are three primary types of SIBO, each categorized by the specific type of gas produced by the bacteria (or archaea) in the small intestine. The type of gas can influence not only the symptoms but also the best approach for treatment.

1. Hydrogen SIBO: This is the most common form of SIBO and is primarily characterized by an overgrowth of hydrogen-producing bacteria in the small intestine. Hydrogen SIBO often presents with symptoms of diarrhea, as the excess hydrogen gas produced during carbohydrate fermentation can speed up gut motility. Other symptoms include bloating, cramping, and gas. Common bacteria associated with hydrogen SIBO include *Escherichia coli*, *Streptococcus*, and *Lactobacillus*.

Bacteria Present In Hydrogen-Dominant SIBO

SIBO can be caused by an overgrowth of various types of bacteria commonly found in the colon, including pathogenic bacteria like *Klebsiella*, but also bacteria that are usually considered opportunistic, such as *E. coli*, and even beneficial bacteria such as *Lactobacillus*. The bacteria set up shop in the usually sterile small intestine and multiply unchecked.

Some of the key bacteria linked to hydrogen-dominant SIBO include:

- *Streptococcus pyogenes:* Known for causing strep throat, this bacteria is often elevated in those with IBS and is frequently linked to hydrogen production in the small intestine.

- *Staphylococcus aureus:* Typically associated with infections, it can also lead to significant digestive issues by contributing to hydrogen gas production in hydrogen-dominant SIBO.

- *Clostridium* spp.: Overgrowth of *Clostridium* is connected to worsening IBS symptoms, partly due to its role in hydrogen production, which disrupts gut function and increases bloating.

- *Klebsiella* spp.: This bacteria is often involved in hydrogen-dominant SIBO and has been implicated in both IBS symptoms and autoimmune issues.

- *Escherichia coli: E. coli* overgrowth is a common culprit in hydrogen-dominant SIBO, leading to excessive hydrogen gas production and digestive discomfort.

A study from *The American Journal of Gastroenterology* identified the most common bacteria associated with hydrogen-dominant

SIBO, including *Streptococcus, Escherichia coli, Staphylococcus, Micrococcus, Klebsiella, Proteus, Lactobacillus, Bacteroides, Clostridium, Veillonella, Fusobacterium,* and *Peptostreptococcus.*

Here's a breakdown of bacteria involved in hydrogen SIBO:

- *Streptococcus* (71 percent)

- *Lactobacillus* (75 percent)

- *Escherichia coli* (69 percent)

- *Bacteroides* (29 percent)

- *Staphylococcus* (25 percent)

- *Clostridium* (25 percent)

- *Micrococcus* (22 percent)

- *Veillonella* (25 percent)

- *Klebsiella* (20 percent)

- *Fusobacterium* (13 percent)

- *Proteus* (11 percent)

- *Peptostreptococcus* (13 percent)

These bacteria drive hydrogen production in SIBO, leading to symptoms like bloating, diarrhea, and discomfort. Hydrogen SIBO is often characterized by its rapid fermentation of carbohydrates, resulting in these troublesome symptoms.

2. Methane SIBO (intestinal methanogen overgrowth, IMO): In this form, the overgrowth is not caused by bacteria but by

archaea, primarily *Methanobrevibacter smithii* (*M. smithii*). These archaea consume the hydrogen produced by other bacteria and release methane as a by-product, which slows down gut motility. As a result, methane-dominant SIBO typically presents with constipation, bloating, and abdominal discomfort. This form can be more challenging to treat and often requires targeting the archaea specifically.

3. Hydrogen sulfide SIBO (sulfur SIBO): This is a rare form of SIBO, where the bacteria produce hydrogen sulfide gas, often leading to sulfur sensitivity. Symptoms can include a rotten egg smell on the breath or in stools, and people may have a sensitivity to sulfur-containing foods (such as garlic, onions, and cruciferous vegetables). Sulfur SIBO can also cause bloating, diarrhea, and abdominal pain.

Understanding which type of SIBO you have is helpful, as each type may require different treatment strategies to effectively clear the overgrowth and resolve symptoms.

Is it SIBO, Histamine Intolerance, or Both?

SIBO and histamine intolerance often go hand in hand, creating a frustrating cycle of symptoms. When bacteria overgrow in the small intestine, some of them produce excess histamine, overwhelming the body's natural ability to break it down with DAO enzymes. This spike in histamine can trigger symptoms such as bloating, stomach pain, cramping, diarrhea, and constipation.

> To make matters worse, SIBO can increase intestinal permeability, allowing even more histamine to slip into the bloodstream, intensifying the reaction. By clearing the bacterial overgrowth and healing the gut lining, you can not only improve your digestive symptoms but also boost your body's ability to tolerate histamine again—restoring balance and giving those DAO enzymes a much-needed break.

Testing for SIBO

SIBO can be tested by your doctor via a small intestine aspirate and fluid culture or using a specialized breath test. The aspirate test is the gold standard, but it is rarely used, as it is more invasive, requiring a flexible tube (endoscope) to be passed down the throat and into the small intestine to sample your intestinal fluid. The sample is then cultured to see if and which bacteria are growing in your small intestine.

Most people prefer using breath tests because they are less invasive (albeit a bit time consuming to complete). Breath tests measure the amount of hydrogen, methane, and/or sulfur gas you breathe out in timed increments after drinking a liquid (usually glucose or lactulose) that is not absorbed in the small intestine unless there are bacteria present. When a rise in gases is seen soon after ingesting the liquid, this may indicate that bacteria are present in the small intestine and going to town on the liquid. Breath tests can be done in a clinic or lab or at home with SIBO breath test kits.

In-home SIBO test options:
- Genova Diagnostics SIBO 3-Hour Lactulose Kit: It is one of the most widely used kits, but tests only for hydrogen and methane SIBO.

- Gemelli Biotech Trio-Smart SIBO Breath Test: It tests for all three types of SIBO.
- Commonwealth Diagnostics SIBO and IMO (Intestinal Methanogen Overgrowth) test: Tests for hydrogen and methane SIBO.

While aspirate/colony tests can provide an exact breakdown of the specific bacteria, breath tests will indicate which gases are elevated and to what degree (in parts per million). The higher the parts per million, the higher the activity of the bacteria in the small intestine.

> **FAQ: Since Hydrogen SIBO is Often Caused by Probiotic Bacteria, Should You Take Probiotics with SIBO?**
>
> While some professionals recommend avoiding *Lactobacillus*- and *Streptococcus*-based probiotics with SIBO, as they can potentially contribute to the overgrowth, *S. boulardii* and spore-based probiotics are generally well tolerated and may help. *S. boulardii* may help clear out an existing overgrowth in the small intestine and prevent antibiotic-caused dysbiosis, while spore-based probiotics can reduce SIBO and increase gut diversity by boosting the growth of other beneficial flora.

Treatment Options
Dietary Approach
Various diets have been studied for SIBO, and some can be helpful for symptom management, while others are meant to be therapeutic options.

Low FODMAP Diet

A diet low in FODMAPs, a group of carbohydrates high in fermentable sugar, cuts off the food supply to any troublesome gut bacteria and has gained a lot of popularity in recent years due to research showing its effectiveness at resolving symptoms. That said, the diet does not cure SIBO! Rather, I like to think of it as a helpful temporary tool to minimize symptoms while treating the overgrowth. Long-term use of the low FODMAP diet can lead to low levels of beneficial bacteria and lower bacterial diversity. For more on the low FODMAP diet, see chapter 4.

The Specific Carbohydrate Diet (SCD)

The SCD eliminates complex carbs that are hard to digest—like grains, sugars, and starches, potential food for pathogenic gut flora—while allowing easily digestible simple carbohydrates such as fruits and honey. It was developed by Dr. Sidney Haas in the 1920s and popularized by Elaine Gotschall to treat what was then called "celiac disease." There is a large body of evidence suggesting it can help reverse IBD, and some practitioners think it can be helpful for treating the symptoms of, and eradicating, SIBO. There's some anecdotal evidence to support this, but no research to support either of these claims. One of the reasons I believe this diet can help is it often starts with an intro phase where an elemental-like diet is consumed, which can reduce SIBO. A similar diet based on the SCD diet is known as the Gut and Psychology Syndrome Diet (GAPS), developed by Dr. Natasha Campbell-McBride.

The Elemental Diet

The Elemental Diet is a liquid diet free of fiber, complex carbs, and protein structures. It provides essential nutrients in a predigested form, absorbed high in the intestine, making it highly effective at starving bacterial overgrowth and treating SIBO. It also promotes bowel rest, which can help with healing and inflammation, benefiting conditions such as IBS, inflammatory bowel disease, and autoimmune disorders.

Used in clinical settings since the 1940s, this temporary diet can lead to lasting symptom relief. In one study, 80 percent of SIBO patients saw breath test normalization and symptom improvement after fourteen days, increasing to 85 percent after twenty-one days.

Dr. Roy and Debbie Steinbock, creators of the Elemental Diet Success Plan, consider it far superior to antibiotics and herbal treatments for SIBO, delivering impressive results when other methods fail. They've seen reductions of over 100 ppm in bacterial overgrowth in two to three weeks—far more than the typical 30 ppm seen with other treatments.

While it can be very effective, the Elemental Diet has its downsides: it's difficult to stick to, not very tasty, and stressful to implement, and it can be expensive. It should be done under medical supervision. Integrative Therapeutics offers a high-quality option, Physicians' Elemental Diet, though homemade versions also exist (with unknown effectiveness).

> ### Peppermint Power for SIBO Success
>
> Peppermint isn't just refreshing—it's also a powerful tool for gut health. With its natural antibacterial properties, peppermint can help combat SIBO. Whether you enjoy a calming cup of peppermint tea or take peppermint oil capsules for a more concentrated effect, it's a gentle, effective way to support your digestion. Just be sure to check the labels, as some capsules may contain soy. This soothing herb is a great addition to your gut-healing toolkit!

Pharmaceutical Approach

The antibiotic rifaximin (Xifaxan) is usually the drug of choice for SIBO because of its ability to stay in the intestines, which limits side effects impacting the rest of the body.

Many of my clients have seen positive results with this medication, but keep in mind that not all insurance covers rifaximin, and it can be expensive out of pocket.

I will share some common dosing protocols, however, your practitioner may provide different dosages depending on your individual circumstances.

- For hydrogen-producing bacteria: 1,200 mg of rifaximin daily, for fourteen days
- For methane-producing bacteria: 1,600 mg of rifaximin per day, for ten days; combined with neomycin (1,000 mg per day, for ten days) or metronidazole (750 mg per day, for ten days)

Herbal Antimicrobials

Many people find herbal antimicrobials as effective, or even more so, than pharmaceuticals. A recent study showed that herbal treatments with oregano oil and berberine blends had a 46 percent success rate, compared to 34 percent for rifaximin. This may be due to the broad-spectrum effects of herbs like oregano and berberine (they also treat protozoa and *H. pylori*). Herbal remedies are also often better tolerated, with fewer side effects like anaphylaxis, hives, or *C. difficile* overgrowth, which can occur with rifaximin.

While prescription medications typically have shorter treatment durations (ten to fourteen days), herbal protocols may take longer (around sixty days), but they tend to be gentler on the gut, sparing healthy bacteria and reducing the risk of digestive issues like diarrhea. For some, they may be more affordable and accessible, as they don't require a prescription. Herbal treatments are also less likely to lead to antibiotic resistance due to their synergistic effects when combined.

Most natural antimicrobial protocols use two to three herbs at a time, depending on the type of SIBO. Berberine and oil of oregano are used for hydrogen SIBO, while berberine, oil of oregano, and garlic oil are used for methane SIBO. Sulfur SIBO, present in 5 percent of cases, requires an entirely different protocol. (See the sulfur protocol on page 105.)

For brand options to consider and dosing protocols of the following herbal antimicrobials, see chapter 15.

Berberine
Berberine has antimicrobial properties against the common pathogens found in SIBO (including *H. pylori*), and can help repair intestinal permeability. It has been found to help clear out pathogenic bacteria overgrowths such as strep and staph.

Oil of oregano
Oil of oregano contains a compound called carvacrol, which has been found to have powerful anti-yeast, antibacterial, and antiviral properties.

Garlic Oil
Particularly effective against methane-SIBO, it can also help in treating strep.

> ## Bacteriophages for *E. coli*–Based SIBO
>
> When dealing with SIBO caused by an overgrowth of *E. coli*, considering natural solutions like *E. coli*-eating bacteriophages can be a game changer. Bacteriophages are benevolent viruses that spe-

cifically target and eliminate harmful bacteria, making them a powerful adjunct to antibiotic therapy. Strains like LH01-Myoviridae, LL5-Siphoviridae, T4D-Myoviridae, and LL12-Myoviridae have been found to selectively target *E. coli*, reducing its overgrowth without harming beneficial bacteria.

Most products on the market, including Designs for Health Probiophage DF, Life Extension FLORASSIST® GI with Phage Technology, and Body Ecology EcoPhage, combine phages and gut-supporting probiotics such as *Bifidobacteria* and a beneficial strain of *Streptococcus* to help displace pathogenic *Streptococcus*.

These products offer a targeted approach that works in harmony with antibiotics or on their own to support gut healing and restore balance.

Treatment Options for Hydrogen Sulfide SIBO

Are you in the rare 5 percent with hydrogen sulfide SIBO? Practitioners have suggested that traditional SIBO protocols don't always work well for hydrogen sulfide SIBO. Potentially helpful protocols used by nutritionist Debbie Steinbock include the elemental diet, bismuth, and oregano oil.

A study from 1998 showed that bismuth subsalicylate (yay, Pepto-Bismol), given at a dose of 524 mg four times a day for three to seven days, could reduce hydrogen sulfide by about 95 percent.

Dr. Greg Nigh suggests that hydrogen sulfide SIBO may be an adaptation to an impaired metabolic sulfate production. Sulfate is required for various important biological functions, such as cell biosynthesis and detoxification of toxins. He suggests that bacteria such as *Desulfovibrio, Staph aureus, E. coli, Campylobacter jejuni, Klebsiella* species, *Bilophila wadsworthia*, and *Helicobacter pylori* overgrow to step in and aid the body in adequate sulfate production.

Dr. Nigh uses a sulfate-activating protocol that includes Epsom salts, molybdenum, hydroxocobalamin, and Korean Red Ginseng to resolve sulfur SIBO. Back in 2016, I independently came to a similar conclusion and have found my sulfur protocol (much the same as his) that I published in my book *Hashimoto's Protocol* and have included in chapter 4 (page 105) helps hydrogen sulfide SIBO as well.

Best Practices for Treating SIBO and Preventing Recurrence

While SIBO is gaining popularity as a diagnosis behind IBS, the antimicrobial protocols to clear it often fall short, with an incomplete resolution, as well as frequent recurrences. This is because SIBO doesn't "just happen." There are often upstream and downstream imbalances that lead to SIBO occurring, and often we need to correct the other imbalances that lead to a SIBO occurrence in order to prevent a relapse.

SIBO recurrence is common, with studies suggesting that it can recur in up to 45 percent to 70 percent of cases within nine months of initial treatment.

Recurrence often happens due to underlying factors like low stomach acid, gut motility issues, or untreated root causes, such as hypothyroidism or other gut infections, so we need to treat these causes!

Low stomach acid, often due to *H. pylori* or from the use of acid-suppressing medications (like Pepcid, Nexium, and Prilosec), contributes to SIBO by impairing digestion and reducing the body's natural defense against bacteria. It allows more bacteria to enter and thrive in the small intestine and slows down gut motility, which gives bacteria more time to overgrow. Additionally, it increases the risk of infections that can further disrupt gut balance, leading to SIBO. If you have both SIBO and *H. pylori*, it's usually best to treat the *H. pylori* first, as that can improve SIBO treatment outcomes. (See the *H. pylori* section in chapter 10 for more details.)

On the other end, parasitic infections like *Blastocystis hominis* and *Giardia* may also slow down motility and can even impact the ileocecal valve, the valve between the small intestine and large intestine. Inflammation and irritation caused by these parasites may lead to dysfunction of the valve, allowing bacteria from the large intestine to move backward into the small intestine, contributing to bacterial overgrowth and increasing the risk of SIBO.

While broad-spectrum antimicrobials can be used if you suspect SIBO and parasites (as we'll discuss in chapter 10), it's helpful to get tested to determine the specific type of SIBO and parasites you may have. This way, treatment can be more targeted.

It's also important to note that in more severe cases, SIBO may require multiple rounds of treatment. One treatment course may "trim" the SIBO, rather than eradicate it, allowing for it to grow back.

Retesting is often recommended about a week after finishing a protocol to ensure you've fully eliminated the overgrowth and not just reduced it.

Think of it like pregnancy—not just because of the bloating—but because even a small overgrowth can cause symptoms such as intestinal permeability and digestive issues.

Another suggestion to prevent recurrence is to try not to snack too frequently. Snacking can prevent the migrating motor complex (MMC), a cyclic wave of movement that clears food out of the small intestine every 90 minutes or so when the stomach is empty (think of it as a street sweeper for the gut), from operating. When food remains in the small intestine longer than it should, this can allow bacteria to grow. Lower frequency MMC is a known cause of SIBO recurrence.

Furthermore, many individuals may also require ongoing motility support, such as thyroid medications in the case of hypothyroidism, or prokinetic support, if slowed motility is an underlying cause.

Gastrointestinal Motility

The journey of food through our digestive system is more than just a mechanical process—it's a finely tuned symphony of organs working together to break down nutrients and keep us healthy. From the moment we take a bite, food begins its trip through a long interconnected tube: the mouth, esophagus, stomach, small intestine, large intestine, and finally, the anus. Along the way, smooth muscles contract in a coordinated, wavelike motion known as peristalsis, pushing food along the digestive tract. Ideally, this process takes about 24 hours, though the timing can vary depending on what and how much we eat.

When everything moves smoothly, digestion feels effortless, and we pass well-formed stool regularly. But when things slow down or speed up, that's when problems arise. If the muscles contract too often, it's called hypermotility, leading to diarrhea. When they don't contract enough, we experience hypomotility, which results in constipation. These disruptions in motility are hallmarks of irritable bowel syndrome (IBS), with diarrhea-predominant IBS linked to hypermotility and constipation-dominant IBS connected to hypomotility.

Hypomotility may be caused by issues such as muscle disorders, nerve damage, vagus nerve issues, low acetylcholine (the main neurotransmitter used by the vagus nerve to help regulate gut motility), stress, nutrient deficiencies, or medications, and can occur anywhere in the digestive tract. When food lingers too long in the intestines, we may experience bloating, abdominal pain, and a cascade of IBS-related symptoms in addition to constipation, and we are vulnerable to bacterial overgrowth and gut infections.

How to Do a Motility Test with Food Markers

The motility test uses food markers, such as red beets, to track bowel transit time. Here's how you do it:

1. Ingest the chosen food marker and record the date and time of consumption.

2. Watch for when your stool presents with the food marker. It can take anywhere from 12 to 48 hours (or longer) to appear.

3. Interpret the results.

Taking less than 18 hours may indicate malabsorption, diarrhea, or parasites. Taking over 24 hours may indicate slowed gut motility or constipation Taking between 18 to 24 hours is considered ideal.

Food marker options I suggest include:

- **Charcoal capsules:** Swallow 4 charcoal capsules with one glass of water. Consider Integrative Therapeutics Activated Charcoal. Avoid eating any black foods, such as black olive tapenade, for a week before doing the test. Note when your stool turns blackish. If constipation is a problem for you, I recommend using another colorant, such as chlorophyll or red cabbage juice, because charcoal can contribute to constipation.

- **Chlorophyll:** Take 2 teaspoons of liquid chlorophyll by mouth. Consider Genestra Brands Liquid Chlorophyll. Note when your stool turns green.

- **Red cabbage juice:** Drink ¼ cup of red cabbage juice prepared using a masticating juicer. Note when your stool turns red/purple.

> • **Red beets:** At least one hour away from other foods, eat one cup of cooked or raw and shredded beetroot. Note when your stool turns red/purple. Beets are high in oxalates, so if you have known issues with oxalates, choose a different marker.

Supporting Motility
Prokinetics
Prokinetics are substances that enhance gastrointestinal motility by promoting smooth muscle contractions and improving communication between the gut and nervous system, essentially retraining it to move more efficiently. These can be prescription, supplemental, or herbal options.

Prescription Prokinetics

- Metoclopramide, bethanechol, and domperidone: They support stomach and intestinal motility by enhancing muscle contractions.

- Low-dose erythromycin: This prescription antibiotic also promotes gastric emptying. It should not be used for longer than four weeks, as it becomes less effective over time.

- Low-dose naltrexone (LDN): Naltrexone, at a standard dose of 50 mg per day, is an FDA-approved medication for opioid withdrawal. However, low doses of this medication (usually 2.5 milligrams per day), have been found used as a prokinetic agent. Additionally, LDN can modulate the immune system, improving autoimmune disease and IBD.

Prokinetic Herbs

These types of herbs enhance motility by increasing the strength or frequency of contractions. Many of them do so by helping the gut to communicate with the central nervous system, essentially retraining it to work more efficiently. In a study of 252 patients with functional digestive symptoms—in particular, pain, bloating, and constipation with or without diarrhea—ninety were identified as having fecal loading and subsequently responded well to prokinetic treatment, diet therapy, and exercise.

- Artichoke extract: Artichoke extract has been shown to be effective in treating patients with dyspepsia and helps to promote gastric emptying. Studies have shown artichoke extract to be an effective prokinetic on its own, but it is often combined with ginger root extract. A 2016 study found Prodigest (OrthoMolecular Products Motility Pro), a formulation containing both artichoke and ginger extracts, significantly promoted gastric emptying in healthy volunteers, with no notable side effects. Another formulation with ginger root extract is Integrative Therapeutics Motility Activator.

- Ginger: This natural prokinetic increases gastric emptying and aids digestion by supporting the production of bile acids and pancreatic acids. It may also have antibacterial, gut-soothing, nausea-relieving, and food-sensitivity-minimizing properties. Ginger is found in various prokinetic supplement blends and in Yogi's Ginger Tea.

- Iberogast: This herbal blend (known as STW 5 in research articles) includes bitter candytuft, which may help improve smooth muscle tone, bloating, and constipation. Medical Futures Iberogast is a potential option.

- D-limonene: A major constituent in several citrus oils (orange, lemon, mandarin, lime, and grapefruit), it supports peristalsis and relieves heartburn and GERD. Consider 1,000 mg twice a day of Integrative Therapeutics D-Limonene or Jarrow Formulas d-Limonene.

Nontraditional Prokinetics Acting on Serotonin Receptors

Supporting healthy gut motility often involves targeting serotonin receptors in the gut, which regulate movement in the digestive system. Research has found people with IBS who experience constipation often have lower levels of serotonin in the gut. Serotonin-focused antidepressants are occasionally used off-label to support gut motility, though their use for motility is rare due to side effects like mood disturbances and sedation.

- Tricyclic antidepressants (TCAs) and selective serotonin reuptake inhibitors (SSRIs), as well as the atypical antidepressant mirtazapine, can influence gut motility by impacting serotonin levels in the gut. These medications are not first-line options for motility support due to their systemic effects, but are more often used for pain management in IBS and refractory cases.

Supplements to Support Serotonin and GI Motility

- 5-HTP (5-hydroxytryptophan): 5-HTP is a precursor to serotonin, naturally boosting serotonin levels in the gut, which in turn promotes peristalsis and smoother digestive transit. Doses of 50 to 300 mg per day may be used, but it's best to start on the lower end and monitor individual responses.

- Vitamin B_6 (as pyridoxine or pyridoxal-5-phosphate or P5P): Vitamin B_6 is an important cofactor for converting 5-HTP into serotonin, and can support motility. Doses of 50 to 200 mg daily are generally recommended. I often prefer the P5P version due to potential of toxicity of the pyridoxine version in doses above 200 mg per day. Consider 50 to 200 mg per day of Rootcology P5P, Designs for Health P5P, Pure Encapsulations P5P 50, or SFI Health P-5-P. Note, vitamin B_6 would not be appropriate for those with gastroparesis or who are experiencing nausea and vomiting, which can be due to too much serotonin.

Mitochondrial Support

Smooth muscles in the digestive tract are responsible for peristalsis, the wavelike contractions that push food through the gut. When mitochondrial function is impaired, the production of ATP (the energy source for muscle contractions) decreases, leading to poor muscle function and slower gut motility. Mitochondrial dysfunction can lead to low muscle tone, including in the gut, contributing to poor gut contractility. Common contributors to mitochondrial dysfunction include exposure to toxins (e.g., mold), chronic inflammation, and nutrient deficiencies. Addressing mitochondrial toxins and utilizing "mito cocktails," made up of mitochondrial supportive nutrients such as B vitamins, CoQ10, d-ribose, magnesium, thiamine, and carnitine, can help with supporting smooth muscle peristalsis. Carnitine, thiamine, magnesium citrate, and alpha-lipoic acid are four nutrients with the most likely benefits for motility.

- Carnitine: Studies have shown a deficiency in carnitine can cause smooth muscle dysmotility in the intestinal tract, resulting in slowed transit time and GI symptoms. In one study, researchers showed L-carnitine levels of the body correlate with the severity of constipation. Several studies have found supplementing with

L-carnitine, a form of carnitine shown to resolve muscle weakness, can promote gut motility and improve constipation challenges as well as support blood sugar balance by optimizing the body's ability to burn fat for energy and a healthy gut microbiome by removing toxic by-products, such as ammonia, from the gut. In several studies, supplementation with 10 to 50 mg per kg per day of carnitine was shown to improve constipation challenges. Carnitine may also help with recurring episodes of severe nausea and vomiting, common in those with gastroparesis. Carnitine is naturally found in muscle meats such as beef, pork, and fish, but higher supplemental dosages (500–2,000 mg per day) may be needed for therapeutic effects. High-quality options include Rootcology Carnitine Blend, Designs for Health Carnitine Synergy, and Pure Encapsulations L-Carnitine.

- Thiamine: A thiamine (vitamin B_1) deficiency can impair peristalsis and lead to slow gut motility, bloating, constipation, and potentially SIBO. Replenishing thiamine can restore motility and resolve constipation. Interestingly, SIBO can lead to a thiamine deficiency, and this can cause a vicious cycle of SIBO. Researchers have noticed that some individuals may require both antimicrobials and thiamine for proper resolution of SIBO and thiamine deficiency, and supplementing with just one may result in ongoing issues. Thiamine helps maintain the proper neurological signaling required for smooth muscle contraction, supporting gut motility. Thiamine is also needed for proper vagal tone and the production of acetylcholine. While RDA doses of thiamine are closer to 1 mg per day, megadoses of thiamine such as 50 to 600 mg have been used to induce peristalsis. For more on how to replenish thiamine, see chapter 6.

- Magnesium citrate: Magnesium helps the muscular valve at the bottom of the stomach to relax, allowing our food to travel to where it needs to go. When we have a deficiency in magnesium, this valve may not function properly, slowing motility and pushing the food and acids in our stomach back up into the esophagus, causing reflux symptoms. Magnesium also helps with constipation because of its stool-softening properties. For more on replenishing magnesium, see chapter 6.

- Alpha-lipoic acid (ALA): ALA has antioxidant properties that protect nerve tissue and improve mitochondrial function. ALA, when combined with other prokinetics, has also been found to improve diabetic neuropathy and gut motility. A high-quality option is Pure Encapsulations Alpha Lipoic Acid.

Vagus Nerve Stimulation

The vagus nerve controls the digestive tract's smooth muscle contractions, facilitating the movement of food through the gut. Stress, inflammation, diabetes, and surgery can damage the vagus nerve or reduce vagal tone, leading to slowed gastric emptying and gut motility. Researchers and biohackers are beginning to find vagal nerve stimulation can also help with constipation.

- Techniques such as deep belly breathing, foot massage, humming, gargling, singing, or cold water face immersion can activate the vagus nerve and improve motility.

- Unlike old-school vagus nerve stimulation implants that were initially developed for epilepsy, devices like Truvaga or Pulsetto are noninvasive tools designed to stimulate the vagus nerve and support motility.

- Electroacupuncture, in which a small electrode at the end of the needle activates the acupuncture point, can stimulate the vagus nerve and improve gastric emptying and could help relieve chronic constipation.

- Acetylcholine (ACh) is the neurotransmitter used by the vagus nerve to signal smooth muscle contractions. Nutrients such as choline and B vitamins (B_1, B_2, B_3, B_5, B_7) are essential for ACh production. Consider Pure Encapsulations Phosphatidylcholine or Vital Nutrients Citicoline (500–2,000 mg/day) to help boost choline levels.

Diabetes and Gastric Hypomotility

One of the most serious complications of diabetes due to consistently high blood sugar is neuropathy, or nerve damage. Neuropathy can impact the nerves throughout the body and cause weakness, pain, and numbness in the feet, legs, and hands as well as damage the vagus nerve and nerves throughout the digestive tract, resulting in slowed gastric emptying and motility. Digestive issues, particularly hypomotility related to delayed gastric emptying, are a common problem for people with diabetes.

Probiotics

Studies on both animals and humans have shown that modifying the gut microbiome with certain probiotic strains can affect motility. For example, one study on rats found a significant delay in intestinal transit time and reduced contractions in the small intestine could be partially reversed by colonizing with *Lactobacillus acidophilus* and *Bifidobacterium bifidum*. In another study on humans with constipation-predominant

IBS, supplementing with the beneficial bacteria *Bifidobacterium lactis* was found to accelerate GI transit time and improve symptoms. For more on probiotics, see chapter 7.

> ## Prokinetic Combination Products
>
> Various supplement manufacturers have created supplements that combine a few prokinetic ingredients to produce synergy benefits.
> High-quality options include:
>
> - Rootcology Carnitine Blend, a combination of L-carnitine in its acetylated form (acetyl-L-carnitine), which supports brain health and acetylcholine levels.
>
> - Pure Encapsulations Motil-Pro contains acetyl-L-carnitine, vitamin B_6 (in the active P5P form), ginger, and 5-HTP.
>
> - Cyto-Matrix GI-Motility Matrix, which contains a number of nutrients to support bowel regularity, including acetyl-L-carnitine, ginger, globe artichoke extract, 5-HTP, zinc, and vitamin B_6 (as P5P).
>
> - Integrative Therapeutics Motility Activator contains artichoke and ginger.
>
> - OrthoMolecular Products Motility Pro (Prodigest motility blend) contains artichoke leaf extract and ginger root extract.

Action Checklist for SIBO

1. Get proper testing.
   - ☐ Schedule a breath test (hydrogen, methane, or both) to determine SIBO type.
   - ☐ Complete any other necessary tests (*H. pylori,* parasites, etc.).

2. Consider adjusting diet for symptom management.
   - ☐ Follow a low FODMAP or SCD diet, or Elemental Diet.
   - ☐ Avoid foods that trigger bloating and gas.

3. Address underlying factors.
   - ☐ Treat any *H. pylori* or other gut infections.
   - ☐ Optimize thyroid hormone levels if you have hypothyroidism. See chapter 13 for more.
   - ☐ Take digestive enzymes to aid proper food breakdown.
   - ☐ Supplement with betaine HCl for low stomach acid.
   - ☐ Use prokinetics to stimulate movement in the gut.

4. Targeted treatment based on SIBO type and level.
   - ☐ Elemental Diet
   - ☐ Antimicrobials tailored to hydrogen/methane SIBO
   - ☐ For hydrogen sulfide SIBO, implement a low-sulfur diet with antimicrobials.

5. Support bowel motility post-treatment.
   - ☐ Consider prokinetics to prevent SIBO relapse.
   - ☐ Avoid frequent snacking to allow the migrating motor complex (MMC) to function properly.
   - ☐ Eat a balanced diet (read: lower in carbs and sugar).

6. Retest and monitor.
   - ☐ Retest one to two weeks after treatment to ensure SIBO is fully eradicated and not just "trimmed."
   - ☐ Monitor symptoms and adjust treatment as necessary.

7. Repeat steps 3 through 6 if necessary.

Intestinal Candidiasis and SIFO

Candida, a yeast naturally found in the gut, typically stays in balance without causing issues. However, when the gut's "good" bacteria are compromised, *Candida* can become opportunistic and overgrow, leading to symptoms such as food sensitivities, bloating, gas, diarrhea, and constipation. In some cases, it can even trigger autoimmune, inflammatory, and neurological symptoms, with recent studies indicating an association between an overgrowth of *Candida* and IBD. When *Candida* overgrows, it shifts from its normal round form into a more invasive, branching form (hyphae). This transformation allows it to weaken and penetrate the intestinal barrier, contributing to food sensitivities, autoimmune disease progression, and systemic inflammation. *Candida* also releases toxins, such as acetaldehyde, which can damage cells and cause brain fog due to free radical activity. Over time, individuals with *Candida* overgrowth may become deficient in molybdenum, a mineral needed to detoxify acetaldehyde.

Additionally, *Candida* can lead to an accumulation of oxalates—compounds that can cause joint pain, thyroid inflammation, and digestive distress. Clearing *Candida* can help reduce oxalate buildup and sensitivity.

Candida overgrowth can occur in both the small and the large intestines. When it overgrows in the small intestine, it's referred to as small intestinal fungal overgrowth (SIFO). Studies show that around 25 percent of people with unexplained GI symptoms, like those associated with IBS, have SIFO, with *Candida* being the cause in 97 percent of cases.

Whether *Candida* is present in the small or large intestine, the treatment approach remains similar. Probiotics, antifungal treatments, and prokinetic support can help restore balance, while addressing underlying issues like mold exposure can prevent recurrence. This section will cover *Candida* in great detail, but for more on how to address mold, see chapter 14.

What Causes a *Candida* Overgrowth?

Anything that imbalances the gut microbiome can promote overgrowth, including alcohol consumption, stress, estrogen dominance, certain medications (antibiotics, proton pump inhibitors, corticosteroids, estrogen, and progesterone, among others), low stomach acid, slow gut motility, pregnancy, a diet rich in carbs (*Candida* feeds on carbohydrates and sugar), ketogenic diets and diets high in saturated fats, a weakened immune system, mold exposure, toxin exposure (especially heavy metals and glyphosate), and parasites and pathogens.

It has been suggested that the presence of parasites and other pathogens in the gut can co-occur with the presence of *Candida,* and in some cases, addressing those pathogens may be a prerequisite for clearing *Candida.*

Though there is limited research on parasites causing *Candida* overgrowth, other colleagues and I have observed the connection to the point that testing for parasites has become a best practice among seasoned functional medicine practitioners. I believe parasites and *Candida* co-occur because parasites can have an impact on bile and bile helps to clear out *Candida* and mold. If you have difficulty getting rid of *Candida* and/or mold overgrowths in the body, it may be beneficial to test for parasites (chapter 14). If your initial *Candida* protocol didn't work, treating parasites, then retreating *Candida* may be needed.

Interestingly, levels of *Candida* in the gut may actually correlate to dental health and presence of *Candida* in the mouth. It's common to find *Candida* in the mouth, and its presence contributes to the formation of plaque and cavities. Research has found that when teeth are brushed after every meal, there is a decrease in *Candida* in the stool, compared to when teeth are brushed just once per day. This suggests oral hygiene may be linked to levels of *Candida* in the gut.

How Do You Know You Have *Candida*?
Risk Factors
Two or more of the following risk factors may indicate a moderate risk. More than four suggests a severe risk.

- History of repeated and prolonged courses of antibacterial drugs
- Prolonged courses of steroids, such as prednisone
- Immune suppression
- History of using the oral contraceptive pill
- Mold exposure
- Parasite exposure
- Heavy metal exposure
- Frequent alcohol and/or sugar consumption

Symptoms
Because *Candida* weakens the intestinal barrier, contributing to intestinal permeability, and releases a variety of toxins, it has a wide-ranging effect on the body. Three or more of the following symptoms may indicate a moderate risk. More than six or recurrent yeast infections suggests a severe risk.

- Recurrent vaginal, prostate, or urinary tract infections
- Feeling sick all over without an apparent cause

- Hormone disturbances
- Sexual dysfunction
- Menstrual irregularities
- PMS
- Low body temperature
- Fatigue
- Multiple chemical sensitivity (tobacco, smoke, perfume, cologne, etc.)
- Trouble with concentration
- Symptoms triggered by foods
- Constipation
- Diarrhea
- Bloating
- Abdominal pain
- Skin rashes
- Sugar cravings
- Tingling, burning, itchy skin
- Food cravings
- Low blood sugar

Testing

Testing can determine the presence of IC.

- Small intestine aspirate and fluid culture, the "gold standard" for diagnosing SIFO and the presence of abnormal fungi growth. However, it is invasive and involves passing a flexible tube (endoscope) down the throat and into the small intestine where a sample of intestinal fluid is taken and tested.
  - Unfortunately, this test is the only option that I am aware of that can pinpoint exactly where the overgrowth is located in your body.

- Organic Acids Test (OAT), which I've found to be the most effective at detecting *Candida* because it not only tests for *Candida* overgrowth in the colon (as stool tests do) but also detects *Candida* metabolites in the body. It can also identify oxalate buildup as well as mold colonization, which can be important co-occurrences of a *Candida* infection.

- Comprehensive stool analysis tests may occasionally pick up a *Candida* overgrowth in the colon, but only in a minority of cases.

Since symptoms of *Candida* are similar to other conditions, such as SIBO and mold toxicity, it's important to get tested to confirm a *Candida* overgrowth.

Treatment Options
Antifungal Diets
When I learned that I had a *Candida* overgrowth in my twenties, I realized that *Candida* loved the same things I did: bread, alcohol, and sugar! Some nutritionists recommend diets that limit the above mentioned substances to starve out *Candida*.

Anti-*Candida* diet
The anti-*Candida* diet is designed to reduce the overgrowth of *Candida* yeast in the body, which can lead to digestive issues, fatigue, and other symptoms. The diet focuses on eliminating foods that feed yeast, such as sugar, refined carbohydrates, and processed foods, while incorporating anti-inflammatory and gut-healing foods. Key components of the diet include nonstarchy vegetables, healthy fats, high-quality protein, and fermented foods rich in probiotics to support gut health. Foods like fruit, alcohol, and gluten are generally limited or avoided, while herbs and supplements that support the body's ability to fight *Candida*, such as garlic and oregano, may be added.

Body Ecology Diet
The Body Ecology Diet was created by Donna Gates and focuses on eating an alkaline, mineral-rich diet, low in sugar and carbohydrates that acidify the body. It includes a minimal consumption of grains

(grains must be soaked to be easily digested) and limited fruits and nuts, with an emphasis on fermented foods to reduce the yeast overgrowth and rebuild microbial balance by supporting the growth of friendly bacteria.

Low-Oxalate Diet

Additionally, I often recommend a low-oxalate diet to help with symptoms of high-oxalate levels (sometimes referred to as oxalate sensitivity, see chapter 4), for some clients with *Candida* and/or mold colonization. While this diet won't starve *Candida*, it's often necessary because *Candida* can produce oxalates, leading to oxalate sensitivity. Please note, oxalate sensitivity is reversible once the cause is resolved.

Pharmaceutical Antifungals

Candida can be treated with antifungal drugs such as fluconazole, amphotericin B, and nystatin. Itraconazole may sometimes be used as a second line. While many antifungal agents have systemic side effects and are associated with liver toxicity and may require monitoring of liver enzymes, nystatin, which works directly in the gut, is generally well tolerated and does not have the same systemic and liver concerns. It is usually prescribed at a dose of 500,000 units per capsule, taken as two capsules, three times per day for thirty to ninety days. Nystatin is also available as a liquid, and when swished and swallowed can be helpful for *Candidiasis* in the mouth, known as oral thrush. Some clinicians prefer to use compounded liquid nystatin because the commercial preparation has sugar, which can feed *Candida*.

Some clinicians may start with a stepwise approach, using nystatin first, followed by fluconazole and perhaps the other antifungals.

Herbal Antifungals

Several broad-spectrum antimicrobial herbs have antifungal properties and can be helpful in controlling *Candida*. Some clinicians use one to three herbs at a time, while others may cycle the herbs for four to seven days at a time to prevent resistance. For brand options to consider and dosing protocols, see chapter 15:

Oil of oregano

Oil of oregano contains a compound called carvacrol, which has been found to have powerful anti-yeast, antibacterial, and antiviral properties. It's often used for *Candida* as well as SIBO.

Berberine

Berberine exhibits significant anti-yeast and antifungal properties. A 2020 study examined the effect of berberine on *Candida* and found it exhibited significant antifungal activity, as well as decreasing the viability of *Candida* biofilms, a collection of microorganisms that house and protect gut pathogens.

Olive leaf

Research has shown olive leaf has antifungal properties and can be effective in reducing *Candida*. One study found it destroyed 15 percent of *Candida* within 24 hours.

Grapefruit seed extract

Grapefruit seed possesses antifungal and antibacterial properties. It works by inhibiting the growth of fungal cells and can also help destroy *Candida* biofilms.

Pau d'arco

Long used in traditional medicine for its anti-inflammatory benefits, pau d'arco also exhibits antifungal activity.

Black walnut
Widely used as an antiparasitic, black walnut is also an antifungal herb. Naphthoquinones, its active compounds, have been shown to have higher antifungal activity than commonly prescribed antifungal drugs.

Undecylenic acid
Classified as an antifungal, undecylenic acid has been shown to disrupt and prevent *Candida* biofilms.

Monolaurin
This chemical derived from lauric acid and glycerin has been shown to exhibit antifungal activity against *Candida albicans,* as well as reduce the pro-inflammatory response.

Garlic oil
Allicin, the main sulfur-containing compound in garlic, exhibits antibacterial, antiviral, and antifungal activity. A study comparing the efficacy of allicin to fluconazole found that while allicin was slightly less effective than fluconazole, it was still able to destroy *Candida* cells.

Black seed oil (*Nigella sativa*)
Studies have shown thymoquinone, one of the active ingredients in black seed oil, exhibits anti-*Candida* activity.

Additional Supportive Supplements
Saccharomyces Boulardii (*S.* boulardii)
This multipurpose beneficial yeast may crowd out pathogenic yeast like *Candida*. Consider taking 5 billion to 15 billion CFUs, 2 to 4 times per day of Rootcology *S. Boulardii*, Pure Encapsulations *Saccharomyces boulardii*, Designs for Health Floramyces, or XYMOGEN Saccharomycin DF.

Biotin

This B vitamin has been shown to either prevent the conversion of *Candida* to the hyphae form or encourage conversion back to its yeast form, rendering it no longer pathogenic. I have found 5,000 to 8,000 mcg (5–8 mg) daily to be a helpful dose. Pure Encapsulations Biotin is a high-quality option.

Molybdenum

Candida can cause a deficiency in molybdenum, a mineral that removes a toxic *Candida*-produced metabolite known as acetaldehyde. Molybdenum is also necessary for proper sulfur metabolism, and a deficiency can lead to symptoms of sulfur intolerance, which include skin rashes, asthma, and gas when eating sulfur-containing foods (e.g., eggs, cruciferous vegetables, garlic, and onions). If this sounds familiar, consider supplementing 500 to 1,000 mcg per day with Biotics Research Mo-Zyme to restore molybdenum levels.

Activated charcoal

Activated charcoal helps bind up yeast toxins. Integrative Therapeutics Activated Charcoal is a potential option. Please note, activated charcoal may deplete magnesium levels and cause constipation. Supplementing with magnesium may help in some cases. It's not a supplement I often recommend to people with IBS-C.

NAC

This amino acid has been shown to exhibit antimicrobial and antifungal properties. One study examining the effect of NAC on fluconazole-susceptible and fluconazole-resistant *Candida albicans* found it reduced the thickness of *Candida* biofilms. Consider taking 1,800 mg daily with food of Rootcology Pure N Acetyl Cysteine, Pure Encapsulations NAC, or Designs for Health N Acetyl-Cysteine.

Systemic enzymes

These contain proteases that can bust through the biofilms that protect pathogens such as *Candida*. Please note that these should be taken on an empty stomach. High-quality options include Rootcology Systemic Enzymes, Wobenzym, Pure Encapsulations Systemic Enzyme Complex, and Designs for Health Inflammatone.

Tips for Preventing a Relapse

Moving forward, there are a few things you can do to help prevent recurrent *Candida* infections:

- Continue eating a balanced diet, limiting the things *Candida* loves . . . alochol, carbohydrates, and sugar.
- Monitor your estrogen levels (high estrogen has been linked to *Candida* overgrowth).
- Consider taking probiotics long term, particularly *S. boulardii*.
- Manage your stress levels. Stress can contribute to the overgrowth of *Candida*. I recommend addressing underlying adrenal issues to help build one's resilience to stress. See chapter 11 for more.
- If you are prone to *Candida* infections in the sinuses, using a neti pot to rinse your sinuses on a daily basis can be helpful.
- Limit your mold exposure as much as possible.
- Replace your toothbrushes and those of family members living with you. In a recent study, *Candida albicans* was identified on toothbrushes. As a general rule, keep toothbrushes clean and change them often.
- Ongoing gut motility support, if hypomotility is an underlying cause.
- If you are struggling to eradicate a *Candida* infection, consider cycling yeast medications and herbs, as yeast organisms can become resistant to these treatments.

Supplements vs. Overgrowths

SUPPLEMENT	TARGETS SIBO	TARGETS SIFO/*CANDIDA*
Activated charcoal		+
Berberine	+	+
Biotin		+
Black seed oil		+
Black walnut		+
E. coli–eating benevolent viruses	+	
Garlic oil (allicin; sulfur-containing)	+(methane-producing)	+
Grapefruit seed extract		+
Molybdenum	+(sulfur SIBO)	+
Monolaurin		+
NAC		+
Oil of oregano	+	+
Olive leaf		+
Pan d'arco		+
Peppermint	+	
S. boulardii	+	+
Spore-based probiotics	+	
Sulfur protocol (page 105)	+(sulfur SIBO)	
Systemic enzymes		+
Undecylenic acid		+

Chapter Summary

- Abnormally high levels of bacteria in the small intestine—a place bacteria do not belong—is known as SIBO and has become increasingly recognized as a potential root cause for IBS.

- If fibrous foods, fermented foods, histamine-containing foods, prebiotics, cruciferous veggies, and/or the use of probiotics seem to cause a flare-up in your digestive symptoms, there's a good chance you have an overgrowth of bacteria in your small intestines.

- A breath test can help tailor your treatment plan by determining which type of SIBO you have (hydrogen, methane, or hydrogen sulfide) and the degree of overgrowth.

- Most natural antimicrobial protocols to treat SIBO use two to three herbs at a time, depending on the type. Berberine and oil of oregano are used for hydrogen SIBO, while berberine, oil of oregano, and garlic oil are used for methane SIBO.

- The *Candida* fungi, an opportunistic yeast, can overgrow in the small or large intestine or both and trigger symptoms, including food sensitivities, bloating, gas, diarrhea, constipation, fatigue, and brain fog.

- Testing is useful for pinpointing exactly where the *Candida* overgrowth is located in your body so you can better tailor a treatment protocol. For example, antifungals (oil of oregano, berberine, olive leaf) should be used for any kind of candidiasis, but motility agents and stomach acid support may be especially important for treating SIFO.

Visit *https://ibsrootcause.com/bonus for notes on this chapter.*

CHAPTER 10

Gut Infections

I've worked with countless people who tried elimination diets in an effort to heal their digestive symptoms. For some, the elimination diets were absolutely the key to restoring health. For others, they produced limited results or results that didn't stick. When digestive symptoms don't subside after a fair amount of root cause digging to remove sensitivities, restore optimal digestion, and utilize nutrients and mucilaginous herbs to heal the gut, there is a good chance an unaddressed gut infection is present. Before you say, "I've been tested for infections," please note that testing methods vary and conventional tests miss all but the most obvious infections.

Gut infections can be caused by parasites, bacteria, viruses, fungi, or sometimes a combination of multiple organisms. When I first began studying functional medicine, IBS, and intestinal permeability, I learned about the role of SIBO (see chapter 9), which was an emerging concept in 2010, but is now more commonly recognized. The research at the time suggested SIBO was the primary cause of IBS, and many professionals still believe it's the sole cause. However, not everyone with IBS has SIBO, elimination of SIBO doesn't always solve IBS, and some people seem to have recurrences, even with treatment.

In the last decade, I learned SIBO seldom happens in isolation, rather it can happen when other factors are present, such as low stomach acid, slowed gut motility, pancreatic dysfunction, an *H. pylori* infection, and most notably, protozoan parasitic infections. In some cases, SIBO may be a contributing cause but not necessarily the main driving cause of IBS symptoms.

My functional medicine training has taught me an infection could also be driving recurrent issues with *Candida*, and much trial and error and personal experience taught me this might be the case with people who have a hard time recovering from mold colonization (see chapter 14) as well.

This is because infections create an environment for overgrowths and colonizations to occur. For example, bile is used to clear out mold, yeast, and bacteria from the small intestine, while *Giardia*, a protozoal infection that colonizes the small intestine, interferes with bile production.

In this chapter, we'll cover IBS-triggering infections, including viral infections, bacterial infections, and parasitic infections including protozoa, the most common drivers on IBS.

Viral Infections

Viruses like norovirus and rotavirus, which cause gastroenteritis (aka the stomach flu), are seldom appreciated triggers for post-infectious IBS (PI-IBS). Those exposed are 4.5 times more likely to develop IBS within a year.

Conventional medicine focuses on rehydration and symptom management, but in some cases, these viruses can linger in the gut, driving persistent IBS symptoms. I've seen cases of chronic norovirus infection many months after the initial illness, especially in people with weakened immunity and low secretory IgA levels.

If IBS symptoms started after a bout of viral gastroenteritis, using immune strengthening supplements including *S. Boualrdii* and Ion Biome can help with recovery. Antiviral therapies, including the herb oil of oregano and the medication nitazoxanide (Alinia) may also help.

Treatment Options for Persistent Viral Infections
Saccharomyces boulardii (*S. boulardii*)
This beneficial yeast can help the body overcome many infections, including those caused by rotavirus and norovirus. Consider 500 mg/day of Rootcology *S. Boulardii*, Pure Encapsulations *Saccharomyces boulardii*, Designs for Health Floramyces, or XYMOGEN Saccharomycin DF.

Serum-derived bovine immunoglobulin (SBI)
Serum-derived bovine immunoglobulin (SBI) has been used for norovirus infections in immunocompromised individuals with excellent results, relieving diarrhea within two days of initiating. It works by binding to norovirus and blocking it from attaching to cells in the intestines, preventing the virus's ability to replicate so the infection can't propagate. It also binds toxic microbial by-products in the gut to eliminate them, preventing intestinal damage/inflammation. Options include the prescription medical food EnteraGam as well as Ortho Molecular Products SBI and Microbiome Labs Mega IGG2000.

Humic acid
Humic acid has antiviral, toxin-binding, and gut-supporting properties. ION* Gut Support is a convenient, tasteless liquid version that can be added to water.

Nitazoxanide (Alinia)
Nitazoxanide has a broad spectrum of activity against protozoa, worms, bacteria, and even viruses, including rotavirus and norovirus. It has

been used successfully for treating persistent norovirus cases in immunocompromised people.

Herbs with antiviral properties

Allicin from garlic oil has been shown to be effective against rotavirus, and carvacrol, a compound in oil of oregano, has been found to have antiviral properties against human norovirus. For brand options to consider, see chapter 15.

Acute Stomach Flu Protocol for Kids (and Adults) from the Mom Files

Norovirus, often called "the stomach flu," is an incredibly contagious virus that causes nausea, vomiting, and diarrhea. Symptoms generally last between three to seven days, but some people may experience digestive issues, appetite loss, and fatigue for weeks afterward, and in some cases, develop post-infectious IBS (PI-IBS).

As a mom, I know firsthand how hard this virus can hit. When my son was just a baby, he needed IV hydration after a severe bout of the stomach flu. More recently, when he was five, he woke up one night with a tummy ache, fever, vomiting, and diarrhea—classic signs of a stomach bug that was going around his kindergarten. Thankfully, with the right tools, we were able to turn things around quickly, getting him recovered within hours (instead of many days like some of his friends) by using the following protocol.

- Prescription Zofran (ondansetron): This antiemetic can help stop vomiting and prevent dehydration by allowing supplements, liquids, and solids to be kept down. Research shows it can shorten the duration of rotavirus by two days. It's dosed by weight for children, every 8 hours as needed, and dissolves in the mouth or in a little bit of water.

- Super grape juice: Some people believe grape juice can treat/prevent the stomach flu. I am not sure if that is true, though surprisingly, it does have some antiviral effects against certain gut viruses. I used it as a tasty option for rehydration and a vehicle for including 1 capsule of SBI, 1 tablespoon of Ion Biome, and one packet of *S. boulardii*. *S. boulardii* has the most research behind it and has been shown to shorten acute gastroenteritis in children. It's safe for use in children three months and older.

I gave him the grape juice concoction before bed and made sure to keep an eye on him throughout the night. The last time he had the stomach flu as a baby, he woke up every few hours vomiting, but this time, he slept through the night and woke up feeling chipper—eating normally, with zero symptoms of the stomach flu.

To keep his recovery going strong, I gave him the grape juice mixture twice a day for the next few days (and took it myself and gave it to my hubby as well). It's now a go-to protocol for our family, and we take these three supplements twice per day (grape juice optional!) as prevention when stomach bugs are going around.

Bacterial Infections That Can Mimic IBS
Foodborne and Waterborne Illness

Stomach cramps, painful bloating, explosive diarrhea, and nonstop vomiting are all-too-familiar signs of food poisoning. Though these acute symptoms tend to pass after a few days once the body flushes out the pathogen, even without treatment, recent studies have shown infections from various bacteria, including *Campylobacter* species,

Clostridium perfringens, Staphylococcus aureus, Bacillus cereus, Shigella, Salmonella, Yersinia enterocolitica, and *Escherichia coli (E. coli),* can increase the risk of post-infectious IBS (PI-IBS).

Some studies have shown PI-IBS develops in 3 to 30 percent of people after this type of bacterial infection, while other research suggests the risk could be six times as great. A 2013 study found a past infection with *Yersinia enterocolitica,* in particular, was most likely to cause IBS later on in life.

Research is ongoing about why PI-IBS develops in these instances, but it's widely thought the infection causes low-grade inflammation and intestinal permeability, which disrupt the gut flora and lead to IBS-like symptoms. However, while most of the bacteria causing food poisoning are thought to pass through, functional medicine testing suggests bacteria may actually linger in the body. Treating the residual bacterial infection, supporting the intestinal lining, and restoring balance in the gut microbiome are the path to healing PI-IBS.

Common bacteria that may mimic IBS symptoms include *Escherichia coli,* including Shiga toxin-producing *E. coli, Shigella, Campylobacter, Salmonella, Yersinia enterocolitica,* enterotoxigenic *Bacteroides fragilis, Clostridium perfringens,* and *Vibrio parahaemolyticus.*

C. Diff Colitis

Another type of bacterial infection that can be misdiagnosed as IBS is *Clostridium difficile,* also known as *C. diff.* This bacteria can cause inflammation in the colon and an imbalance in gut microbiota. Symptoms may include persistent diarrhea, abdominal cramps, and fever. It is often associated with excessive antibiotic use and is treated conventionally with *other* antibiotics and even fecal microbial transplants (see page 219). It can be challenging to treat, but thankfully *S. boulardii* can be very helpful. Consider taking 5 billion to 15 billion CFUs, two to four times per day for sixty days. Options include Rootcology *S.*

Boulardii, Pure Encapsulations *Saccharomyces boulardii*, Designs for Health Floramyces, and XYMOGEN Saccharomycin DF.

Signs and Symptoms of a Lingering Bacterial Infection
I consider the following red flag symptoms that warrant urgent stool testing to determine if you have a lingering bacterial infection:

- Weight loss
- Severe, excessive, or prolonged diarrhea (lasting more than several days)
- High fever
- Bloody stool (This may be seen in infections like *E. coli* or *Shigella*.)
- Recent travel to areas with a known risk of foodborne or waterborne illnesses
- Severe or persistent abdominal pain or vomiting with diarrhea

Testing and Treatment for Bacterial Infections
If you show red flag symptoms, I urge you to see your practitioner and request a stool test for bacterial infections. Fortunately, the stool tests used conventionally are pretty great at detecting these infections rapidly, allowing for timely treatment.

It's important to note that while red flag symptoms are often acute symptoms of a bacterial infection, some of us may just experience IBS symptoms while still having these infections! I have seen these infections on comprehensive stool analysis tests of people with digestive symptoms. In general, antibiotics are used for acute bacterial infections, but please note that in some cases, too many antibiotics can worsen diarrhea (such as in the case of *C. diff.* colitis) by upsetting the microbial balance in the gut.

Probiotics (including *S. boulardii* for *C. diff.*), bacteriophages (for *E. coli* such as Designs for Health Probiophage DF), and herbal remedies including Biocidin Botanicals Biocidin Liquid and berberine may be used as complementary therapies to treat the infection.

Lyme Disease and *Borellia Burgdoferi*

Another very important and potential bacterial trigger of IBS and IBD is *Borrelia burgdorferi,* the bacteria that causes Lyme disease. Lyme disease can mimic the symptoms of IBS such as abdominal pain, acid reflux, chronic diarrhea, and blood in the stool.

Lyme disease is one of the more serious infections that can lead to some debilitating symptoms, if not found and addressed accordingly. The condition is progressive, leading to more and more symptoms.

Lyme has been primarily thought to be a tick-borne infection triggered by a tick bite (ticks carry the *Borrelia* bacteria), so I always ask my clients if they had spent time in the wilderness camping, hiking, or trail running before their diagnosis. However, according to Lyme advocates, the bacteria may also be acquired through other methods, including mosquito bites, and from mother to child. Lyme is also a zoonotic disease, meaning it can be transferred between us and our furry family members (most likely due to them carrying infected ticks into our homes, but direct transmission has not been ruled out).

How Do You Know You Have Lyme Disease?

Red flag symptoms include a tick bite and a rash that slowly spreads from the tick bite site (though a rash is not always present). Other symptoms include:

- Fever
- Headache
- Extreme fatigue
- Joint stiffness
- Muscle aches and pains
- Swollen lymph nodes

Testing for Lyme disease can be done by testing for the presence of antibodies produced by the immune system to fight off the *Borrelia* bacteria or its genetic material (known as PCR testing). Options include:

- IGeneX Lyme ImmunoBlot IgG: a blood antibody test
- Vibrant Wellness Tickborne Disease Panel: a blood antibody and PCR test
- GeneX Tick Borne Disease Panel 7 (TBD7): a urine PCR test

Treatment Options

Lyme treatments can get complicated, and I often recommend working with a Lyme-literate practitioner. Oftentimes people with chronic Lyme have some degree of immune suppression, which can be caused by mold. Therefore mold testing should be done with chronic Lyme (see chapter 14).

> ### Lyme and IBD
>
> Lyme disease may be an underrecognized trigger for gastrointestinal systems, and some researchers believe it is an underlying trigger for inflammatory bowel diseases, including Crohn's disease. A 2023 case report found that a fourteen-year-old male with a diagnosis of Crohn's disease actually had Lyme disease caused by *Borrelia burgdorferi*. When treatment was targeted to the underlying infection, his Crohn's disease went into complete remission.

H. pylori and IBS

Helicobacter pylori (*H. pylori*) is a common yet underappreciated infection when it comes to IBS (and also autoimmunity), with some estimates placing the worldwide infection rate at 50 percent.

People with an *H. pylori* infection are nearly three times more likely to develop IBS than those who have not been infected, and people with IBS have significantly higher rates of *H. pylori* infection. Furthermore, research shows that treating *H. pylori* infections can lead to improvement or disappearance of IBS symptoms.

H. pylori can be transmitted orally, from person to person via kissing, sharing utensils, and breastfeeding, as well as potentially between people and their pets (via those doggie kisses!). It can also be transmitted through contaminated food or water.

H. pylori burrows into the stomach lining, releasing urease, which neutralizes stomach acid and triggers inflammation. This leads to:

- Intestinal permeability, which can set off immune responses tied to various autoimmune conditions.
- Low stomach acid, leading to poor digestion, low iron levels, food sensitivities, and increased risk of parasitic infections and SIBO.
- Damage to the stomach lining, increasing ulcer risk and autoimmune gastritis, which can cause nutrient deficiencies and pernicious anemia.
- Chronic inflammation linked to stomach cancer.
- Destruction of parietal cells of the stomach, leading to autoimmune gastritis, pernicious anemia, and B_{12} deficiency.

How Do You Know You Have *H. pylori*?
Risk Factors
If you have two or more of the following risk factors, you are at moderate risk for *H. pylori* issues. Four or more, suggest a severe risk.

- History of taking antacids, proton pump inhibitors, or other medications for heartburn
- History of ulcer

- Having a period of high stress recently/around my diagnosis
- Family member diagnosed with *H. pylori*
- Graves' disease or Hashimoto's thyroiditis
- Exposure to mold
- Personal or family history of stomach cancer

Symptoms

Three or more of the following symptoms indicates a moderate risk. Six or more indicates a severe risk.

- Acid reflux
- Anemia or low ferritin
- Need for digestive enzymes
- Food sensitivities
- B_{12} deficiency
- Difficulty tolerating meat
- Nausea
- Belching
- Bloating
- Prolonged fullness after eating
- Feeling full soon after eating
- Thyroid nodules
- Thyroid (TPO/TG) antibodies over 500 IU/mL
- Pernicious anemia
- Headaches or migraines
- Histamine issues
- Hair loss
- Belching or burping after some supplements
- Muscle pains or weakness
- Reactive hypoglycemia
- Waking up at night, hungry

Testing

I have found stool antigen tests for *H. pylori* are the least invasive, most helpful, and reliable tests for an active infection. Please note, they may be less reliable in people with loose stools. The *H. pylori* stool antigen test is available through various comprehensive stool tests.

Conventional doctors may recommend breath tests, but a positive result will be found only in severe cases, while blood tests to screen for antibodies to *H. pylori* may not differentiate between past and current infections.

Treatment Options

H. pylori can be a tough cookie to eradicate. In recent years, it has begun to show resistance, not just to conventional antibiotics, but also to herbal antimicrobial protocols as well. Some people may need a combination of therapies, and I always encourage treating all family members and then retesting to ensure that the infection has been cleared.

Dietary Approach

While I don't believe diet can eradicate *H. pylori*, it may play a supportive role in clearing it and reducing symptoms. Some experts recommend avoiding foods, drinks, or substances that stimulate the secretion of gastric acid and/or can irritate the stomach lining, including coffee, alcohol, smoking, spicy foods, fizzy drinks, sour fruit, and pepper. That said, there are conflicting studies on coffee and alcohol!

The foods and culinary herbs that have been shown to suppress *H. pylori* include cabbage juice, turmeric, garlic, broccoli sprouts, ginger, black cumin seed, and oregano. Cranberries (and their juice) have been found to inhibit the growth of *H. pylori* and prevent its adhesion to the stomach. Besides being able to kill *H. pylori*, borage can also inhibit the adhesion of *H. pylori* strains to the stomach walls.

H. pylori can contribute to a multitude of food sensitivities, and eliminating reactive foods can reduce symptoms and create a healing environment for the gut. Keep in mind, removing foods will not clear the infection, but doing so may resolve some of the symptoms caused by the *H. pylori*–induced food sensitivities, such as acid reflux.

Rx: Triple and Quadruple Therapy Approach

Pharmacologic treatments combine two to three antibiotics—or as I like to call them, "the big guns"—with an acid-suppressing medication that allows the antibiotics to reach the infection. Multiple drugs are used due to the possibility of antibiotic resistance, and bismuth subsalicylate (the ingredient in over-the-counter Pepto-Bismol) may be a helpful option for resistant strains. Please note that the "triple" or "quadruple" antibiotic therapies may disrupt gut health. To mitigate this, pairing antibiotics with *S. boulardii* can help reduce gut dysbiosis during treatment. Following up treatment with probiotics may also help.

Herbal Antimicrobials

Herbal antimicrobials may also be effective for suppressing some stains of *H. pylori*, but the protocols are longer compared to prescription protocols. That said, they are often gentler on the gut flora.

The most common *H. pylori* protocol used by functional medicine practitioners utilizes mastic gum and deglycyrrhizinated licorice (DGL), dosed three times per day, for a period of sixty days. Mastic gum has been used traditionally to help treat stomach pain, and modern research has shown it to be effective against multiple strains of *H. pylori,* while DGL coats and soothes the intestinal lining and promotes the healing of ulcers, a common complication attributed to *H. pylori*.

Antimicrobial herbs—including oil of oregano, berberine, black seed oil, monolaurin, and garlic oil—also have antimicrobial activity for *H. pylori*. See the Antimicrobial Herbs for Infections box on page 332 for more.

> ## Tummy Tea for Two?
>
> Herbal remedies have been used for centuries for healing, and some herbs can be made into delicious tea. Two teas have come to my attention for use in treating *H. pylori:*
>
> - Matula tea is a blend of flowers, stems, and leaves from several different plant species: olive tree leaf, deglycyrrhizinated licorice, honeybush leaves, rooibos leaves, and the fruit and leaves from wild guava. Many of these herbs are reported to have antimicrobial properties against *H. pylori*. A number of individuals and plenty of anecdotal evidence confirm the effectiveness of these herbs in dealing with *H. pylori*.
>
> - Herbs of the Saints is another company that makes an *H. pylori* tea blend that includes purple coneflower, chamomile, thyme, and peppermint. Purple coneflower (also known as echinacea) is well known for its immune-supporting and antibacterial properties. Thyme has long been used in traditional medicine for its antibacterial properties, and chamomile and peppermint are known for their digestion-soothing properties.
>
> Though I can't confirm the 98 percent success rate touted by the Matula tea website, these teas offer a tasty complement (and perhaps sometimes an alternative) to other therapies.

Soothing Support

Aloe vera inner gel, known for its soothing benefits, was also found to be effective against fifteen strains of *H. pylori* (both susceptible to antibiotics and resistant). The natural alkaline properties of the aloe vera plant help balance the pH of the colon, which can be helpful. Consider Rootcology Aloe, Designs for Health Aloe/200x, or Nature's Way Organic Aloe Vera Whole Leaf Juice.

Zinc carnosine is also often recommended due to its ability to repair the stomach lining and inhibit *H. pylori* activity. Fish oils have in vitro antibiotic activity against *H. pylori,* and have also been studied for their anti-inflammatory activity and ability to protect against ulcer formation. For more on these, see chapter 6.

Probiotics to Help

While *S. boulardii* won't take care of an *H. pylori* infection by itself, it bolsters the body's immune defenses in fighting gut infections and can counterbalance the overgrowth of opportunistic bacteria and yeast, from antimicrobial therapies. It can also minimize side effects from triple therapy such as nausea, discomfort, bitter taste, and diarrhea. Consider 500 mg twice per day of a high-quality option such as Rootcology *S. Boulardii*, Pure Encapsulations *Saccharomyces boulardii*, Designs for Health Floramyces, or XYMOGEN Saccharomycin DF.

Another probiotic, *Lactobacillus rhamnosus* GG, when used concurrently with seven-day triple therapy significantly minimized gastrointestinal side effects of the medications, including diarrhea, nausea, and taste disturbance.

Lactobacillus reuteri DSM 17938 has been shown to significantly reduce the amount of *H. pylori* in the stomach. It can work on its own and in conjunction with antibiotic therapy, leading to higher eradication rates than antibiotics alone. One study showed that combining *Lactobacillus reuteri* DSM 17938 with omeprazole resulted in eradication of *H. pylori* in 60 percent of people over the course of thirty days (compared to 0 percent with omeprazole alone). Microbiome Labs PyloGuard contains this specific probiotic strain.

H. pylori and Ulcers

Doctors once thought stress was the sole cause of ulcers, and while stress does play a role, we now know that *H. pylori* bacteria are the primary culprit. This bacteria thrives in the stomach's lining, especially when stress weakens our immune defenses. Transmitted through close contact or contaminated food and water, *H. pylori* triggers inflammation, low stomach acid, and intestinal permeability, all of which can lead to ulcers, food sensitivities, and even autoimmune issues. Antibiotics are now a standard treatment, thanks to the pioneering work of researchers like Barry Marshall and Robin Warren, who connected *H. pylori* to ulcers. Despite early skepticism, their discovery revolutionized ulcer treatment and earned them the 2005 Nobel Prize in Physiology. I hope the role of gut infections in causing IBS will soon become more prominent as well.

Biofilm Busters

When *H. pylori* embeds itself in the stomach lining, it forms a biofilm that shields it from stomach acid and the immune system. This biofilm also makes *H. pylori* resistant to treatments, such as antibiotics and herbal antimicrobials. Biofilm busters can be helpful for clearing *H. pylori,* making it easier for antimicrobials to reach the bacteria. NAC can act as a biofilm buster and also supports gut healing, offering gastro-protective effects by thickening the mucus layer in the stomach, which can help with ulcers. A daily dose of 1,800 mg with food is recommended. Consider the following brands: Rootcology Pure N-Acetyl Cysteine, Pure Encapsulations NAC, or Designs for Health N-Acetyl-Cysteine. Systemic enzymes, when taken on an empty stomach, can also help with breaking down biofilms. However, if you suspect an ulcer, avoid systemic enzymes until it's healed.

Gut Infections

A Note About Stomach Acid Support and *H. pylori*

A big part of creating a healthy gut and microbiome for many people is using digestive enzymes, including stomach acid support. However, people with an *H. pylori* infection/ulcer/acid reflux will benefit from treating *H. pylori* before they utilize digestive enzymes containing betaine with pepsin to increase stomach acid. Using betaine with pepsin can make an active infection worse.

Root Cause Research Corner: On Resistance

Due to extremely high rates of resistance to antibiotics and even to herbal antimicrobials, it's wise to combine a few different therapies at once for best results with eradicating *H. pylori*. Both aloe vera and berberine have been shown to be effective against antibiotic-resistant *H. pylori* strains.

Another helpful option for resistant *H. pylori* strains may be the popular over-the-counter product Pepto-Bismol, which contains the antimicrobial bismuth subsalicylate. Bismuth has biofilm-busting properties against various gut microbes, including *H. pylori* and *Klebsiella*.

A small observational study of 39 people reported a 74 percent success rate in eradicating *H. pylori* through using a combination of bismuth subsalicylate (the study participants took four to six Pepto-Bismol tablets daily in divided doses between meals), oil of oregano, mastic gum, a broad-spectrum probiotic, and a 5:2 blend of soluble-to-insoluble fiber over the course of two weeks.

Parasitic Infections of the Gut

In my humble opinion, parasitic infections are the elephant in the room when it comes to IBS! You might think that parasites affect only people in developing countries (and certainly not those of us in the United States or Europe), but parasitic infections are incredibly common in IBS (and autoimmune conditions). You may also have heard that parasites (most notably whipworm), are used to help with autoimmune conditions and IBD, so they can't be "bad." But here's the thing, just as is the case with bacteria, not all parasites are created equal—some are pathogenic, some beneficial, and others cause problems only when the body is out of balance.

By definition, a parasite is "an organism that lives in or on an organism of another species (its host) and benefits by deriving nutrients at the other's expense." There are many different types of parasites that can infect humans, and they are classified into three main types: ectoparasites (such as ticks, fleas, mites, and lice), helminths (worms, visible to the naked eye), and protozoa (microscopic single-celled organisms not visible to the naked eye).

Most of the parasites I have seen personally and in research that can trigger IBS are protozoa, and as many as 70 percent of people with IBS may have one.

Parasites are often overlooked in conventional medicine, especially in the U.S., where many doctors are trained to think parasites are primarily a concern in developing countries. This gap in education means that the presence of protozoa and other organisms can be ignored or downplayed as harmless. However, I, along with other functional medicine practitioners, have found these organisms to be much more common—and pathogenic—than conventional medicine recognizes.

I believe everyone with IBS, IBD, and autoimmune disease should be evaluated for parasitic infections. Unfortunately, parasites can be challenging to diagnose, and some are challenging to treat. False negatives in stool tests are common, and in my experience, comprehensive stool testing is crucial for uncovering these hidden infections. Some parasites can be resistant to conventional treatments, and others may need a few treatment cycles.

I've found that treating these infections can significantly reduce inflammation, help autoimmune conditions like Hashimoto's and IBD, and yes, resolve IBS!

Protozoa: A Potential Root Cause of IBS?

One of the main reasons I wanted to write this book is to shed light on a particular type of infection seldom considered a driving factor in common digestive conditions: protozoal gut infections.

Protozoa are single-celled organisms that can multiply and live in the gut, blood, and tissues of humans. They most often spread through contaminated food and water, insect bites, and person-to-person contact. Protozoa are some of the most prevalent parasitic infections observed in humans and can trigger digestive symptoms and even autoimmunity. One of the main ways protozoa cause digestive and immune system issues is by loosening the intestinal tight junctions. They also break down secretory IgA (the GI tract's first line of defense) and the immune system of their infected host.

It's also worth mentioning that in my experience, they can cause many of the other patterns seen in IBS, such as food sensitivities, intestinal permeability, *Candida* and SIBO, digestive enzyme disturbances, and even nutrient deficiencies, so they really can be at the root of the root.

There are thousands of protozoa that can affect people, but the main types include amoebas, ciliates, flagellates, and sporozoans.

Numerous studies have found a higher rate of protozoan infections in people with IBS, with one Iranian study finding 30 percent of participants with IBS had at least one intestinal parasite. People with IBD may also have a higher prevalence of protozoan infections, with one study reporting that the *Giardia* parasite in approximately 60 percent of people with Crohn's disease! The types of infections detected and the rates of infections do vary across the studies, and I think it's worth mentioning that there are various types of parasite detection methods that can be used, and some are more helpful than others.

The most common type of protozoa tied to IBS is *Blastocystis hominis* (*Blasto*). Other common protozoal infections implicated in IBS include *Entamoeba histolytica, Giardia intestinalis,* and *Cryptosporidium.*

Blastocystis hominis

A meta-analysis conducted in 2017 found a *Blastocystis hominis* infection to be a significant risk factor for IBS. In study after study, this microscopic single-cell organism is more prevalent in people with IBS compared to controls. Different studies indicate that between 13 and 73 percent of people with IBS, in particular diarrhea-predominant IBS, may have *B. hominis.* As parasite detection methods are not 100 percent reliable (and can give many false negatives), these rates could be even higher.

Many conventional physicians will say there is no need to treat *Blasto.* However, studies indicate that eradicating *Blastocystis hominis* in cases of IBS often leads to the remission of the condition (as long as the correct treatments are used). To further complicate things, many strains of *Blastocystis hominis* show resistance to the usual drug of choice for protozoal infections, metronidazole.

Additionally, I've found *Blastocystis hominis* notorious for causing multiple food sensitivities. A true food sensitivity, such as celiac disease, usually results in a resolution of symptoms once the triggering food is removed, but people with *B. hominis* infections will have multiple food sensitivities, often to gluten, dairy, soy, sugars, starches, grains, caffeine, fruit, and carbonated beverages, and will keep getting more. While removing reactive foods to lower inflammation and support gut healing can improve symptoms, an exclusion diet will not eradicate the pathogen. Furthermore, in my clinical experience, I find this particular protozoa commonly in those with Hashimoto's.

Blasto can be treated with antiprotozoal medications, and/or herbs with antiprotozoal activity, and/or the beneficial yeast *Saccharomyces boulardii*. (More on these under Treatment Options.)

> ### Connecting the Dots on *Blastocystis hominis*
>
> When I was first researching the causes of intestinal permeability and autoimmunity to recover my own health, I came across information on how SIBO can trigger IBS. I thought for sure it was my root cause, as I had bloating. But testing revealed otherwise, and in fact I had another type of infection I had never heard of: *Blastocystis hominis*.
>
> In reading the medical literature about *Blastocystis hominis* I read a mix of things. Some researchers believed it was commensal and not harmful to humans. Others were convinced it was pathogenic and an important cause of chronic hives and IBS. More research revealed there were as many as twenty-two subtypes (nine are known to infect humans), and perhaps only a few of them were pathogenic. At the time, there was nothing in the literature that suggested it could be connected to Hashimoto's, yet treating this infection helped me reduce my digestive symptoms, food sensitivities, thyroid symptoms, and even thyroid antibodies (a marker of how aggressive the autoimmune condition is)!
>
> When I began to work with clients with Hashimoto's and utilize stool testing, I made a peculiar observation that around 30 percent of my Hashimoto's clients had this infection. One client happened to have the early stages of Hashimoto's but also intense IBS, and she sought out my help for the IBS, having come across my book and website. Since her symptoms were so profound, I suggested that

she undergo various tests, including stool and SIBO. To my surprise she didn't have SIBO but did have *Blastocystis hominis*. Treatment resolved her IBS completely, as well as her thyroid symptoms.

Since that time, three studies have found treating *Blastocystis hominis* can reduce TSH and thyroid antibodies and lead to Hashimoto's remission. Of course it's also been recognized as a significant treatable cause of IBS!

The Chronic Urticaria, Hashimoto's, IBS, and *Blasto* Connection

The connection between chronic urticaria, Hashimoto's, IBS, and *Blastocystis hominis* is both fascinating and often overlooked. As a health researcher, I'm always struck by how much research is available, yet how few are connecting the dots.

- Those with Hashimoto's are more prone to chronic spontaneous urticaria (chronic hives), characterized by itchy, swollen rashes. In fact, forty-two studies have linked Hashimoto's to chronic hives, and thyroid hormone treatment can sometimes clear up these hives.

- Clinically, I've also seen that people with Hashimoto's are more likely to develop IBS.

- One study in Egypt found that 61 percent of people with chronic hives had *Blastocystis hominis*, compared to only 8 percent of healthy controls.

- One U.S. review of over 53 million people found that IBS was four to five times more common in those with urticaria.

- Research has found that between 13 and 73 percent of IBS cases involve *Blasto*.

> • Emerging research is showing that eradicating *Blastocystis hominis* in cases of urticaria, Hashimoto's, and IBS often leads to the remission of the conditions.
>
> After reading hundreds of studies like this, it became clear to me that all these conditions are connected. A *Blastocystis hominis* infection may be at the root of IBS, hives, and Hashimoto's, and eradicating this pathogen can lead to an elimination of symptoms!

Additional Protozoa That Are Known Pathogens

There are a few well-known protozoal infections that most clinicians recognize as causing acute digestive symptoms. These infections are often linked to post-infectious IBS and IBD. However, there's a common misconception that once the acute symptoms subside or a person completes one round of antiparasitic treatment, the pathogens are gone. Many researchers now believe these parasites may cause lasting changes in the gut, but they miss the fact that the parasites are still actively multiplying. While most researchers don't even test for the presence of these parasites, in many cases the tests they're using may miss them anyway. In my experience, I've seen these infections still present on lab tests years after the acute symptoms have resolved, even after the initial antiparasitic treatments. If I see one of these infections on a stool test, I definitely recommend treating them, potentially with multiple rounds of treatment and doing retests to ensure they're gone.

Giardia (Giardia spp.)

Giardia is a microscopic parasite that can cause a diarrheal illness known as giardiasis, commonly referred to as "Beaver Fever" (not to be mistaken with "Bieber *Fever*"). This nickname stems from its association with infected beavers, which can contaminate natural water sources with the parasite. It's one of the most common causes of waterborne diseases worldwide, especially in areas where water sanitation is poor, and can be transmitted via childcare settings, untreated river water, swimming pool water, and occasionally well water and tap water! *Giardia* cysts can survive in cold water for months! People who have had a *Giardia* infection are about four times more likely to be diagnosed with IBS than those without *Giardia*. While most doctors may believe that the infection will "go away on its own" or "after a short course of treatment," the parasite can persist and lead to ongoing symptoms. A 2017 study found the *Giardia* parasite present in 8.3 percent of those with IBS! This parasite is also associated with malabsorption of Vitamin A, B_{12}, and folate, fructose and fat malabsorption (the latter presents as foul-smelling, greasy stools). One of the reasons for its persistence is that *Giardia* can lead to crypt hyperplasia, or more prominent, "deeper" holes within the intestinal lining that can hide infections and may require multiple rounds of healing protocols.

The Impact of Crypt Hyperplasia

Crypt hyperplasia are more prominent, "deeper" holes within the intestinal lining that can hide infections and may require multiple rounds of healing protocols.

A person with crypt hyperplasia may need to go through a few rounds of treatment to heal their gut. Eliminating inflammatory foods and using healing nutrients/herbs may improve symptoms, but symptoms quickly return as layers of the mucosa heal and expose parasites. Antiparasitic treatment will be required to clear the parasites, followed by gut-supportive interventions, sometimes followed by another round of antiparasitics. In my experience, most people need one round of antiparasitics, but I have personally seen some complex cases requiring two to three rounds, and

> colleagues have mentioned seeing up to seven rounds in very sick individuals!

Entamoeba histolytica

In studies on IBS patients, *Entamoeba histolytica* was detected in anywhere from 3 to 7 percent of patients; it may also contribute to or be mistaken for inflammatory conditions such as IBD. Though this infection may sometimes be asymptomatic, it can cause abdominal pain, tenderness, intense diarrhea, constipation, nausea, and weight loss. It can also become systemic, leading to lung and liver abscesses that can be mistaken for tumors. An attempted biopsy of an *E. histolytica* could potentially lead to death from a disseminated infection. Unfortunately, this is one of the most challenging infections to treat, as the cyst form is resistant to many treatments. This infection often requires prolonged multidrug protocols, including the medication paromomycin to clear cysts.

Cryptosporidium

In a study of 109 people with IBS, *Cryptosporidium* was detected in 9.2 percent, while the control group had zero incidence of *Cryptosporidium*. *Cryptosporidium parvum* is often linked to contaminated food or contact with farm animals and is known for causing watery diarrhea.

Additional protozoal infections that are controversial, in terms of whether they are pathogenic or not, but may still contribute to IBS include:

Chilomastix mesnili

This parasite can create symptoms, including diarrhea, when it overgrows or becomes opportunistic. Although it is considered a commensal organism (meaning it naturally exists in our digestive tract), individuals can become infected if they ingest contaminated water.

Pentatrichomonas hominis
This parasite can lead to low levels of inflammation if it overgrows, and has been linked to IBS, gastrointestinal cancer, rheumatoid arthritis, and lupus. I've noticed it causes fat malabsorption. *Pentatrichomonas hominis* is contracted through the fecal-oral route and may be passed between humans and cats.

Cyclospora spp.
Research has shown the *Cyclospora* species can persist in individuals who are immunocompromised or have an autoimmune condition, leading to symptoms such as persistent diarrhea for months. Interestingly, researchers have hypothesized this infection may be related to celiac disease and gluten-related disorders.

Endolimax nana
This parasite is implicated in increasing intestinal permeability, causing persistent and chronic inflammation, worsening autoimmune conditions over time and rheumatoid arthritis. One case study reported on a person who was experiencing IBS symptoms for ten months had symptom resolution after being treated with metronidazole, after tests revealed *Blastocystis hominis* and *Endolimax nana*. Personally, *Endolimax nana* caused the most awful bloating, full body inflammation, and new onset food sensitivities!

Dientoamoeba fragilis
This parasite can cause diarrhea, abdominal pain, and flatulence and has been linked to IBS, histamine issues, and ulcerative colitis. It may also be associated with pinworms.

Worldwide, the incidence of *Dientamoeba fragilis* may range from 0.5 to 16 percent, and has been implicated as a notable cause of gastrointestinal disease and colitis. A 2010 study found up to 4 percent of IBS patients were infected with *D. fragilis* and suggested those infected may be "misdiagnosed" with IBS.

Notably, there's some evidence of an intimate relationship between *D. fragilis* and pinworms, as the two often co-occur, and experimental pinworm infections also resulted in *D. fragilis* infections. A study on 35 children with *Dientamoeba fragilis* found that 91 percent of them had gastrointestinal symptoms, with diarrhea being the most common in children with acute symptoms, and abdominal pain more common in children with chronic symptoms.

Treatment with diiodohydroxyquin or metronidazole was found to be effective, with the children's symptoms significantly lessened or eliminated. Nitazoxanide is also an effective option.

What About Parasitic Worms?

The most relevant parasites I see in terms of IBS are protozoal infections, but in some cases, worms may be behind IBS symptoms as well, especially in people who have celiac disease that's not responsive to the gluten-free diet. Celiac disease can increase the risk of parasitic worm infections, which can lead to ongoing malabsorption and inflammation, despite eating a gluten-free diet. Out of 300+ GI-MAP tests I reviewed from people with autoimmune and digestive issues, only 14 had worms, and those individuals often had celiac disease. (Please note, the GI-MAP test produces many false negative results for parasites.)

While we may tend to think of worms as undesirable souvenirs from travel to developing countries, please know these worms can be acquired close to home, including in the U.S. and Europe.

People can have intestinal worms for years without noticeable symptoms, but common signs to watch for include abdominal pain, fatigue, and gastrointestinal issues such as diarrhea with or without blood or mucus, gas, bloating, nausea, or vomiting. In some cases, worms may lead to more severe symptoms such as anemia, neurological issues, itching around the rectum or vulva, and allergic reactions such as sneezing, runny nose, or elevated IgE levels. Visible worms in the stool and unexplained weight loss are more definitive signs. Worm infections increase the risk of anemia and intestinal blockages, especially in older adults or those with weakened immune systems.

It's important to note that most stool tests don't screen for the most common worms, pinworms, which are common in children, affecting 20 percent of U.S. children between the ages of five and ten. These worms can spread easily, often resulting in infections that mimic IBS. Children are particularly susceptible to pinworms and may be the vectors who bring worms to the rest of the family, because they may play in environments with contaminated soil, such as sandboxes and school playgrounds. They tend to put their hands in their mouths and not wash their hands, despite persistent parents who insist otherwise.

How Do You Know You Have a Protozoan Infection?

Protozoa are a common cause of IBS, and even though some people may be asymptomatic, I generally assume most people with IBS have some sort of protozoan parasitic infection. In people who have celiac disease that has not 100 percent resolved on a gluten-free diet, I suspect protozoa and/or parasitic worms.

Risk Factors
Having a compromised digestive system and stomach acid issues is a risk factor, as stomach acid is thought to be naturally protective. If you have two or more of the following risk factors, you are at moderate risk for a protozoa. Four or more suggest a severe risk.

- Foreign travel
- Eating raw fish, including sushi
- Eating undercooked food from an infected animal, such as a cow, pig, or fish
- Consumption of contaminated water (drinking water from ponds)
- Contact with contaminated feces
- Living with pets
- History of food poisoning
- Wilderness camping
- Having attended group childcare
- Having children in group childcare
- Working in childcare
- Growing up in an orphanage or in a multiple family setting

Though tests are best for determining what's living inside your intestines, the following symptoms have been associated with parasitic infections.

Signs and Symptoms of Parasitic Infections
Three or more of the following symptoms indicates a moderate risk. Six or more indicates a severe risk or recurring parasite issues.

- Anal itching
- Anemia
- Autoimmune disease

IBS

- Asthma
- Chin acne, or acne around forehead
- Constipation
- Diarrhea
- Elevated eosinophils (disease-fighting white blood cells) on lab test
- Food sensitivities
- Gas
- Histamine issues (for more on histamine, see the box on page 179)
- Hives
- Allergies
- Joint/muscle aches
- Malabsorption
- Plant fibers in bowel movements
- Rashes
- Raw foods are irritating
- Skin ulcers
- Symptoms worsen around the full moon
- Teeth grinding

Teeth Grinding, Full Moon, and Parasites... Fact or Fiction?

Two seemingly odd indications of parasitic infections in integrative communities are teeth grinding at night and symptoms that worsen around the full moon. As open-minded as I am, these symptoms seemed like a stretch to me, so I needed to research them a bit!

Teeth Grinding and Parasites

There's some evidence that teeth grinding, or bruxism, may be linked to parasitic infections—particularly worms. A study found that 11 out of 50 children with bruxism had a parasitic infection, most commonly with pinworms (*Enterobius vermicularis*). While the exact cause isn't fully understood, one theory is that the stress parasites place on the body or the gut-brain axis disruptions could lead to teeth grinding. Parasites also secrete metabolites that might have toxic effects, which may contribute to this symptom.

Parasites and the Full Moon

In alternative medicine circles, it's been proposed that parasites might be more active around the full moon, and there could be some truth to this. All living beings are influenced by the moon's cycles, and parasites have their own biological rhythms. During a full moon, serotonin production increases, and since parasites have serotonin receptors that help them move, they may become more active. At the same time, melatonin (which helps modulate the immune system) decreases, potentially allowing parasites to replicate more easily. If you notice disrupted sleep or symptoms worsening during a full moon, supplementing with melatonin might help.

Testing for Parasites

Parasite testing isn't foolproof. Parasites may not show up in every stool sample, and different detection methods yield different results. Parasites are often missed on Ova and Parasite tests ordered by conventional labs, and even missed by many functional medicine stool tests.

In 2015, I analyzed my Hashimoto's clients using the BioHealth 401H test (which required four samples and used microscopy). I found that 35 percent had *Blastocystis hominis*. When using the GI-MAP DNA test (which uses only one stool sample), only 16 percent tested positive. Unfortunately, the BioHealth Lab has closed, but ParaWellness Research, a lab that specializes in finding parasites, uses similar detection methods and has found parasitic infections in my clients missed by other tests. The limitation of this test is that it tests only for protozoa, not for other digestive markers that may be out of balance in IBS. From the comprehensive stool tests, the Gut Zoomer test, at the time of writing this book, has yielded more parasitic infections in my clinical experience compared to other tests.

Additionally, some comprehensive stool tests offer an Ova and Parasite add-on test that collects multiple stool samples over several days for analysis. This increases the chances of detecting parasites or their eggs. Please note, I don't believe any of the aforementioned tests actually test for pinworms!

For detecting parasites:
- Cellophane tape test for pinworms (see below).
- ParaWellness Research Comprehensive Parasite Test: A stool test that uses microscopy to detect various protozoa, amoebas, and worms.
- Comprehensive stool analysis tests. These can screen for a range of parasites. The Gut Zoomer seems to be the most helpful.
- Ova and Parasite x3 Tests: This test collects three stool samples over separate days, increasing the chances of detecting parasites. It can be added on to many comprehensive stool tests, such as Genova Diagnostics GI Effects.

Pinworms

Pinworms, also called threadworms, are small, thin roundworms that typically reside in the colon and rectum. The female pinworm lays eggs around the anus at night, causing symptoms like disturbed sleep, irritability, and itching (pruritus ani). Infection can spread through direct contact by scratching the itch and ingesting the eggs, or indirectly via contaminated bedding or clothing, as pinworm eggs can survive on surfaces. Pinworm infections are more common in young children but can affect anyone.

Pinworms often do not come up on comprehensive stool analysis tests, but a simple home-based butt inspection and a "butt tape test" are the most reliable ways to test specifically for pinworms, which like to come out to play at night.

- Butt inspection: Upon inspecting the anus with a flashlight, you might notice white quarter-inch threadlike worms that move. Eek!

- The tape test: Press the sticky side of a piece of cellophane tape against the area around the anus—this is where pinworms lay their eggs at night—for three consecutive nights. The tape can then be taken to a doctor to be examined under a microscope to confirm it contains pinworm eggs.

Treatment Options

- Pyrantel is an over-the-counter antiparasitic medication often marketed as a pinworm treatment (such as Pin-X or Reese's Pinworm Medicine) that can be purchased in most pharmacies in the U.S. This treatment paralyzes the worms so that they come out of the body. If you use this treatment and you indeed do have pinworms, consider this fair warning that you may see them in your next bowel movement! A second dose is recommended after fourteen days to target newly hatched worms. If you have any neuromuscular conditions like myasthenia gravis, consult your doctor before taking Pyrantel, as

> the medication can have mild paralytic effects in humans as well.
>
> - Washing all bedsheets, undergarments, and towels in hot water daily is recommended to kill eggs. Frequent hand washing and keeping kids' fingernails short is also helpful to prevent reinfection. Additionally, cleaning toilets and bathroom surfaces regularly is important.
>
> - Since reinfection is easy, it's recommended that the entire household be treated if one person is infected.
>
> - Pinworms spread the protozoal parasite *Diantoamoeba fragilis,* which can lead to histamine issues, IBS, and IBD. If pinworms are found, it might be wise to also do a treatment for *D. fragilis.*

Treatment Options for Parasitic Infections

Knowing which pathogen is present can be the key to figuring out the correct treatment protocol. Different bugs respond to different drugs! This is why I generally advocate for testing, though broad-spectrum protocols may be helpful, too, if a parasite test is not an option or comes up negative. Parasites have complex life cycles, often involving stages like growth, reproduction, and transmission. This can make them tricky to treat, as different stages may be more resistant to antimicrobials.

For example, *Blastocystis hominis* has four forms, including a tough cyst stage that can survive in harsh conditions. To fully eradicate parasites, treatments must last long enough to cover multiple life cycles—typically two to three months for herbal remedies or multiple courses of prescription medications. Understanding the parasite's life cycle is key to ensuring the treatment is effective. As there are likely thousands (literally, if not more) of these critters in a given infected person, a percentage of them will likely be in cyst form on any given day. In my functional medicine training, I was taught most parasites have thirty-day life cycles, however research is still ongoing about the exact length. It does seem it may vary depending on the infection. Some protozoa, such as *Giardia*, may have short life cycles (as in days), while others may have longer ones. Studies on cattle done in the 1980s reported it takes one hundred days to break a parasitic cycle (at least in cattle).

Treatment Options for Protozoa

While some people advocate diet to manage symptoms of infections, in my experience, diets don't solve parasitic infections. That said, diets can be used to help with managing symptoms, as protozoa are notorious for causing inflammatory reactions to foods.

We generally need an antimicrobial intervention such as a medication or an herb to clear the infection. However, if a person has low secretory IgA, the beneficial yeast *S. boulardii* has become my treatment of choice for many protozoa. Sometimes it is all that's needed to clear an infection; sometimes it's part of the treatment plan.

Diet

Polyphenol-containing foods

Polyphenols are antioxidants that promote the growth of good gut bacteria and stimulate the immune system to fight off infections. A high-polyphenol diet won't clear the parasitic infection but may support healing gut diversity. For more, see chapter 8.

Pharmaceutical Approach

There are many different pharmaceuticals available to eradicate protozoal infections, but most often, the medication metronidazole is used. It's generally well tolerated, though it can sometimes cause unpleasant side effects such as confusion, peripheral neuropathy, nausea, and vomiting. People who are taking it need to completely avoid alcohol while taking it and for 48 to 72 hours after taking the last dose due to a very unpleasant drug-alcohol interaction (a derivative of the drug is given to alcoholics to deter them from drinking). Sadly, many pathogens have become resistant to it.

A newer and often better tolerated, albeit more expensive, choice is the broad-spectrum antimicrobial nitazoxanide (Alinia). It is effective for a variety of protozoa, including *Giardia, Entamoeba, Cryptosporidium, Cyclospora, Trichomonas, Encephalitozoon intestinalis, Isospora belli, Blastocystis hominis, Balantidium coli,* worms, including *Ascaris, Trichuris trichura, Taenia saginata, Hymenolepis nana,* and *Fasciola hepatica.* It also has antimicrobial activity against a number of anaerobic bacteria including *H. pylori.* It's important to note that both medications can cause a depletion of thiamine, and I often recommend Benfotiamine 600 mg per day after completing treatment.

Other commonly used medications with antiprotozoal activity include albendazole, mebendazole, paromomycin, tetracycline, tinidazole, and trimethoprim-sulfamethoxazole.

Antimicrobial Herbs

A variety of antimicrobial herbs including oil of oregano, berberine, nigella sativa, garlic oil, cat's claw, and monolaurin have various levels of antiparasitic activity. I generally combine two to three antimicrobial herbs and use them for sixty days to ensure at least two parasitic life cycles are covered. See the Antimicrobial Herbs for Infection box on page 332 for more details.

Probiotics

My top choice for clearing many common protozoa, especially if a person is found to have low secretory IgA levels, is the beneficial yeast,

S. boulardii, which raises secretory IgA and can help the body overcome the infection of many protozoa. Research shows *S. boulardii* is beneficial for eradicating *Blastocystis hominis* infections—even as a stand-alone treatment—and can significantly reduce related symptoms. In one study of *B. hominis* in children, *S. boulardii* produced an outcome similar to the anti-parasitic medication metronidazole and in one month reversed symptoms/normalized stool tests in 94.4 percent of the study group. Please note, while the study used the probiotic for just ten days, I often recommend using it for at least sixty days. It has also been shown to be effective against *Giardia, Blastocystis, Chilomastix, Entamoeba,* and has a general effect of reducing the number of parasitic cysts. Interestingly, while this probiotic is usually used once per day for most indications, I have found that it tends to work best when used two to three times per day, sometimes in higher than standard doses. Studies using *S. boulardii* for protozoal infections including *Giardia, Blastocystis,* and *Entamoeba* use 250 mg two to three times per day. High-quality options include Rootcology *S. Boulardii*, Pure Encapsulations *Saccharomyces boulardii*, Designs for Health Floramyces, and XYMOGEN Saccharomycin DF. I sometimes use it as a stand-alone, but most often in combination with other treatments.

Systemic Enzymes
When taken on an empty stomach, systemic enzymes (also known as proteolytic enzymes) can bust through the biofilms that protect pathogens such as bacteria and parasites, allowing for clearing more effectively. High-quality options include Rootcology Systemic Enzymes, Wobenzym, Pure Encapsulations Systemic Enzyme Complex, and Designs for Health Inflammatone.

Antimicrobial Herbs for Infections

For brand options to consider and dosing protocols, see chapter 15.

Oil of oregano: Oil of oregano contains carvacrol, a compound with powerful anti-yeast, antiprotozoal, antibacterial, and antiviral properties. It can also help heal ulcers, likely by way of its anti-inflammatory properties. It's often used for parasitic infections and is particularly effective for treating *Blastocystis hominis, Cyclospora, Dientoamoeba, Entamoeba histolytica,* and *Endolimax nana* infections.

Berberine: Berberine compounds have powerful antimicrobial properties and can be used for a variety of infections. It can help clear out protozoa such as *Blastocystis hominis, Dientamoeba, Giardia, Pentatrichomonas,* and *Entamoeba histolytica* and has been shown to be effective in treating *H. pylori* strains, including those resistant to antibiotics. In certain cases of *B. hominis* infections, I pair berberine with oil of oregano and *S. boulardii*.

Black seed oil (Nigella sativa): Black seed oil has been called a cure for everything but death and has a powerful antimicrobial profile. Research has shown black seed (or black cumin seed) oil to have antiparasitic effects on a variety of protozoa (and parasitic worms), and it is particularly effective for treating *Blasto, Giardia, Entamoeba histolytica,* and *Pentatrichomonas* infections. Black seed oil is well demonstrated to have antibacterial properties, and these may play a role in the treatment of *H. pylori* as well. Thymoquinone (TQ), one of the active compounds found in black seed oil, acts as a biofilm disruptor, meaning it can break free from the protective coating *H. pylori* uses to protect itself, allowing antibacterial components to reach the *H. pylori* bacteria and eradicate it. It also has gastro-protective properties, possibly due in part to its inhibiting effect on acid hypersecretion, that may help with issues like gastritis, ulcers, and acid reflux.

Cat's claw (Uncaria tomentosa): Studies have shown cat's claw to be effective against a multitude of pathogenic infections such as *Plasmodium* and *Babesia*.

Monolaurin: It has antiparasitic properties against *Blastocystis hominis*, *Giardia*, and *Entamoeba histolytica* and activity against *H. pylori*.

Cat's claw and monolaurin work in synergy to support the body in clearing and suppressing a multitude of pathogenic infections.

Garlic oil: Allicin is a sulfur-containing compound that lends garlic to its antimicrobial properties. It's used for methane SIBO, and also inhibits the replication and invasion of protozoa such as *Blastocystis hominis*, *Babesia*, *Dientamoeba*, *Giardia*, *Endolimax nana*, and *Entamoeba histolytica*. It also has antimicrobial activity against *H. pylori* and has been shown to be protective against ulcers.

S. boulardii and Antimicrobial Herbs vs. Infections

Viruses	S. boulardii	Oil of Oregano	Black Seed Oil	Garlic Oil	Berberine	Monolaurin
Norovirus	+	+			+	
Rotavirus	+			+		
Bacteria						
C. difficile	+					
H. pylori	+	+	+	+	+	+
Protozoa						
Blastocystis hominins	+	+	+	+	+	+
Giardia	+		+	+	+	+
Cyclospora		+				
Dientamoeba		+	+	+	+	
Chilomastix	+					
Pentatrichomonas			+		+	
Endolimax nana		+		+		
Entamoeba histolytica	+	+	+	+	+	+

Treatment Options for Worms

While veterinarians commonly deworm pets, some practitioners suggest humans may benefit from deworming, too—though thankfully, we don't share the same social or dietary habits as our ahem four-legged butt-sniffing family members!

The antiparasitic medication you'll receive, along with the dosage schedule, duration of treatment, will depend on the type of worm you have. In very severe cases in which parasites may affect other parts of the body, additional treatments such as surgery and other medications to address additional problems caused by the parasites may be necessary.

Here are a few human deworming options:

- Over-the-Counter: Pyrantel is an OTC antiparasitic, often used for pinworms, but can also target *Ascariasis,* hookworms, *Trichostrongyliasis,* and *Trichinella.*

- Prescription Medications: Mebendazole, effective against a range of worms, including pinworms, whipworms, roundworms, and hookworms infections. It is available OTC in Europe but requires a prescription in the U.S. Other common prescription options include albendazole, ivermectin (not just for horses!), praziquantel, nitazoxanide (Alinia), and metronidazole (Flagyl).

- Natural Treatments: While I may prefer natural remedies for many conditions, worms are probably the biggest exception. The issue I have with natural treatments is they tend to be broad spectrum and systemic, which is great for targeting foreign pathogens such as viruses, bacteria, yeast, and even protozoa, as they have unique biologic features we can target while leaving our own bodies virtually unaffected. However, when it comes to worms, they're technically animals, just like us, so the broad-spectrum treatments that are effective for worms may affect us as well! Herbal treatments, like sweet wormwood (*Artemisia annua*), can be effective but carry risks, including liver injury. I recommend using natural options only under supervision with careful monitoring.

Tips for Preventing a Relapse

Follow these best practices to prevent parasitic infection and re-infection:

- Wash your hands regularly, especially after using the bathroom and before handling food.
- Keep your fingernails short and clean. Long fingernails can trap protozoa and parasite eggs, making them easier to spread.
- Pathogens are known to live on toothbrushes. Discard and replace all your toothbrushes frequently (every two weeks) and after treating an infection.
- Regularly wash clothing, undergarments, bedding, and other personal items.
- Handle food safely:
    - Thoroughly cook poultry, pork, beef, and other red meats.
    - Never eat undercooked or raw meat.
    - Use separate cutting boards for meats and vegetables.
    - Thoroughly wash all fruits and vegetables.
- Avoid swimming in waters that may be contaminated.
- Only drink filtered or bottled water, especially when traveling or camping.
- Support your secretory IgA levels with *S. boulardii*, L-glutamine, and/or reishi.
- Wear shoes when you walk outdoors. Parasites, such as hookworms, can penetrate your skin when you come into contact with soil that contains their larvae.
- If you suspect or find out you have parasites, test all family members, pets, and childcare providers. Chances are you all

have them and everybody should be treated at the same time.

- Low stomach acid can cause recurrent infections, so be sure to maintain optimal digestion and take digestive enzymes if you are deficient, particularly betaine with pepsin.

Chapter Summary

- When digestive symptoms don't subside after a fair amount of root cause digging to remove sensitivities, restore optimal digestion, and utilize nutrients and mucilaginous herbs to heal the gut, there is a good chance an unaddressed gut infection is present.

- Infections can be caused by parasites, bacteria, viruses, fungi, or other microorganisms that cause a reaction in the body.

- Viral infections thought to be self-limiting can persist in immunocompromised individuals and may cause IBS symptoms. Treatment options include immune support and antivirals.

- *Borrelia burgdorferi,* the bacteria that causes Lyme disease, is a potential bacterial trigger of IBS and IBD.

- *Helicobacter pylori* (*H. pylori*) is a common yet underappreciated bacterial infection when it comes to IBS and autoimmunity. I have found stool antigen tests for *H. pylori* to be the least invasive, most helpful, and reliable. The most common *H. pylori* protocol used by functional medicine practitioners is mastic gum and deglycyrrhizinated licorice (DGL).

- Protozoa, a type of parasite, are the most common drivers of IBS, and as many as 70 percent of people with IBS may have one. The most common is *Blastocystis hominis* (*Blasto*).

- To clear a protozoan infection, we generally need an herbal or prescription antimicrobial. When a person has low secretory IgA, the beneficial yeast *S. boulardii* can often support the body in eliminating many protozoan infections and reduce related symptoms.

Visit https://ibsrootcause.com/bonus for notes on this chapter.

CHAPTER 11

Alterations in Stress Hormones

When I first began having IBS symptoms, my old-school physician told me stress was likely a contributing factor. He wasn't the first person to make that connection. In the early days, the predominant theory behind the cause of IBS was that the condition was "psychogenic" or rooted in mental health.

It's true that up to a third of people with IBS also experience anxiety or depression, which seems to support this idea. But as you'll discover in this book, there's more beneath the surface.

IBS can be triggered by many factors, including physical ones, but stress plays a big role too. My doctor wasn't wrong—but I wish he had offered more tangible advice. In functional medicine, we know stress is a major root cause of many health conditions, including digestive issues.

I remember the first time I experienced the profound impact of the gut and brain connection. It was the day after Christmas and I was in my first year of pharmacy school. My parents received an early morning call that my uncle had been hit by a drunk driver on his way home from our family Christmas celebration the night before and was in the emergency room. Both of my parents were scheduled to work that day, and since I was on break from school and the most fluent English speaker (and practically a qualified health care professional in my own mind), I drove to the hospital to look after my uncle, talk to the medical team, and sign off on forms.

I knew his injuries were quite serious and he was in the Intensive Care Unit, but I was unprepared for the scene that greeted me when I arrived: blood, bruising, bandages, beeping monitors, and the scuffle of healthcare professionals monitoring his vital signs and looking out for his needs.

Seeing him in a fragile, semi-conscious state was not just emotionally upsetting, it was physically overwhelming as well. I recall needing to run to the bathroom with cramping and diarrhea before being able to talk to his doctors.

This was my first glimpse into just how impactful stress can be to our digestive function. When the body is under stress, we tend to be shifted toward the sympathetic "fight-or-flight" state, where survival is prioritized over digestion. Over time, this can diminish digestive function. Instead, we need to be in the relaxed, parasympathetic, "rest and digest" state for the optimal release of stomach acid, digestive enzymes, and bile, among other functions of good digestion.

In the early 19th century, IBS was thought to mainly affect hysterical, hypochondriac, or depressed women, and sadly, this psychosomatic view still lingers today. This can lead to digestive symptoms being dismissed as "all in your head," making it difficult to get proper medical support to address the real root causes behind IBS.

But depression, anxiety, stress, and other mood issues could certainly play a role in symptoms because the brain and gut are in constant communication, forming a fascinating two-way street known as the gut-brain axis. Through channels like the vagus nerve, immune system, and hypothalamic-pituitary-adrenal (HPA) axis, the gut talks to the brain and vice versa. It's why if you're feeling stressed out by a deadline, you may have stomach cramps and diarrhea. But it's important to understand that IBS-related symptoms are not the result of an overactive imagination, rather there is a strong research-backed mind-body connection.

Stress and mood can shift the gut microbiome, while an imbalanced gut microbiome can cause anxiety, depression, and even inflammation. It's a cycle—gut health impacts the brain, and our mental state can alter the gut's balance. Think of it as your gut and brain constantly influencing each other, with disruptions in one often stirring up trouble in the other.

How Does Stress Impact IBS?

Stress can disrupt gut function in many ways. It affects gut motility (as I experienced during the stress of seeing my uncle), increases gut sensitivity, alters secretions like stomach acid and bile, and raises intestinal permeability. Stress also reduces mucosal blood flow, weakens the gut's ability to repair its lining, weakens the gut's internal defenses, and negatively impacts gut bacteria. When stress becomes chronic, this can lead to the development of any number of gastrointestinal disorders such as IBS, food intolerances, ulcers, and GERD. Stress can also trigger an IBD flare and exacerbate IBD symptoms.

Cortisol is the most important hormone in terms of helping the body adapt to stress. You may have heard that cortisol is "bad." This is misleading. While high levels of cortisol are problematic, low levels of cortisol (hypocortisolism) are just as troublesome (if not more so), and can lead to debilitating (and even life-threatening) symptoms. We absolutely need cortisol—*in the right amounts.*

Chronic stress can lead to both high and low cortisol levels, each with different implications for IBS. Initially, high cortisol increases gut permeability, disrupts digestion, and fuels inflammation, often worsening IBS symptoms like diarrhea, constipation, and heightened gut sensitivity.

Over time, prolonged stress can deplete cortisol, leaving the body less able to manage inflammation and stress. Low cortisol is linked to increased gut permeability, inflammation, and worsened IBS symptoms, as well as mood disorders like anxiety and depression.

Overall, chronic stress has been found to be a strong predictor of symptom intensity in people diagnosed with IBS and an impaired stress response has been found to predict IBS symptom severity. The good news is that reducing stress can ease symptoms over time.

Root Cause Research Corner: The Many Manifestations of Stress on Digestion

Let's take a closer look at some of the ways stress can impact digestion:

- Stress lowers stomach acid, digestive enzymes, and bile, leading to malabsorption of foods. Large food particles enter the gut, triggering immune responses that can cause acid reflux, bloating, constipation, nutrient deficiencies, and even autoimmune conditions.

- Stress depletes glutamine, which is essential for repairing the gut lining. This weakens the gut barrier, leading to inflammation, gut imbalances, and a higher risk of infections.

- Stress hormones such as adrenaline can make harmful bacteria more aggressive, allowing them to form biofilms that shield them from being eliminated.

- Stress disrupts the balance of good and bad bacteria in the gut, leading to dysbiosis.

- Stress can cause the immune system to attack the gut microbiome and trigger an IgA immune response to commensal (friendly) bacteria.

- Stress lowers the number of anti-inflammatory gut bacteria, increasing inflammation and susceptibility to illness.

- Stress affects digestive muscles, leading to constipation or diarrhea. In "fight or flight" mode, digestion stalls, slowing stomach and small intestine activity (causing constipation), while speeding up the colon to clear out potential toxins (causing diarrhea).

- Stress weakens SIgA, an immune protein that protects the gut from pathogens, leaving the body more vulnerable to infections such as *H. pylori* and protozoa. It also loosens tight junctions in the gut lining, allowing infections to take hold.

Parasympathetic vs. Sympathetic Nervous System

Isn't it amazing how our body does things, without us having to think about them? The autonomic nervous system, which I liked to call the "automatic" nervous system during pharmacy school to help me remember its function, runs vital functions like breathing, digestion, and heart rate behind the scenes. It has two modes that work like yin and yang:

The parasympathetic nervous system is our "rest and digest" mode. This is when the body relaxes, heals, and supports digestion. It triggers the release of saliva, digestive enzymes, bile, and insulin, helping our body break down food, absorb nutrients, and store energy for later. It also keeps things moving smoothly through the intestines with peristalsis. When you're calm, your body is able to focus on these tasks—helping digestion work like a well-oiled machine.

On the flip side, the sympathetic nervous system is our "fight-or-flight" mode. When activated, digestion is put on the back burner. Blood is redirected to your muscles, heart rate spikes, and energy is pulled from sugar and fat to handle immediate stress. Your body is ready to run from a tiger, not digest a meal.

Too much time in fight-or-flight can leave your gut neglected, slowing digestion and repair and contributing to constipation. But we can't be in rest-and-digest all the time either. The key is balance—being able to rev up when needed and relax to support digestion and healing when the coast is clear.

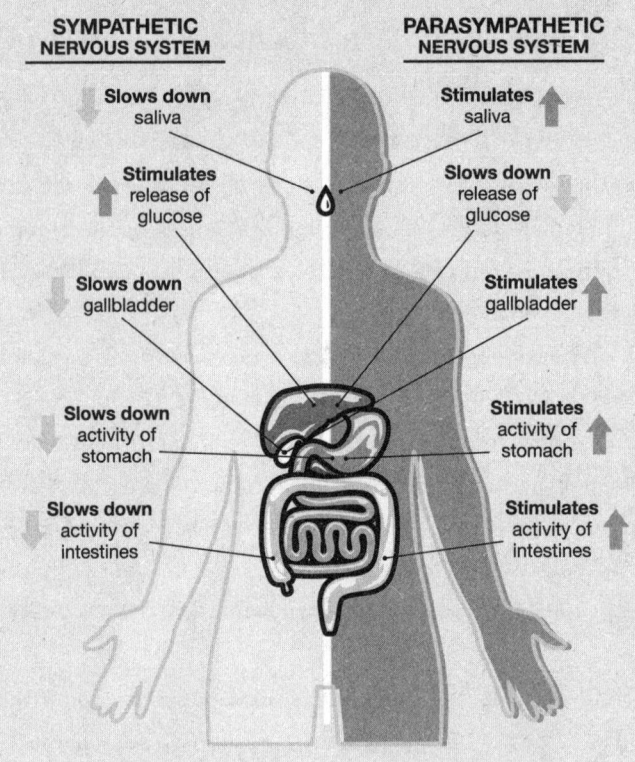

So What is Stress Exactly?

We've all heard that we should be "less stressed," but before we get into how to be less stressed, let's first define what the body perceives as stress. Stress, broadly defined, is anything that throws the body's natural equilibrium, or homeostasis, off course. Here are the main culprits that trigger an overactive fight-or-flight response:

- Psychological Stress: Emotions like grief, fear, anxiety, and even excitement can trigger stress—especially in situations that are new, unpredictable, or feel out of our control. Major life events like a breakup, financial strain, or the loss of a loved one are obvious stressors, but even positive changes (marriage, a new baby, grad school) or daily frustrations (a messy house, a text from your boss, or a tech failure) can activate the stress response.

- Trauma: A history of trauma, especially early in life, can leave the nervous system stuck in fight-or-flight mode, impairing the body's ability to rest and heal. Research shows people with IBS are significantly more likely to have experienced trauma or Adverse Childhood Experiences (ACEs), which are linked to long-term hormonal and digestive imbalances.

- Sleep Deprivation: Lack of sleep is one of the fastest ways to stress the body. In my own experience, missing sleep triggered cramps and diarrhea. One study even found that women with IBS had worse symptoms the day after poor sleep. It's no coincidence I developed IBS during pharmacy school while living on 3–4 hours of sleep and taking multiple exams per week!

- Circadian Rhythm Disruption: It's not just how much sleep you get, but when you sleep. The circadian rhythm regulates not only sleep-wake cycles, but also digestion, microbiota, gut motility, and inflammation. Night shifts and irregular sleep can throw off this internal clock, leading to fatigue, insomnia, and worsening gut symptoms.

- Chronic Inflammation: While short-term inflammation helps us heal, chronic inflammation- often driven by gut dysbiosis, infections, poor diet, toxins, or overexertion-can overwhelm the body. I often see it underlying IBS symptoms, especially in people also dealing with injuries, obesity, overwork, or sleep apnea.

- Nutrient Deficiencies: The adrenals need nutrients like healthy fats, protein, B vitamins, iron, sodium, magnesium, and vitamins A, C, and D to make stress hormones. When these nutrients are depleted, the body struggles to adapt to stress—leaving you more reactive and symptomatic.

- Blood Sugar Swings: A high-carb meal can spike blood sugar and trigger an insulin surge, often followed by a crash. That drop (reactive hypoglycemia) prompts a cortisol release to stabilize blood sugar—but it can also activate the stress response and worsen IBS symptoms like cramping, bloating, or diarrhea. Repeated swings also impair gut motility and microbiome balance.

How Do You Know You Have Stress Hormone Imbalance?

Symptoms

Symptoms may include the following:

- Feeling overwhelmed
- Feeling tired despite adequate sleep
- Trouble falling asleep or staying asleep

- Difficulty getting up in the morning
- Dependency on caffeine
- Cravings for salty foods (a.k.a. the "I just ate a whole bag of chips syndrome")
- Cravings for sweet foods
- Increased effort required for everyday activities
- Intolerance to exercise
- Low blood pressure
- Feeling faint/dizzy when getting up quickly
- Easily startled
- Mental fog or trouble concentrating
- Alternating diarrhea/constipation
- Low blood sugar (often presenting as feeling angry when hungry, or as I like to call it "hangry")
- Decreased sex drive
- Decreased ability to handle stress
- Longer healing time
- Mild depression
- Less enjoyment in life
- Feeling worse after skipping meals
- Increased PMS
- Reduced ability to make decisions
- Reduced productivity
- Poor memory

In addition to looking at your symptoms, you can determine if you have stress hormone imbalance by utilizing the following self-assessments.

Are you irritable?
Irritability and overwhelm are two cardinal signs of imbalance.

Do you have low blood pressure?
People with adrenal dysfunction often have low blood pressure and/or a drop in blood pressure after standing up from a lying down or sitting position (orthostatic hypotension).

Do you have light sensitivity?
Usually our pupils dilate (enlarge) in the dark and contract (get smaller) in the light. People with low adrenal function may often have difficulty contracting their pupils and experience light sensitivity, difficulty seeing in bright lights, or having to wear sunglasses on most days.

Is your body temperature unstable?
Morning temperatures that are fluctuating and on the low side may be suggestive of adrenal insufficiency. Hypothyroidism or an underactive thyroid will also present as low temperatures, however, the low temperatures will be daily and stable.

Do you crave the whole bag of chips?
Cravings for salt and salty foods like crackers, chips, pretzels, and olives are a cardinal sign of adrenal issues.

Do you sometimes feel "hangry"?
If you skip a meal or go too long without eating, do you become angry or irritable? That combination of hunger and anger is "hanger" and a sign of the blood sugar imbalances associated with adrenal dysfunction.

Testing
I've found symptom self-assessments are excellent indicators of an impaired stress response and provide the information we need to start providing the body with the right kind of support. However, testing

may help with determining other potential interventions more specific to your individualized hormone levels and patterns.

- Precision Analytical DUTCH (Dried Urine Test for Comprehensive Hormones) Complete, to assess adrenal function through urine testing. It measures four or five samples throughout the day to measure cortisol levels, providing a good sense of the daily cortisol rhythm. You don't have to stop any supplements or protocols in order to do the test.

- ZRT Laboratory Adrenal Stress Test Kit, to measure four cortisol readings throughout the day, cortisol sum, and DHEA. You may need to stop caffeine and some supplements to ensure accurate testing.

> ### Signs of Acute Adrenal Failure or Addisonian Crisis
> Seek emergency medical treatment if you experience extreme weakness, mental confusion, dizziness, severe abdominal pain, vomiting, and diarrhea, fever, sudden pain in your lower back or legs, nausea, extremely low blood pressure, or reduced consciousness or delirium. These may indicate Addison's disease or damaged adrenals that are unable to produce enough cortisol. Dangerously low levels of cortisol can be life-threatening.

Supporting the Parasympathetic State

Addressing your stress response will be incredibly helpful in shifting you into the parasympathetic rest and digest state. I've already shared some strategies on how you can shift into that state around mealtimes in chapter 5, but you may require more support for chronic stress dysfunction.

Many of the strategies that address stress will help you spend more overall time in the parasympathetic state. Some strategies also have research-backed connections to impacting digestion as well.

All of the following methods have the potential to help, as do interventions focused on burnout and adrenal healing.

Neurotransmitter approach

There is a body of emerging research exploring the complex connection between neurotransmitters and IBS. IBS patients with altered gut motility patterns and visceral hypersensitivity also tend to have altered levels of neurotransmitters, such as serotonin, "the feel good" neurotransmitter, and GABA, a neurotransmitter known for its calming effect.

Conventional doctors may prescribe antidepressants to manage IBS because they can reduce pain and improve gut function through their impact on serotonin receptors. Tricyclic antidepressants, such as amitriptyline or desipramine, block the reuptake of serotonin and have anticholinergic effects, which can help relieve pain and diarrhea. SSRIs like Zoloft can ease pain while blocking serotonin reabsorption, which can help relieve constipation.

The dopamine/norepinephrine reuptake inhibitor bupropion (Wellbutrin) may be used for IBS and has even been found to induce remission in IBD.

Newer medications that modulate serotonin receptors in the gut are also available (see page 410).

5-HTP is the precursor to serotonin and is available as a supplement. It may improve rectal pain in some IBS patients because of how it affects serotonin production.

Low levels of GABA are associated with chronic pain and anxiety. The GABA system in those with IBS has been shown to be irregular, and the use of GABA as a supplement may improve abdominal pain, bloating, diarrhea, and reduce visceral hypersensitivity.

Mind-body practices for IBS

Many experts view mind-body practices as a cornerstone of IBS management, and for good reason. Stress strongly impacts gut function, and research shows these techniques can significantly reduce symptoms by activating the parasympathetic (rest-and-digest) response.

Yoga

Combining movement, breathwork, and meditation, yoga has been shown to reduce IBS symptom severity, improve mental health, and enhance quality of life. One study even found hatha yoga to be as effective as the low FODMAP diet for symptom relief.

Mindfulness Meditation

A systematic review found that mindfulness improves quality of life and significantly lowers pain in adults with IBS.

Breathwork

Practicing slow, deep breathing strengthens vagal tone and supports digestion. One study found six weeks of breathwork helped improve IBS-C symptoms. A favorite technique is 4-7-8 breathing: inhale for 4 counts, hold for 7, exhale for 8.

Cognitive Behavioral Therapy (CBT)

CBT helps reframe negative thought patterns and improve stress resilience. It's one of the most well-studied psychological tools for IBS, with effects lasting up to a year after treatment.

Other helpful approaches

Hypnotherapy, biofeedback, psychodynamic therapy, acupuncture, and massage have also shown benefits for symptom reduction.

A meta-analysis found no one approach is best, many mind-body therapies work. The key is choosing the practices you enjoy and can stick with regularly.

Balance blood sugar

Stabilizing blood sugar is key to restoring stress hormone balance and digestive health. For most people with mild blood sugar imbalances, simple diet and lifestyle changes can make a big difference (such as eating more protein, fat and fiber, and fewer simple carbohydrates), often without the need for medications. However, as blood sugar issues progress to insulin resistance, prediabetes, or diabetes, more support may be needed. Those with diabetes can still benefit from lifestyle changes but may require a more intensive functional medicine approach to achieve balance. To get my Blood Sugar Balance Toolkit, go to ibsrootcause.com/bonus.

Replenish electrolytes

Electrolytes, such as sodium and potassium, play a key role in muscle function, fluid balance, and overall digestive, nervous, and cardiovascular health, especially when it comes to regulating blood pressure. They're also great for gut motility, helping to pull water into the colon and keep things moving—making them useful for addressing constipation. You can find electrolytes in foods such as meat, fish, bone broth, fruits, veggies, sea salt, sea vegetables, and teas. Stress tends to deplete sodium the most (those salty cravings are your body's way of saying it needs more!), so adding high-quality sea salt to your daily routine can be helpful.

An electrolyte supplement can also support you. Rootcology's Electrolyte Blend includes sodium, potassium, chloride, and magnesium, plus adrenal-supporting ingredients such as vitamin C, which gets depleted during times of stress, and D-ribose, a mitochondrial nutrient that helps with fatigue.

Circadian rhythm reset

Having a healthy circadian rhythm is a key and often overlooked component of a happy and healthy gut. The circadian rhythm can become unbalanced due to a lack of natural light during the day stimulating our energy production and the artificial lights of modern living that make nighttime as bright as daytime so the body doesn't get the "power down" message to prepare for sleep.

Studies have found blue lights, emitted from electronic devices (cell phones, laptops, tablets), can significantly impact the circadian rhythm, increase alertness, and contribute to sleep problems when used at night.

To restore circadian rhythm balance:

- Get regular exposure to sunlight during the day, especially bright, outdoor light first thing in the morning (or consider bright light therapy boxes if going outside is not an option).

- Limit artificial light at night, especially blue light. Avoid electronic devices (TV, phone, computer) for one to two hours (the more the better!) before bedtime. If you need to use a device, consider putting it in "nighttime" mode or wear blue light blocking glasses, such as True Dark eyewear. Put black tape over appliances with lights, such as humidifiers, chargers, and smoke detectors.

- Practice good sleep hygiene by developing a calming bedtime routine (try a soothing Epsom salt bath or journaling), sleeping in a cool (between 60 and 67 degrees Fahrenheit), dark environment, and avoiding caffeine eight hours before bedtime.

Reduce inflammation

Reducing inflammation helps support healthy adrenal (and gut) function. For more on inflammation and ways to address it, see chapter 13.

Boost oxytocin

Doing what makes us feel good prompts the release of the "love" hormone oxytocin, which can quickly shift the body into a parasympathetic, healing state. Oxytocin has been found to provide anti-inflammatory and pain-relieving effects by reducing pro-inflammatory cytokines and blocking pain signals while stimulating the release of the body's natural pain relievers. Studies have shown it can reduce abdominal pain and increase visceral pain thresholds in patients with IBS. Incorporate some of these natural oxytocin-boosting activities into your daily routine:

- Hugging, touching, cuddling, affectionate caressing, or even sitting close to someone we care about boosts oxytocin. Petting an animal companion counts, too!
- Give yourself a butterfly hug: cross your arms, place your fingers on your chest, just under the collarbone, and tap your hands left-right-left-right, like fluttering butterfly wings, for at least eight rounds, until you feel more relaxed.
- Massage therapy for as little as 15 minutes has been shown to boost oxytocin levels and increase relaxation.
- Laugh more! Laughter has been found to raise oxytocin levels and help counter the negative effects of our stress hormone, cortisol.
- Unplug from negative news, music, and other media and dial up healing music and messages.

Address trauma

Unprocessed trauma can act like a toxin in the body—contributing to digestive issues, anxiety, depression, pain, and poor sleep. Reprocessing past events may be the missing link in healing your gut and overall health.

Therapies like cognitive behavioral therapy (CBT) are effective for both mood and IBS symptoms. Somatic experiencing, which taps into the mind-body connection, and practices like deep breathing and yoga can also help release stored emotional tension. EMDR (Eye Movement Desensitization and Reprocessing) is particularly useful for addressing trauma and has been shown to reduce chronic pain. Personally, EMDR once helped me resolve a lingering case of acid reflux when nothing else worked.

Supplement Recommendations for Stress Support
ABC Blend

The ABCs of adrenal support are Adaptogens, B vitamins, and vitamin C. Adaptogenic herbs are any natural herb products that support the body's ability to deal with stressors, normalize the HPA axis, and subsequently may improve stress-related IBS symptoms. In order to be considered an adaptogen, an herb must possess three main qualities:

1. It must be non-toxic to the patient at normal doses.
2. It should help the entire body to cope with stress.
3. It should help the body to return to "normal" regardless of how stress is currently affecting the person's functioning. In other words, an adaptogenic herb needs to be able to both tone down overactive systems and boost underactive systems in the body.

You can get adaptogens as stand-alone products but for convenience, improved efficacy through synergy, and so you don't have to pop 20 different pills a day, I usually recommend taking an adrenal support blend that contains a mix of synergistic adaptogens (the A's) as well as the common vitamins that become depleted due to chronic stress (the Bs and C).

I created Rootcology Adrenal Support Blend to include five carefully chosen, synergistic adaptogens: ashwagandha, American ginseng, eleuthero, licorice, and Rhodiola rosea due to their unique, multi-purpose properties. When used together, they address several stress and digestion related issues: Low cortisol levels (rhodiola, licorice), blood sugar metabolism, mitochondrial function (rhodiola, eleuthero), viral infections (licorice), and gut inflammation (licorice). The blend also contains the B vitamins and vitamin C for complete adrenal ABC support.

Please note, this blend has been specially formulated with licorice, which helps us increase our cortisol levels, and is excellent for people with low cortisol or experiencing fluctuations in the cortisol rhythm, such as excessively low cortisol in the morning and too much later in the day. People with high blood pressure and/or high cortisol levels should avoid it and instead consider Pure Encapsulations Daily Stress Formula.

Magnesium

The body requires magnesium for a healthy stress response, and it can become depleted due to chronic stress. Magnesium deficiency is also a common cause of gut motility issues and constipation as magnesium helps draw water into the intestines, softening stool and stimulating peristalsis. Because magnesium is often difficult to obtain from foods, most people will benefit from long-term supplementation. For more on magnesium, see chapter 6.

For Additional Adrenal Support: *Adrenal Transformation Protocol*

To restore stress hormone balance, you may find the four-week program in my book *Adrenal Transformation Protocol* helpful. Based on a program that has helped thousands of participants dramatically improve their health, *Adrenal Transformation Protocol* is designed to make it easy for you to get at the root cause of your symptoms, balance your stress response, and gradually build up your resilience to prevent excess stress from overwhelming your adrenals now and in the future. This comprehensive plan is based on a few simple lifestyle changes to address your healing from every angle and help you feel more calm, energetic, clear-headed, happier, and alive each day.

Chapter Summary

- Chronic stress can impact digestion by shifting the body into the sympathetic "fight-or-flight" state in which survival is prioritized over digestion.

- Stress can increase IBS symptom intensity.

- Insufficient sleep, circadian rhythm balance, inflammation, nutritional imbalances, blood sugar imbalance, psychological stress, and trauma can contribute to an overactive sympathetic response.

- Self-assessments are useful indicators of an impaired stress response but functional medicine tests like the Precision Analytical DUTCH and ZRT Laboratory Adrenal Stress Test Kit can measure your specific cortisol levels and help identify interventions tailored to your unique situation.

- Adrenal support strategies include neurotransmitters (5HTP and GABA), mind-body practices (including yoga, deep breathing, and cognitive behavioral therapy), balancing blood sugar, replenishing electrolytes, restoring circadian rhythm balance and optimizing sleep, reducing inflammation, boosting oxytocin, addressing trauma, and supplementing with an adrenal support blend and magnesium.

Visit https://ibsrootcause.com/bonus for notes on this chapter.

CHAPTER 12

Thyroid Hormones and Autoimmunity

The gut and thyroid connection is a subject near and dear to my heart; I struggled with IBS for many years before getting a Hashimoto's thyroiditis diagnosis. One of the reasons this IBS book is a natural evolution of my work with Hashimoto's is because many people with thyroid issues have IBS and vice versa. It's my educated guess that IBS-D often develops first and then leads to malabsorption of vital nutrients required for thyroid function, resulting in hypothyroidism, which can eventually lead to constipation.

Many of the same strategies that resolved my IBS symptoms helped me reduce my Hashimoto's symptoms and markers and helped many of my clients and readers as well.

My hope is figuring out the root cause of your IBS will help you prevent and/or improve your thyroid condition. Just as most things in the body, it's important to note that the gut and thyroid hormones are bidirectional. Helping balance thyroid hormones can help the gut and vice versa.

What Is the Thyroid Hormone and IBS Connection?

Thyroid hormones regulate every metabolic process in the body, so an imbalance is going to throw the digestive system way off track.

When it comes to hypothyroidism, not enough thyroid hormone for the body to function optimally slows everything down. Inadequate amounts of digestive enzymes and bile are produced to support the proper breakdown and absorption of food, contributing to poor digestion, food sensitivities, gut dysbiosis, and intestinal permeability (adding fire to the immune system attack!). Thyroid hormones also regulate transit time, which slows down in hypothyroidism, often leading to constipation—a common GI symptom in Hashimoto's and a frequent complaint among my clients. This slower transit can disrupt the microbiome and increase the risk of gut infections. Chronic infections caused by certain bacteria, protozoa/parasites, and fungi/yeast, are common in those with Hashimoto's (some studies indicate SIBO may be present in as many as 50 percent of people with hypothyroidism), and they can lead to diarrhea. Food sensitivities, thyroid medication imbalances, and viruses can also be a reason for loose stools.

Symptoms of hypothyroidism and IBS resemble each other so closely that many people with thyroid dysfunction are diagnosed with IBS prior to getting their thyroid adequately tested. An interesting report from Nepal found 18.5 percent of people who have IBS actually have thyroid dysfunction, most of them subclinical hypothyroidism (the early stages).

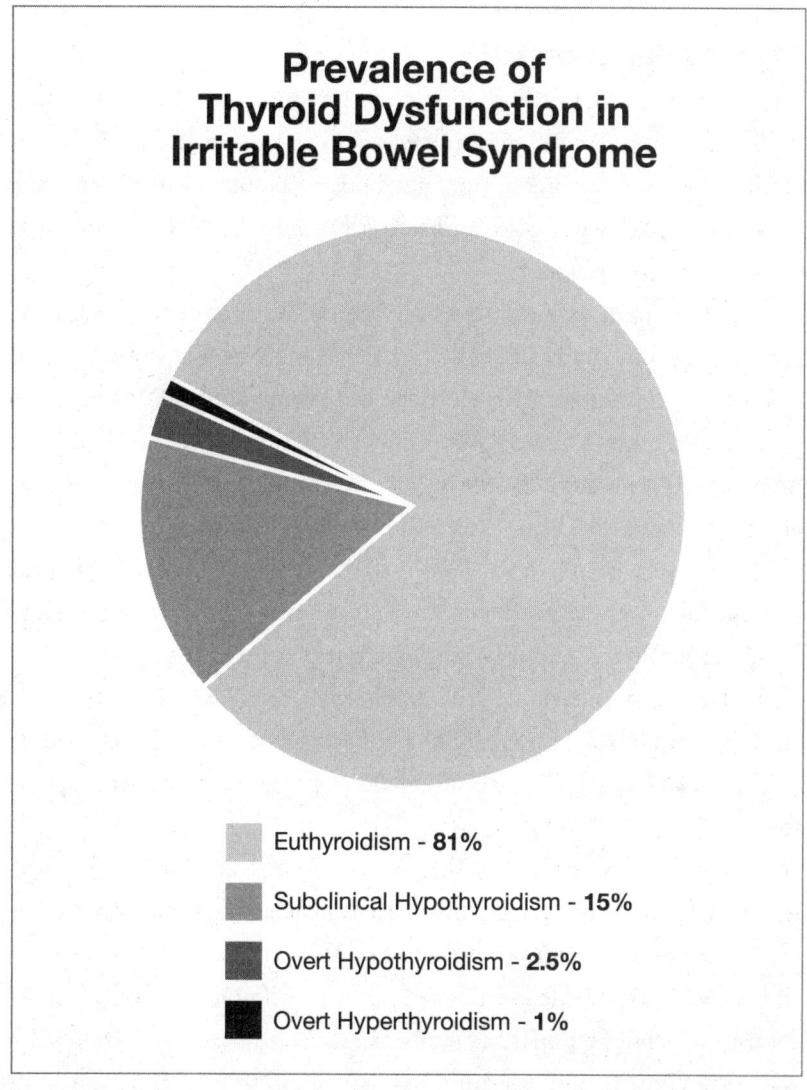

In the case of hyperthyroidism, too much thyroid hormone speeds everything up, increasing transit time and often causing diarrhea. Excess thyroid hormone is also associated with low stomach acid and fat malabsorption issues which can cause acid reflux, stomach pain, gas, and bloating.

Thyroid Function 101

The thyroid is a butterfly-shaped gland in the front of the neck that produces hormones vital to nearly every organ system. These hormones regulate heart rate, breathing, metabolism, blood pressure, and the menstrual cycle, while also supporting hormone production and nervous system development.

The two main biologically active thyroid hormones are triiodothyronine (T3) and thyroxine (T4). T3 is the more potent hormone and has a more immediate effect on the body's metabolism, while T4 is produced in larger amounts but is converted into T3 in tissues to exert its effects. Both are crucial for regulating various bodily functions, including metabolism, heart rate, and body temperature.

Low levels of T3 and T4 signal the release of TSH (thyroid stimulating hormone produced in the pituitary gland), while high levels of circulating T3 and T4 stop the release of TSH. In people with normal thyroid function, TSH levels may fluctuate at times when the body requires more thyroid hormone to be consumed, such as during periods of stress, illness, lack of sleep, pregnancy, or low temperatures.

The two most common thyroid conditions are Graves' disease, when the thyroid makes too much thyroid hormones (the most common cause of hyperthyroidism) and Hashimoto's thyroiditis, when the thyroid makes too little hormone (the most common cause of hypothyroidism which may impact as many as 1 in 8 women).

Both Graves' and Hashimoto's are autoimmune conditions, in which the immune system

has identified thyroid cells as foreign or harmful substances and developed antibodies to attack these cells. This attack causes inflammation and damage to the cells that produce thyroid hormones. In the case of hypothyroidism, this causes an underproduction of thyroid hormone while in Graves, it causes an overproduction.

Most diseases of autoimmunity are linked to gut health in some way because the gut controls the immune system and digestive symptoms can be one of the first signs of an autoimmune thyroid condition.

How Do You Know You Have Thyroid Hormone Imbalance?

Symptoms

COMMON SYMPTOMS OF HYPOTHYROIDISM	COMMON SYMPTOMS OF HYPERTHYROIDISM
Cold intolerance	Anxiety
Constipation	Eye protrusion
Depression	Fatigue
Dry skin	Hair loss
Fatigue	Heart palpitations
Forgetfulness	Heat intolerance
Hair loss	Increased appetite
Joint pain	Irritability
Loss of ambition	Menstrual disturbances
Low libido	Muscle loss and pain
Menstrual irregularities	Sleep disturbances
Muscle cramps	Tremors
Stiffness	Weight loss

While symptoms of hyperthyroidism (like anxiety, irritability, insomnia, and palpitations) are commonly attributed to Graves' disease, it's important to note they can also occur when someone is overmedicated with thyroid hormones and in the early stages of Hashimoto's.

When the thyroid is initially under attack by the immune system, thyroid cells are broken down, and release thyroid hormones into the bloodstream. This causes thyroid hormone surges (or a transient hyperthyroidism known as thyrotoxicosis or Hashitoxicosis), as well as mood alterations, followed by an onset of hypothyroidism. Hypothyroidism, in turn, is connected with brain fog, depression, fatigue, low libido, and pain.

Also, because Graves' and Hashimoto's are autoimmune inflammatory conditions, thyroid antibodies and inflammation can lead to numerous symptoms even when thyroid hormones are normal. Thus it is not uncommon for my thyroid clients to report feeling moody, depressed, anxious, and irritable when their thyroid hormone levels and/or thyroid antibodies are out of balance.

Testing

In my clinical experience, I've seen many cases of thyroid problems go undiagnosed (or misdiagnosed) because most doctors don't perform a comprehensive test panel.

I spent almost a decade undiagnosed because I only had my TSH, thyroid stimulating hormone, tested. My thyroid condition was missed, leading me to deal with needless "mystery" symptoms such as chronic fatigue, depression, anxiety, and many others, for far too long! For this reason, it's important to have a full thyroid panel done.

Full thyroid panel:

- For suspected subclinical hypothyroidism (most commonly associated with IBS), I recommend a full thyroid panel, which includes TSH, T4, T3, and the two most common Hashimoto's antibodies, thyroid peroxidase antibodies (TPO) and thyroglobulin antibodies (TG). The antibodies are often elevated before changes in other thyroid markers are seen and they indicate an autoimmune process within the thyroid gland.

- Graves' disease, which causes hyperthyroidism, is less common than Hashimoto's but still important to rule out as a cause of IBS. Graves' disease also presents with antibodies. The lab tests used to check for Graves' antibodies are the thyroid-stimulating immunoglobulin (TSI) test and the TSH receptor-binding inhibitor immunoglobulin (TBII) test.

Full Thyroid Panel with Optimal Reference Ranges

TEST	STANDARD REFERENCE RANGE	OPTIMAL REFERENCE RANGE
TSH	0.4- 5.5 µIU/mL	0.5-2 µIU/mL 0.5-2.5 µIU/mL in elderly
Free T4	9-23 pmol/L	15-23 pmol/L
Free T3	3-7 pmol/L	5-7 pmol/L
Reverse T3	11-21 ng/dL	11-18 ng/dL
TPO Antibodies (Hashimoto's)	<35 IU/ml	<2 IU/ml
TG Antibodies (Hashimoto's)	<35 IU/ml	<2 IU/ml
TSI (Graves')	0-0.55 IU/L or <130 percent	<0.55 IU/L or <80 percent
TBII (Graves')	0-1.75 U/L	0-1 U/L or 16 to 100 percent inhibition of TSH binding

Understanding your labs:
TSH

- If your TSH is elevated, this may mean you need to talk to your doctor about starting or increasing thyroid hormones. An elevated TSH means you do not have enough thyroid hormone on board and you are hypothyroid.

- If your TSH is low, and you take thyroid medications, your doctor may need to lower your dose.

- If your TSH is under 0.4 µIU/mL and/or you have symptoms of hyperthyroidism (and don't take any thyroid medications), you may also want to test for Graves' antibodies.

- I have found that I, as well as many other thyroid patients, feel best when my TSH is between 0.5 and 2 µIU/mL (for elderly clients, up to 2.5 µIU/mL). Research has shown that a healthy person, without a thyroid condition should have a TSH right around one. I suspect thyroid dysfunction if I see a TSH above 3 µIU/m.

Free T4

- Measures the levels of T4 hormone available to be converted to T3, the active thyroid hormone. Low levels may indicate hypothyroidism.

Free T3

- Free T3 measures the levels of active T3 hormone available for use in the body. Inadequate or excess amounts of the active thyroid hormone T3, may also lead to issues with mood, fatigue, brain fog, and pain.

- If free T3 is low or free T3 is low *and* free T4 is optimal or above the reference range, you may not be converting T4 into active T3 properly. Your body is not making enough T3 hormone from the T4. This can happen for a variety of reasons, including nutrient deficiencies, stress, infections, and genetics. If you are taking a T4-only thyroid medication, you may wish to speak to your doctor about switching medications to a T3-containing version or adjust the dose of your current medication.

- High T3 can cause pain, including carpal tunnel syndrome and may mean you need to lower your dose of thyroid medication.

Reverse T3

- Reverse T3 measures how much of the active free T3 hormone is able to bind at thyroid receptors. Reverse T3 is produced in stressful situations and binds to thyroid receptors, but turns them off instead of activating them.

- The reverse T3 test is sometimes used to identify cases of poor T4 to T3 conversion (under stressful situations, T4 gets converted to reverse T3 instead of to T3) as well as thyroid symptoms due to adrenal stress instead of thyroid malfunction or autoimmunity.

- If reverse T3 is too high, you may want to talk to your doctor about switching to a thyroid medication that contains T3 to ensure the right hormone is getting to the right receptors (or adjusting the dose).

Thyroid antibodies
- It is important to pay attention to thyroid antibodies because they are going to be the first indication of a thyroid problem in many cases. They can be elevated for as many as 10 to 15 years before a change in TSH is even detected. The presence of thyroid antibodies also means your thyroid is being actively destroyed.

- An ultrasound test can be used to help diagnose thyroid disease that may not be indicated by bloodwork (research suggests 10 to 50 percent of people with Hashimoto's may not test positive for antibodies). Physical changes to the thyroid could indicate Hashimoto's (rubbery thyroid, shrunken thyroid, enlarged thyroid, or abnormal growths in the thyroid) or another autoimmune process as well as benign or cancerous nodules or lumps.

Interpreting Thyroid Test Results

The handy chart below explains what your thyroid lab numbers may mean.

RESULT 1

TSH	FREE T3	FREE T4	TPO/TG Antibodies
Normal	Normal	Normal	-

Interpretation: Normal Thyroid Unless Symptomatic

The person has thyroid function within the normal level, with a low risk of Hashimoto's/Graves'. (If you have thyroid symptoms, double check the reference ranges for optimal levels, test reverse T3, and do a thyroid ultrasound.)

RESULT 2

TSH	FREE T3	FREE T4	TPO/TG Antibodies
Normal	Low	Low	+/-

Interpretation: Central Hypothyroidism

The thyroid and the pituitary are not communicating. There are low levels of thyroid hormone around, but the pituitary is not sending out a message to make more. Hashimoto's may be present.

RESULT 3

TSH	FREE T3	FREE T4	TPO/TG Antibodies
Normal	Normal	Normal	+

Interpretation: Euthyroid Hashimoto's

The thyroid is still making enough thyroid hormone, but is under attack.

RESULT 4

TSH	FREE T3	FREE T4	TPO/TG Antibodies
Elevated	Normal	Normal	+/-

Interpretation: Subclinical Hypothyroidism

The thyroid is losing its ability to make enough thyroid hormone. This is considered Stage 2 of Hashimoto's, especially if antibodies are positive. (However, some people with seronegative Hashimoto's don't test positive for antibodies, despite their thyroid being under attack.) A thyroid ultrasound can be helpful for diagnosing Hashimoto's at this point.

RESULT 5

TSH	FREE T3	FREE T4	TPO/TG Antibodies
Elevated	Low	Low	+/-

Interpretation: Hypothyroidism

This is an indication that the person is euthyroid (has thyroid function within the normal level), with a low risk of Hashimoto's/Graves'. I recommend double checking the reference ranges for optimal levels, testing reverse T3, and doing a thyroid ultrasound if you still have thyroid symptoms.

RESULT 6

TSH	FREE T3	FREE T4	TPO/TG Antibodies
Low	Normal	Normal	+/-

Interpretation: Subclinical Hyperthyroidism

This is an indication that the person is euthyroid (has thyroid function within the normal level), with a low risk of Hashimoto's/Graves'. I recommend double checking the reference ranges for optimal levels, testing reverse T3, and doing a thyroid ultrasound if you still have thyroid symptoms.

RESULT 7

TSH	FREE T3	FREE T4	TPO/TG Antibodies
Low	High	High	+/-

Interpretation: Hypothyroidism

The pituitary is telling the thyroid to make less thyroid hormone, as it has detected excess levels of thyroid hormone. (This often indicates Graves' disease or overmedication.) If Graves' disease is suspected, test for TSH receptor antibodies.

This chart explains thyroid lab results.

A Client Story from Dr. Izabella's Files

Anna reached out to me in 2013, after her blood work indicated Hashimoto's antibodies. She was tired, losing hair, and anxious, although her biggest complaint was chronic diarrhea. She had actually been diagnosed with IBS about a year prior.

Her diarrhea began on her honeymoon in Mexico, where she experienced a bout of "food poisoning. She was treated with antiparasitic and antibiotic medications—unfortunately, to no avail. The diarrhea continued, multiple times per day.

Anna experienced some relief after having read my book *Hashimoto's thyroiditis* and starting the gluten-free diet, but felt stuck and needed more help. Because I learned all autoimmune disease is associated with impaired gut health, we decided to focus there. Since we caught the beginning stages of Hashimoto's I was hopeful that if we found what was causing her IBS, we would be able to prevent the progression of her thyroid condition.

We removed gluten, grains, and dairy, as well as lettuce, which came up positive on her food sensitivity test. She saw a little bit of improvement, but was not 100 percent well. Since she had already been gluten free for over six months, I knew it was time to dig deeper.

I was convinced Anna's new onset IBS was connected with her trip abroad and a parasite she picked up while traveling. When we eat foods in a foreign country, our bodies may not have the same resistance the locals have, especially if we are under stress.

To test Anna for parasites, we used the BioHealth Labs 401H Test, which was the test I preferred at the time. Anna and I were both disappointed when the test was negative. She was a newlywed, not feeling well, and paying out of pocket, so I felt bad she

> had to spend more money, but I also suggested she get the Genova Diagnostics GI Effects test.
>
> The GI Effects test showed she had *Blastocystis hominis,* a one-celled protozoan parasite. Anna worked with her doctor to receive targeted prescription medications for *B. hominis* and continued a grain-free diet and gut support nutrients for two months after the treatment.
>
> Her IBS went into remission and she regained her energy levels. No more multiple trips to the bathroom! Her thyroid antibodies began to drop as well! She has regained most foods but still maintains a gluten-free diet. Last I heard from her, she was studying for an exam to get into an MBA program and planning a trip to Europe with her husband.

What Causes Thyroid Hormone Imbalance?

The most common reasons for thyroid hormone imbalance are:

- Physical damage to or removal of the thyroid: Surgery to remove all or part of the thyroid, radiation to treat cancers of the head and neck, or damage to the thyroid gland caused by an infection or accident, can slow or eliminate the thyroid's ability to make thyroid hormones, leading to hypothyroidism. In rare cases, people may be born without a thyroid gland.

- Iodine deficiency or excess: Iodine is a nutrient required to make thyroid hormones, however the amount needs to be just right. Iodine deficiency is the leading cause of hypothyroidism in developing nations yet due to widespread use of iodine fortified salt and other foods in the U.S. and other western nations, the main cause of thyroid issues for most people in those areas is related to autoimmunity. In developed nations, excess iodine has been found to increase the risk of thyroid autoimmunity.

- Autoimmune attack: When the immune system is triggered to attack the thyroid gland as a foreign invader, the thyroid gland will eventually be compromised so much it is unable to function properly. It may either be unable to produce enough thyroid hormones (hypothyroidism) or produce too many (hyperthyroidism). Remember, autoimmunity develops when three things are present: the right genes, exposure to a trigger (trauma, stress, toxins), and intestinal permeability. Many gut-related issues, such as food intolerances and sensitivities, pathogenic infections, and nutrient deficiencies, have been implicated as triggers in cases of autoimmunity, as well as contributors to intestinal permeability. Hyperthyroidism may also result from overactive thyroid nodules.

What do all of these triggers have in common? According to my Safety Theory of Hashimoto's, they send a message to the body that the world we are living in is not a safe place and it should go into energy-conservation mode to help us survive. One very effective way to do that is to slow down the thyroid gland. Based on my work with thousands of people with Hashimoto's and the study of biology, medicine, the concept of adaptive physiology, and the leading theories of autoimmune disease, I believe early humans developed the propensity toward autoimmune thyroid disorders because they helped us survive and that "survival advantage" has been passed on to those of us with thyroid disease as a predisposition for developing thyroid disorders in times of danger. One way to outsmart autoimmune thyroid disease—and IBS—is to make your body understand it's safe by eliminating these triggers.

If you have both IBS and thyroid issues, consider a few common causes:

- SIBO: Because GI motility is disturbed in hypothyroidism, this can lead to SIBO. SIBO has been reportedly found in up to 50 percent of people with hypothyroidism and up to 56 percent of pregnant women with subclinical hypothyroidism. Additionally, the use of levothyroxine is considered a risk factor for SIBO. So if you have IBS and hypothyroidism, you may need to focus on restoring thyroid hormones and clearing SIBO (see chapter 9).

- Celiac disease: Celiac disease could be a source of your IBS-related symptoms and thyroid issues. Celiac disease is more common in people with an autoimmune thyroid condition with some studies indicating the risk is five times higher than in the general population. Studies estimate anywhere between 1.2 to 15 percent of people with Hashimoto's and 4.5 percent of people with Graves' disease also have celiac disease. A higher prevalence of celiac disease has been found in people of caucasian ethnicity, especially in Scandinavian countries, Ireland, the UK, Scotland, and Italy.

- *Blastocystis hominis:* If you have both IBS and Hashimoto's, you may want to look at chapter X, where I discuss *B. hominis,* a pathogen identified as a potential trigger for both (and also for chronic hives).

  I have worked with numerous people in the early stages of Hashimoto's where IBS was their biggest complaint and treating the cause behind IBS helped prevent the need for further thyroid intervention.

  I was so excited to see researchers reporting similar stories with treatment of *Blastocystis hominis* leading to a remission of Hashimoto's.

  A case study on a 49-year-old man with chronic urticaria (hives) and Hashimoto's found eradicating his *Blastocystis homi-*

nis infection resolved his hives and normalized his thyroid function. During the four years of follow-up, the man remained symptom free with normal thyroid function.

A study published in 2020 measured the free T3, free T4, TSH, anti-TPO, and Interleukin-17 (IL-17) (which mediates inflammation) levels of 20 people with Hashimoto's, 20 people with Hashimoto's and a *Blastocystis hominis* infection, and 20 people with neither condition. IL-17 was significantly higher in those with Hashimoto's who were infected with *B. hominis*, compared with Hashimoto's patients who were not infected. After *B. hominis* was eradicated, TSH, anti-TPO, and IL-17 were significantly decreased. Researchers concluded the treatment of *B. hominis* infections improves Hashimoto's through reductions in IL-17, anti-TPO, and TSH levels.

- *H. pylori* infections: Both Graves' disease and Hashimoto's have been tied to *H. pylori* infections. A 2013 Chinese study found a rate of *H. pylori* infection in 66 percent of people with Graves' disease and 37.7 percent of people with Hashimoto's. As the rate of *H. pylori* in controls was 32 percent, the researchers concluded *H. pylori* was not likely a causative factor for Hashimoto's—but of course, they did not perform deeper tests such as genetic tests on the controls to determine if the controls had the correct genetic predisposition to develop autoimmune thyroiditis after an infection. Additionally, the researchers didn't perform antibody studies, conduct before and after studies of thyroid function, or test for autoimmune markers after treating *H. pylori*. Other studies have shown cross-reactive antibodies between *H. pylori* and Hashimoto's, improved thyroid hormone absorption, reduced thyroid antibodies (up to 2,000 points!), and even normalized TSH levels after *H. pylori* eradication

Over a three-year period, I reviewed around 300 GI-MAP stool tests from clients and readers with Hashimoto's. I found that 21 percent tested positive for *H. pylori*, and when I included lower levels, 33 percent had the pathogen. Many of my clients saw significant improvements in their Hashimoto's symptoms after treating *H. pylori*, with several even experiencing a reduction in thyroid antibodies—some put their Hashimoto's into remission!

While spontaneous remission is more common in Graves' disease, treating *H. pylori* can sometimes lead to remission in both conditions. Personally, I've had *H. pylori* multiple times, and treating it helped lower my thyroid antibodies, reduce acid reflux, eliminate food sensitivities, improve my voice hoarseness, and get rid of headaches.

For more, see chapter 10.

Treatment Options

Balancing thyroid hormones can help with digestive symptoms and addressing the autoimmune component of the illness can often help even further. You will note that many of the recommendations for autoimmunity are also helpful for gut health.

Treatment Approach for Thyroid Hormone Balancing

In addition to looking into the root causes of thyroid issues, focusing on proper thyroid hormone balance using medications and/or nutritional therapies is often required for restoring the health of the body and the digestive tract.

For Hashimoto's

Prescription thyroid hormones can be an important part of restoring thyroid hormone balance and getting well. There are several different types of thyroid medication options and it's important to know what they are and how they work.

- T4-containing medications (including Synthroid, Levoxyl, Levothyroxine, and Tirosint) will need to be converted to the active thyroid hormone, T3, in the body.

- T3-containing medications (like Cytomel and compounded T3) are available, though not often prescribed as a stand-alone therapy because they have a short half life which may lead to fluctuating levels. They're often used as an add-on to T4-containing meds.

- Combination T4/T3 medications, sometimes called Natural Desiccated Thyroid when derived from animal thyroid glands (Armour, NP Thyroid, and compounded T4/T3 medications) may be a helpful alternative for people who are taking T4 medications, but still have unresolved thyroid symptoms.

Medication selection is both an art and science for people with hypothyroidism and many people do say thyroid hormones are life changing for them. That said, I see many people who do not feel well on thyroid medications because of these three issues:

- Poor conversion: In my experience working with thousands of people with Hashimoto's, some of them just don't feel great with T4 only options and feel significantly better with an addition of a T3 containing medication and/or switching to a combination T4/T3 medication. Oftentimes their lab results might show they are not converting T4 to T3 correctly, leading to their T4 levels being in the top of the reference range and their T3 levels toward the bottom (or beneath the reference range).

- Poor absorption: People with gastrointestinal issues such as gastritis can have issues absorbing thyroid medications and some people have issues with the fillers (such as lactose) in thyroid meds. One medication which comes in a gelcap and liquid formulation, Tirosint, has been shown to be better absorbed, allowing for improved thyroid symptom control in people who didn't see improvement on other medications.

- Dosage: Thyroid medications can be of tremendous benefit, yet it's important to know that thyroid medications are goldilocks hormones, which means they need to be used in just the right dose—and there are risk factors of being under- and overmedicated. Your optimal thyroid numbers are going to be different from your mother's optimal thyroid numbers, which are going to be different from your neighbor's optimal thyroid numbers. I personally feel best with a TSH a bit under 1 µIU/mL, and like a sloth with a TSH of 4 µIU/mL (which is considered an acceptable range by some), but you may need some trial and error to find your personal best TSH. I and other functional medicine practitioners generally recommend a TSH between 0.5 and 2 µIU/mL for most. Work with your doctor to find a type and dose of medication that works for you.

For Graves' disease

The three traditional treatments for Graves' disease include pharmaceutical options (antithyroid medications and beta-blockers), radioactive-iodine therapy, and thyroidectomy (surgical removal or partial removal of the thyroid).

Methimazole and propylthiouracil are antithyroid medications that may help control the symptoms of hyperthyroidism by reducing the production of thyroid hormones. Researchers have found that in some cases the autoimmune attack in Graves' may be self-limiting and temporarily suppressing thyroid function with antithyroid meds can restore a euthyroid state that continues even after the medications have been stopped. Unfortunately not everyone is a candidate for antithyroid medications. There is a risk of liver damage or significantly depressed white blood cell count, as well as a number of other side effects and drug interactions. Furthermore, some people just don't feel well on these medications, and methimazole is contraindicated during the first trimester of pregnancy.

Beta-blockers (which lower blood pressure by causing the heart to beat more slowly) are sometimes used to address heart palpitations and other cardiac symptoms associated with hyperthyroidism, though they do not address thyroid or immune system health.

If a person does not get into remission spontaneously or with antithyroid medications, doctors may recommend radioactive iodine or surgery. These conventional treatments are irreversible thyroid treatments that will cause permanent hypothyroidism and lead to a requirement for thyroid hormones for life.

As a potential complement or alternative to anti-thyroid medications, herbs with antithyroid activity such as bugleweed, motherwort, and lemon balm may be recommended by integrative health care professionals, including Dr. Eric Osansky, who is an expert on Graves' disease and the author of books about integrative approaches to treating it. Dr. Osansky explains bugleweed has antithyroid activity and prevents thyroid antibodies from binding to the thyroid. Motherwort is used more for the cardiac symptoms seen in Graves', and works as an herbal beta blocker. It can alleviate symptoms such as heart palpitations, anxiety, sleeplessness, and reduced appetite. Lemon balm appears to block hormone receptors, preventing TSH from binding to thyroid tissue and keeping antibodies from attaching to the thyroid.

Please note, most of these herbs are not safe during pregnancy and have their own set of side effects. Herb Pharm Thyroid Calming Liquid Herbal Formula contains bugleweed, motherwort, and lemon balm.

Autoimmune Treatment Options

If your test results suggest you have a thyroid condition, figuring out the underlying reasons *why* your thyroid hormones are imbalanced can be the key to your healing. In the case of the two most common thyroid conditions, Hashimoto's and Graves' disease, an immune system imbalance is at the root. So while your thyroid function will likely benefit from some type of thyroid hormone replacement medication (or hormone suppressant medication in the case of Graves'), medication won't address the "root causes" of your autoimmune disease or the reason why your immune system is attacking your thyroid.

Take a root cause approach

This means addressing immune system imbalance by avoiding autoimmune triggers and building up the body's strength, healing capacity, and resilience alongside relevant conventional approaches such as thyroid medications.

In my personal experience and work with those with Hashimoto's, I've realized symptoms can be greatly improved by supporting a healthy gut. By addressing the main root causes of IBS and digestive distress, the chapters in this book may help you restore thyroid hormone balance and find relief from gastrointestinal symptoms.

However, after following the thyroid-supporting recommendations in this chapter and gut-healing ones in *IBS Root Cause,* you may find you need to do additional digging to get at the root of the immune system attack. I have a website dedicated to helping people optimize their hormones and get into remission from Hashimoto's hypothyroidism, www.thyroidpharmacist.com, and wrote an entire ebook on how to optimize thyroid hormones titled, appropriately enough, *Optimizing Thyroid Hormones.*

You may also benefit from my three books on Hashimoto's, which contain detailed guidance on the root cause of Hashimoto's and protocols so you can take charge of your thyroid health.

- *Hashimoto's Thyroiditis: Lifestyle Interventions for Finding and Treating the Root Cause:* My findings on the dietary changes, supplements, and medications that helped me feel better and how you can use them to identify your own root causes.

- *Hashimoto's Protocol: A 90-Day Plan for Reversing Thyroid Symptoms and Getting Your Life Back:* A step-by-step, streamlined plan of the most effective interventions to reverse the autoimmune damage at the root of Hashimoto's.

- *Hashimoto's: Food Pharmacology: Nutrition Protocols and Healing Recipes to Take Charge of Your Thyroid Health:* A cookbook featuring 125 delicious recipes with thyroid-supporting nutrients, strategies for making dietary changes an easy part of one's life, and protocols that can help transform the body into a safe place so it can receive the foods needed to heal.

If you have Graves' disease, consider these titles by Dr. Eric Osansky:

- *Natural Treatment Solutions for Hyperthyroidism and Graves' Disease 3rd Edition*

- *The Hyperthyroid Healing Diet: Reverse Hyperthyroidism and Graves' Disease and Save Your Thyroid Through Diet and Lifestyle Changes*

With a root cause approach, you will see improvements in your health with each trigger you address!

> ## The Root Cause Approach to Hashimoto's
>
> - Utilize comprehensive thyroid tests to determine diagnosis and the need for thyroid-hormone therapy.
> - Use optimal and functional ranges of thyroid hormones instead of outdated reference ranges.
> - Optimize thyroid hormone absorption and conversion when necessary (all are produced by the thyroid gland, but only T4 is present in levothyroxine, the most commonly prescribed thyroid drug.)
> - Optimize nutrition by eliminating reactive food and addressing deficiencies and digestion.
> - Address the stress response.
> - Address the health of the detoxification system.
> - Address the state of the gut.
> - Identify the person's unique triggers such as chronic infections, toxins, or traumas.
> - Track thyroid antibodies every three months to see if the interventions are making the condition less aggressive.
> - Appreciate the person's experience and always utilize the person's symptoms as a guide for adjusting treatment.

Gluten-free diet

Because celiac disease frequently co-occurs with thyroid conditions, a gluten-free diet may be helpful. An Italian study focused on people who had subclinical hypothyroidism, Hashimoto's, and celiac disease, but who had not been following a gluten-free diet. With the implementation of a gluten-free diet, participants improved both their intestinal symptoms and their thyroid function. About 71 percent of people who had subclinical hypothyroidism (a mildly underactive thyroid) and who had strictly followed a one-year gluten withdrawal (as confirmed by intestinal mucosa recovery), saw a return in normal thyroid function. Additionally, 19 percent of people who followed the gluten-free diet were able to normalize their thyroid antibodies, no longer testing positive for Hashimoto's.

Healing, nutrient-dense diet

Even in those without celiac disease, removing various dietary triggers can help address thyroid symptoms and thyroid markers. Multiple diets have been reported to reverse Hashimoto's and other autoimmune conditions, including the Specific Carbohydrate diet, Paleo diet, Autoimmune Paleo (AIP) diet, Low FODMAPs diet, and Body Ecology diet, as well as gluten-, soy-, dairy-, and iodine-free diets. The connecting thread behind these diverse diets is that they all remove various reactive foods. Most of the diets also include animal proteins, are more nutrient-dense than the Standard American Diet (S.A.D.), and remove processed foods.

In analyzing the diets that have worked for my clients and readers, I've found the following three diets to be especially helpful: gluten-, dairy-, and soy-free diet, the Paleo diet and the Autoimmune Paleo (AIP) diet.

Grain-Free Diets (Paleo, Autoimmune Paleo)

Grain-free diets, like Paleo and Autoimmune Paleo (AIP), aim to reduce inflammation and heal intestinal permeability, which can help reverse IBS-like symptoms and support autoimmune conditions such as Hashimoto's, rheumatoid arthritis, lupus, multiple sclerosis and IBD.

The Paleo diet removes gluten, soy, dairy, grains, nightshades, legumes, and processed foods. The AIP diet goes further, eliminating additional foods known to trigger inflammation. AIP avoids gluten, grains (corn, quinoa, buckwheat, rice), dairy, eggs, soy, alcohol, caffeine, legumes, nightshades (like tomatoes and peppers), sweeteners, canned/processed foods, high-glycemic foods, and nuts/seeds (except coconut).

In contrast, the AIP includes organic vegetables (excluding nightshades), fermented foods, grass-fed meats and organ meats, wild-caught fish, healthy fats/oils, low-glycemic fruits, coconut products, and hydrolyzed beef protein.

If the full AIP diet feels overwhelming, start with gluten-free, and gradually eliminate other food groups. My book *Hashimoto's Food Pharmacology* is a detailed nutrition guide on diets for Hashimoto's (and other autoimmune conditions), including the gluten, dairy, and soy-free diet, the Paleo Diet, and the AIP diet and has over one hundred delicious recipes.

Low-dose naltrexone (LDN)

Naltrexone is an FDA-approved medication that has been used since the 1980s for opioid withdrawal. Low doses of this medication (hence, low-dose naltrexone or LDN) have been found to modulate the immune system and have shown promise in improving cases of autoimmune disease, including IBD, Graves, and Hashimoto's. It has also been studied for its potential benefits for gastrointestinal disorders. A 2006 clinical trial on 42 people with IBS found four weeks of treatment with LDN improved symptoms in 76 percent of participants, with the biggest improvement in pain scores.

Selenium

Selenium deficiency is incredibly common in people with Hashimoto's and is a known trigger for autoimmune thyroid conditions. Fortunately, supplementing with selenium can reduce thyroid antibodies, ease symptoms, and improve overall well-being. In just three months, selenium can lower thyroid antibodies by 40 percent. Research also shows that combining selenium with myo-inositol significantly improves thyroid antibodies and elevated TSH.

Selenium offers similar benefits for hyperthyroidism, helping manage Graves' disease and improving symptoms when used with conventional treatments. A meta review of treatments used to manage Graves' orbitopathy showed selenium is an effective therapy for those with milder forms of the disease. Studies even suggest selenium can reduce anxiety which is very common in autoimmune thyroid disease. Doses of 200–400 mcg per day are generally safe and effective, but keep in mind that selenium has a narrow therapeutic range. Doses under 100 mcg (when used without myo-inositol) may not be effective, while over 800 mcg can be toxic.

L-carnitine

L-carnitine has been found to be incredibly helpful for thyroid issues, potentially due to its ability to modulate thyroid hormones within our cells. Studies have shown benefits in both hypothyroidism and hyperthyroidism. With regard to hyperthyroidism, it seems to work as a peripheral antagonist, preventing thyroid hormone receptors from excess thyroid hormone and ameliorating symptoms such as palpitations, tremors, insomnia and even muscle wasting. It's also been used extensively to resolve hypothyroid-related fatigue and constipation. High-quality options include Rootcology Carnitine Blend, Designs for Health Carnitine Synergy, and Pure Encapsulations L-Carnitine.

Synergistic nutrients: L-carnitine and selenium for hyperthyroidism

Using multiple nutrients together can have a synergistic effect. In one study on subclinical hyperthyroidism, patients with low TSH (0.1-0.4

mIU/L) and positive antibodies took 500 mg of L-carnitine and 83 mcg of selenium daily for a month. The result? A 50 percent reduction in symptoms, while thyroid hormones and antibodies moved in the normal range.

Synergistic nutrients: myo-inositol and selenium for Hashimoto's

Myo-inositol (a type of natural sugar alcohol with anti-inflammatory effects) can be helpful for Hashimoto's as a stand-alone or alongside selenium. Research has shown a combination of selenium and myo-inositol can have a synergistic effect that maximizes the benefit to thyroid function. Consuming both of these together may not just reduce thyroid antibodies, but can also reduce TSH by an average of 30 percent. In some cases of subclinical hypothyroidism, this combo can normalize TSH levels, reduce the risk of developing overt hypothyroidism, and improve overall well-being.

The synergistic doses studied were 600 mg of myo-inositol and 83 mcg of Selenium, so I created Rootcology Selenium + Myo-Inositol with that exact amount to maximize the benefits of these nutrients.

Aloe vera (*Aloe barbadensis*) (for Hashimoto's)

Aloe vera is a nutrient-rich plant packed with vitamins A, C, E, B-complex, and key minerals like selenium, zinc, magnesium, and copper, all of which support healthy T4 to T3 conversion and are often deficient in Hashimoto's.

It offers anti-inflammatory, antibacterial, antiviral, and adaptogenic benefits, making it helpful for infections that can trigger autoimmunity. Aloe also supports digestion, liver function, blood sugar balance, and helps relieve acid reflux and constipation, common in hypothyroidism and IBS.

Aloe has immune-modulating effects that may reduce thyroid inflammation and increase T4 levels. In one study, daily Aloe barbadensis juice led to a 54 percent reduction in TSH, lower TPO antibodies, and higher free T4 in women with subclinical Hashimoto's—not on thyroid meds.

Caution: Some people may be sensitive to anthraquinones in whole leaf aloe. Rootcology's Aloe is tested to contain <0.1 ppm. Aloe should be avoided during pregnancy, breastfeeding, or with diabetes or bowel obstruction. Always consult your practitioner before use.

Chapter Summary

- Many people with thyroid issues have IBS and vice versa. Figuring out the root cause of your IBS will help you prevent and/or improve your thyroid condition.

- Many cases of thyroid problems go undiagnosed (or misdiagnosed) because most doctors don't perform a comprehensive test panel.

- The two most common thyroid conditions are autoimmune conditions: Hashimoto's (hypothyroidism) and Graves' disease (hyperthyroidism).

- Celiac disease is more common in people with an autoimmune thyroid condition and can be a source of IBS-related symptoms and thyroid issues.

- Hypothyroidism can cause SIBO.

- *Blastocystis hominis* can be a trigger for both Hashimoto's and IBS.

- Both Graves' disease and Hashimoto's have been tied to *H. pylori* infections.

- Thyroid-supporting supplements include selenium, L-carnitine, myo-inositol, and aloe vera.

Visit https://ibsrootcause.com/bonus for notes on this chapter.

CHAPTER 13

Inflammation and Inflammatory Bowel Disease (IBD)

The date was April 17, 2018 and it was 5 a.m., two days before my due date. I woke up with cramping in my stomach and knew I was likely going into labor. I let my husband know and labored at home in my bed for a few hours until I felt it was a decent enough hour to call my doula.

The doula recommended I go to the hospital. I had a peaceful morning, showered, put on a dress, and ate a lovely oxytocin breakfast of banana pancakes, strawberries, and date balls made by my sweet mom, who was staying at our home and had been anxiously awaiting the arrival of her first grandbaby.

We drove to the hospital, and on the way there, my husband mentioned, "I don't want to worry you, but I had some blood in my poop this morning." I remember being so focused on my laboring, I just thought he must be having sympathy pains. Or perhaps a hemorrhoid.

The next 72 hours were the most incredible and difficult and life-changing hours of my life. After 16 hours of labor, our beautiful son

Dimitry was born. I remember holding him and wondering how it was possible to love someone you just met in such an intense way. He was perfect and I wanted to spend all of eternity holding him in that little hospital room, overlooking the Boulder mountains.

But things weren't going according to plan . . . as I later learned happens sometimes due to the elevation, our little one struggled with breathing. The NICU team whisked him away to provide oxygen, and we spent three scary days in the NICU before we were discharged.

At home, our sweet son struggled with nursing and I didn't seem to have a milk supply, so we started him on donor breast milk with a bottle, and I made a new friend: the breast pump.

During all of this, my husband again mentioned that his bowel movements were streaked with blood—and all of a sudden, my ultra-marathon running husband who was up at 5 a.m. was sleeping in until 11 a.m. Did I mention we had just had a baby?!

We called our wonderful physician, Dr. David Tusek, who immediately requested Michael get a colonoscopy. We bought the colonoscopy prep and I ran a GI-MAP stool test on my husband, a test I had used with clients with Hashimoto's to uncover the root cause of their issues.

It all happened in a blur. When our son was just two weeks old, I drove my husband to a clinic to get the colonoscopy. We were shocked to hear the diagnosis: ulcerative colitis, and my husband was prescribed three medications, including Canasa suppositories.

I immediately got to work to see what we could do to get him to feel better and reverse the condition. Fortunately, during my pregnancy, I had been invited to speak on thyroid health during an Institute for Functional Medicine seminar, and a big bonus of being a speaker is that I was also allowed to be an attendee, and the course happened to be one on gut health which included targeted lectures on IBD.

We were also in luck, as three of our dear friends from Boulder were world-renowned inflammatory bowel experts, two of them having reversed their own Crohn's disease: nutritionist Debbie Steinbock of Mindful Nutrition, whose husband Dr. Roy, happened to be our son's pediatrician, Steven Wright, founder of the Healthy Gut Project and SCD Lifestyle, and Dr. Jill Carnahan, a functional medicine doctor. I'm grateful to say that thanks to my functional medicine training, the help of some great friends and practitioners, and my husband's commitment to healing, we were able to get my husband into remission within a month of his UC diagnosis. I've seen these same protocols help others reach remission too and I'm excited to share them with the world in this book.

Is it IBS or IBD?

In recent years, scientists have begun to appreciate the role of inflammation in IBS. Studies have focused on the presence of mucosal inflammation in IBS, increased recruitment of mast cells, inflammatory cytokines in post infectious IBS, as well as the overlap between IBS and inflammatory bowel disease.

Inflammation can be a part of the overall presentation in a person with IBS, but it's important to note that some people with IBS may have another medically distinct inflammatory condition such as ulcerative colitis (UC) or Crohn's disease, which are both autoimmune conditions commonly referred to as inflammatory bowel disease (IBD). Inflammatory bowel disease may have some of the same causes as IBS, but due to the degree of intestinal inflammation, it requires a different treatment approach.

There are a lot of overlapping digestive symptoms, but IBD is considered a "structural" disorder by medical professionals, meaning physicians can use a scope to see damage to the intestines.

In contrast, IBS is considered a functional disorder. There's no "visible" damage to the structure of the intestines—at least not with the current methods used to examine the intestines—rather the disorder is thought to simply affect the *function* of the digestive tract.

While a good doctor will usually recognize red flag symptoms of IBD such as rectal bleeding, fever, and chronic diarrhea and refer a patient for a diagnostic work up, I have seen too many people receive the IBS label when indeed they had IBD. In fact, up to 10 percent of people diagnosed with IBS may have Crohn's disease or ulcerative colitis, while up to 23 percent may have microscopic colitis. Additionally, IBD patients are three times more likely to have had a previous diagnosis or treatment for IBS than controls. In some cases, the misdiagnosis wasn't discovered for five or more years!

It's important to have a correct diagnosis because IBD is considered the third-highest risk condition for colorectal cancer and can potentially progress into very serious conditions requiring intestinal surgery if not treated properly.

Red Flags for IBD: Pregnancy and Digestive Symptoms

When I was pregnant with my son, I spoke with a professional surrogate who mentioned she had severe IBS. As I waddled around, exhausted, I admired her for carrying other people's children. She said she loved giving that gift, and surprisingly, she felt better than usual during pregnancy. I asked if she had been fully evaluated, as remission of digestive symptoms during pregnancy is often linked to IBD. Sure enough, she was later diagnosed with IBD.

While most pregnant women experience constipation due to hormonal changes, some see their digestive symptoms worsen or improve, which can be a red flag for immune-mediated conditions like ulcerative colitis or Crohn's disease. Pregnancy shifts the immune system, lowering certain immune responses while boosting

> others, like natural killer cells. This shift from Th1 to Th2 cytokines may explain why some women with IBD improve or even go into remission during pregnancy.

Inflammatory bowel disease (IBD) is a term used to describe three types of chronic inflammation of the digestive tract, including ulcerative colitis, Crohn's disease, and microscopic colitis. Ulcerative colitis is characterized by inflammation and ulcers (sores) along the lining of the colon and rectum, Crohn's disease involves inflammation throughout the digestive tract, and microscopic colitis refers to inflammation of the colon and rectum that is only visible under a microscope. All three are considered autoimmune conditions.

Please note that while bloody stools are a red flag for IBD, not everyone with IBD has them.

Ulcerative colitis symptoms include:
- Chronic diarrhea, sometimes bloody*
- Fatigue, fever, weight loss, anemia*
- Rectal bleeding*
- Frequent, small bowel movements
- Abdominal cramping
- Joint pain
- Skin sores, rashes
- Mood swings
- Constipation (though diarrhea is more common, one third to one half of patients with UC experience the opposite problem)

Crohn's disease symptoms include:
- Rectal bleeding*
- Fissures, fistulas, and abscesses*
- Fever*

- Cramping and abdominal pain, especially on the right side
- Fatigue
- Prolonged diarrhea
- Weight loss*
- Feeling of fullness on the right side of abdomen
- Constipation (though not as common as diarrhea, constipation does occur in some people)

Microscopic colitis symptoms include:
- Watery diarrhea
- Abdominal cramping
- Weight loss*
- Fecal incontinence

*These are "red flag" symptoms that should be immediately addressed with your health care provider.

Do You Have Hemorrhoids or IBD?

People with IBS, especially those who experience persistent constipation, are likely to develop hemorrhoids and may not be surprised by a little bit of blood with their bowel movements. However rectal bleeding can also be a sign of IBD. Hemorrhoids have symptoms limited to the rectal area but rectal bleeding accompanied by changes in bowel habits or stool color and consistency and other symptoms such as abdominal cramps, fever, and weight loss could indicate a condition other than hemorrhoids, including IBD, colorectal cancer, or anal cancer, and should be discussed immediately with a health care provider.

See chapter 7 for what to do about hemorrhoids.

Can You Have IBS and IBD?

Both IBS and IBD can cause similar digestive symptoms such as diarrhea, cramping, abdominal pain, and even constipation. As I mentioned, some people who are labeled with IBS may actually have undiagnosed IBD, and ongoing research suggests these conditions may exist on a continuum, rather than being entirely separate issues.

While inflammation is key in IBD, it's important to note that some people with IBS also have low-grade intestinal inflammation. These individuals may benefit from some of the anti-inflammatory, gut-healing strategies I share in this chapter. Research shows that IBS and IBD share similar underlying mechanisms, such as intestinal permeability, gut dysbiosis, and immune activation, indicating there's more to IBD than just inflammation. In fact, about 28 percent of people with ulcerative colitis in remission still experience IBS-like symptoms, likely due to issues with gut motility and dysbiosis—two common root causes of IBS that persist even when IBD is in remission.

Although more research is needed to fully understand these connections, I believe addressing the overlapping root causes of IBS can benefit people with IBD. However, it's important to prioritize healing the structural damage to the intestines first and foremost in cases of IBD. This chapter is focused on healing that damage.

What Causes IBD?

Various theories have been proposed as to why a person may develop IBD. Anything that activates the immune system and triggers inflammation could be at the root of IBD, including gut dysbiosis, food sensitivities, and an underlying infection or overgrowth. There also appears to be a genetic component to IBD, so someone with a family history of IBD may be more likely to develop the condition themselves. The FUT2 gene has been associated with lowered amounts of *Bifidobacteria* which contributes to IBS and linked to IBD, with studies finding an increased risk of developing Crohn's disease in people with the non-secretor phenotype (about 20 percent of Caucasians). Environmental triggers like certain medications, smoking, stress, and depression may also be potential root causes of IBD.

Steve Wright, a gut health expert and founder of the Healthy Gut Project, believes IBD can be related to hormone levels and chronic stress and likely starts developing long before the onset of symptoms. Dr. Jill Carnahan, a functional medicine expert, says other potential root causes of IBD may include mold exposure, SIBO, Lyme disease, and Epstein-Barr virus (EBV).

Research supports a lot of what they are saying!

Protozoal infections

Various protozoal infections can trigger and/or exacerbate inflammatory bowel disease. One study from 1998 found *Giardia* in 61.6 percent of people with Crohn's disease and reported that treatment can result in significant clinical improvement. A 2023 study found protozoal infections in $^{107}/_{152}$ people with ulcerative colitis, *Blastocystis* in 52.33 percent of cases, *Giardia lamblia, Cryptosporidium, Entamoeba histolytica/dispar,* and *Endolimax nana* in 20.56 percent, 14.95 percent, 6.54 percent, and 1.86 percent of cases respectively. While a 2012 study found much lower rates of *Blastocystis* in IBD and questioned its relevance in the pathogenesis of IBD, it's important to note that detection methods may vary and treatment can often help. A different small study of 6 patients with refractory ulcerative colitis and *Blastocystis hominis* reported that *Blasto* could be a relevant infection. The researchers reported: "All six almost completely recovered three weeks later" after a 10-14 day treatment with metronidazole! Interestingly, metronidazole has a long history of use in IBD. Its benefits were thought to be due to its antibacterial effects, but I personally wonder if the main benefits are due to the antiprotozoal effects in relevant infections. For more on protozoan infections, see chapter 10.

Epstein-Barr Virus (EBV)

There is increasing evidence of the role of Epstein-Barr virus (EBV) in the pathogenesis of IBD, due to EBV's ability to evoke a severe immune response in the colon. IBD patients who are found to have a reactivated EBV infection may experience more severe symptoms, and there may be overlapping symptoms between the two conditions. Additionally, patients with IBD who are prescribed immunosuppressant drugs may be at an increased risk of reactivated EBV, so there is a bit of a bidirectional relationship here Additionally, the common IBD prescription sulfasalazine has also been implicated in EBV reactivations, perhaps because it prevents proper absorption of folate, an important nutrient for managing EBV.

Mold toxin exposure

Mold exposure is associated with the development of a number of autoimmune diseases, including Crohn's disease and ulcerative colitis. Exposure to mold toxins may increase pro-inflammatory markers and the immune response, which may be one explanation for its link to IBD. Mycophenolic acid is a mycotoxin that is produced by many different types of molds, and acts as an immunosuppressant, increasing the risk of opportunistic infections like *Candida*. Interestingly, mycophenolic acid, also used as an immunosuppressant drug for transplants and autoimmune conditions, has been shown to cause GI symptoms in about 30 percent of users, ranging from mild diarrhea to severe bleeding ulcers. For more on mold, see chapter 14.

Lyme and IBD

Borrelia burgdorferi, the bacteria that causes Lyme disease, has been shown to trigger an autoimmune response and some researchers believe it is an underlying trigger for IBD. For more on Lyme, see chapter 10.

Other potential origins and drivers of IBD include:

Iron overload

Recent research shows a link between excess iron in the body and the development of IBD. There is a close association between ferroptosis, which is characterized by high iron levels, and Crohn's disease and ulcerative colitis. Excess iron may also induce colitis and change composition of the gut microbiota.

Food additives

Food additives are incredibly common in our food supply today, used to improve the taste, texture, and shelf-life of packaged foods, and many have been associated with IBS and IBD, with researchers suggesting that food additives are an environmental trigger for IBD. Research has connected carrageenan, erythritol, sucralose, and saccharin, among others to the development of IBD. For more, see what to avoid with IBD on page 403.

Pathogenic *E. coli*

Various pathogenic *E. coli* species have been implicated in triggering IBD and new research suggests toxins produced by the bacteria can trigger inflammation and IBD. Shiga-like toxin–producing *Escherichia coli* (STEC) can produce symptoms that mimic ulcerative colitis such as bloody diarrhea and abdominal pain. For more on infections, see chapter 10.

Certain medications

Antibiotics, non-steroidal anti-inflammatory drugs (NSAIDs), oral contraceptives, mycophenolate mofetil (an immunosuppressant drug with action similar to mycophenolic acid), etanercept, ipilimumab, rituximab, and sodium phosphate have been linked to and may increase someone's chances of developing IBD.

Candida

Recent research has associated an overgrowth of *Candida* with IBD and has found a higher proportion of *Candida* in stools of IBD patients compared with healthy subjects. For more on *Candida*, see chapter 9.

MAP

Mycobacterium avium, subspecies *paratuberculosis* (MAP), is a bacteria that is very common in livestock and can be transmitted through the feces and milk of an infected animal. It is well established that MAP causes Johne's disease in cows, an inflammatory bowel disease in animals very similar to Crohn's disease. MAP is difficult to detect in people, but has been reported to be extremely common in those with Crohn's disease. One study found MAP was present in the digestive tracts of 92 percent of people with Crohn's disease, compared to 26 percent of controls. There is still some debate about the presence, etiology, and treatment of MAP in Crohn's disease patients, and more research is necessary to support the use of anti-MAP therapy for treatment.

Various other infections

Various infections including *Klebsiella*, *Clostridia*, CMV, measles, *Salmonella*, and *Campylobacter* may trigger or exacerbate IBD. For more, see chapter 10.

High protease activity

A pattern of decreased levels of beta glucuronidase (potentially due to dysbiosis or artificial sweeteners) that causes high levels of circulating proteases and can damage the intestinal mucus layer has been found in patients with IBD.

How Do You Know You Have IBD?
Testing
Proper diagnosis of IBD typically requires consultation with a gastroenterologist or a health care specialist experienced in treating these conditions.

Diagnostic Tests
Endoscopic procedures, in which a tube-like instrument with a camera is used to visually examine the digestive tract, such as a colonoscopy, endoscopy, sigmoidoscopy, and capsule endoscopy, and biopsy are used to diagnose IBD. X-rays, CT scans, and MRIs may also be utilized.

> *Additional Helpful Tests:*
> - Anti-*Saccharomyces cerevisiae* antibodies: Crohn's disease is associated with anti-*Saccharomyces cerevisiae* antibodies (ASCAs), so testing for ASCAs through a blood test or a stool test can be useful in diagnosing Crohn's disease.
>
> - Perinuclear anti-neutrophil cytoplasmic antibodies (pANCA): More common in ulcerative colitis and sometimes used alongside ASCA to distinguish between IBD subtypes.
>
> - Fecal calprotectin: Comprehensive stool analysis tests may show elevated calprotectin, a protein that may indicate inflammation in the gut. Elevated levels could indicate ulcerative colitis or Crohn's disease, but they could also come from food reactions, celiac disease, cancer, NSAIDs, poor blood supply, or infections.
>
> - C-reactive protein: Elevated levels of this protein in a blood sample indicate inflammation, though not necessarily in the gut.

- Erythrocyte sedimentation rate (ESR): Another nonspecific inflammation marker often elevated in active disease.

Treatment Options
Conventional Approach
Prescription drugs are often used to lower systemic inflammation to allow the intestines to heal. These may include anti-inflammatory drugs, courses of corticosteroids, and/or drugs that suppress the immune system. A newer option is biologics, which are drugs that target the proteins in the body causing inflammation.

My opinion is medications can be helpful in getting into remission, although please be mindful of the long-term side effects, especially with biologics.

Anti-inflammatory Drugs
For mild to moderate IBD, anti-inflammatories are often used. They include aminosalicylates, such as sulfasalazine (Asacol, Pentasa), mesalamine (Delzicol, Rowasa, others), balsalazide (Colazal) and olsalazine (Dipentum). Please note that aminosalicylates may interfere with folate absorption, so supplementing extra folate may be needed. Corticosteroids may also be used. These drugs work by reducing the inflammation in the colon. Side effects may include headaches, nausea, abdominal pain, cramping, vomiting, rash, or fever. In a very small number of people, these medications may cause diarrhea.

Some of these medications are available as a suppository, which may be more effective for some people, as they have a localized effect on inflammation. For example, mesalamine is available in suppository form (Canasa) to treat mild to moderate ulcerative colitis, and works to reduce inflammation directly inside the intestines, which I always love as a pharmacologist, as it helps to make the drug more effective and have fewer systemic effects.

Immunosuppressants

These drugs suppress the immune response, leading to lowered inflammation in the digestive tract. Options are azathioprine (Azasan, Imuran), mercaptopurine (Purinethol, Purixan), and methotrexate (Trexall). Newer, small molecule drugs are also used to reduce inflammation in IBD by targeting specific parts of the immune system, such as tofacitinib (Xeljanz), upadacitinib (Rinvoq), and ozanimod (Zeposia). Side effects of immunosuppressants can vary greatly, but may include nausea, allergic reactions, and an increased risk of infection. Please note, the USDA issued a warning of an increased risk of blood clots and cancer with tofacitinib.

Biologics

This newer class of drug therapy works by neutralizing proteins in the body that can drive inflammation. They are administered either through an IV infusion or self-administered injections. Biologics (sometimes called monocolonal antibodies), include infliximab (Remicade), adalimumab (Humira), golimumab (Simponi), certolizumab (Cimzia), vedolizumab (Entyvio), ustekinumab (Stelara), and risankizumab (Skyrizi). Side effects may include increased risk of infection, allergic reactions, and reactivation of viruses such as Hepatitis B or tuberculosis. Less common side effects are cardiac issues and central nervous system disorders.

Antibiotics

Antibiotics such as ciprofloxacin (Cipro) and metronidazole (Flagyl) are sometimes used in addition to other medications for IBD, or if there is a concern about infection. Common side effects can include nausea, diarrhea, yeast infections, dizziness, or rash.

OTC medications

Fiber supplements such as psyllium powder (Metamucil) or methylcellulose (Citrucel) may be used to treat mild to moderate diarrhea by adding bulk to the stool. The antidiarrheal (Imodium A-D) is sometimes recommended for diarrhea in Crohn's, however it should be avoided in acute flares, with strictures, fever, bloody diarrhea and in severe ulcerative colitis as it can lead to a life-threatening complication known as toxic megacolon.

In extreme cases, surgery may be recommended. This may include a partial or total colectomy (removal of the colon), a proctocolectomy (the removal of the rectum and colon), or a J-pouch surgery (where a pouch connecting the small intestine to the rectum is created).

Immune Suppression and Modulation for Inflammation

Many of the medications work by *modulating* the immune system, rather than healing the cause of the inflammation in IBD. Essentially, they cut off the chemical messengers sent out by the body in response to inflammation.

I personally believe that modulating the immune system isn't a bad thing in the short term, it can be incredibly helpful in buying us time to find the cause as it can help the gut lining and any ulcerations heal. However, some immune modulating medications can lead to highly undesirable side effects and/or shut down certain pathways that fight cancers and infections making people more susceptible to both.

Additionally, many people with IBD who experience structural intestinal healing by using these drugs can still have IBS-like digestive symptoms. Research has found the prevalence of IBS symptoms in patients in remission from IBD is anywhere between 11 and 64 percent!

It's important to note that people with IBD are at greater risk for developing bile acid diarrhea, SIBO, or sub occlusive crisis, and in some cases, more than one treatment approach is needed to have a full resolution of the residual IBS symptoms.

I do also want to note that people with IBD will need to follow anti-inflammatory recommendations, *and* they may have other drivers of digestive issues. While many of the IBS strategies used can be helpful for IBD, some can actually be harmful, especially in the early stages of healing simply because the intestinal lining may be too inflamed. I'll share more in the coming pages.

Strategies to Lower Inflammation

In addition to addressing root causes, diet, supplements, and strategic medications may be used to lower body and gut inflammation and can help induce and maintain remission in inflammatory bowel disease.

Low Dose Naltrexone (LDN)

In my work with autoimmunity, I have found one medication incredibly helpful, inexpensive, and with a minimal side effect profile (aka a pharmacists' dream) is naltrexone. When used off-label in small doses (1.5-4.5mg per day, usually prepared by compounding pharmacists), low-dose naltrexone (or LDN as those of us in the know call it), can help with various inflammatory and autoimmune conditions, including IBD.

LDN reduces inflammation in the intestinal mucosa and improves epithelial barrier function by improving wound healing and reducing stress on the mucosa. Naltrexone may be helpful in getting IBD into remission, maintaining remission, and preventing certain types of cancer, including colorectal cancer.

- Getting well: One study found that after 12 weeks of treatment with LDN, 74.5 percent of people with IBD who were not responding to traditional therapy experienced clinical improvement in their symptoms, and 25.5 percent had total remission of IBD.

- Staying well: Because people with IBD are at greater risk for colon cancer, and research has shown LDN can slow or stop the progression of colorectal cancer, I advocate for the long term use of LDN for people diagnosed with IBD, to induce and sustain remission and potentially prevent colorectal cancer.

In addition to calming gut inflammation, LDN has been linked to reduced pain and swelling throughout the body. It's also been shown to be safe and effective in a number of other autoimmune conditions because of its ability to enhance immune function and reduce inflammation.

Dietary Strategies To Induce Remission

Diet can be an incredibly helpful tool for inducing remission. My dear friend Debbie Steinbock, gut expert, nutritionist, and co-creator of the Elemental Diet Success Plan Course, uses a combination of a "soft and mushy" diet, devoid of fibrous, difficult to digest foods as well as a semi-elemental diet, combined with mucilaginous, gut-healing herbs to lower inflammation and support the mucosal healing in IBD as a first step. I'll summarize additional potential diets studied for IBD.

The Soft and Mushy Diet

A soft and mushy diet free of reactive foods can relieve symptoms, support gut healing, and be helpful in bringing about remission in IBD. The most common reactive foods in a person with an inflamed gut tend to be high in fiber, foods that have a rough texture (like raw vegetables), fried foods, spicy foods, nuts, seeds, and legumes. The "soft and mushy" diet includes soft, well-cooked foods that are easy to chew, and in some cases foods that are pureed and liquid only. Think soups and stews.

The Semi-Elemental Diet

The Elemental Diet is a liquid diet free of non-digestible substances such as fiber, complex carbohydrates, and protein structures. Researchers first began to use this method in hospitals in the 1940s, after they noticed that avoiding oral food and instead giving patients IV nutrition gave the digestive tract a chance to heal. They hypothesized mucosal healing occurred thanks to bowel rest.

Because the elemental diet is pre-digested, it offers the opportunity for bowel rest while consuming the nutrients needed to heal (and live) orally.

The elemental diet is primarily used in SIBO, but it has also been shown to be effective at inducing remission in Crohn's disease and ulcerative colitis. One study showed that four weeks of an elemental diet resulted in remission for 71 percent of participants with Crohn's disease. Another study showed 56 percent of people with ulcerative colitis went into remission on the elemental diet, and 46 percent of these people remained in remission for seven to twenty-eight months.

Using the elemental diet for all meals for four weeks can be a challenge for most people (it's typically used for two weeks in SIBO), so Debbie uses it in a "semi-elemental fashion." For example, she may recommend two to three days of a full elemental diet (where every meal is an elemental shake), followed by elemental shakes for breakfast and/or lunch for a few weeks until remission is attained. The remainder of the day's meals would consist of soft and mushy foods.

Specific Carbohydrate Diet (SCD)

The specific carbohydrate diet can get up to ⅓ of people with IBD into remission in about two months, and that number increases to 42 percent after six months.

The SCD diet was originally developed by Dr. Sidney Haas in the 1920s to help manage symptoms in children with "celiac disease" (a term that was then used more broadly as a catchall for chronic digestive issues and not yet linked specifically to gluten) through eliminating certain sweets and starches. While it's fallen out of favor for people with celiac disease, it has been widely studied for IBD and can be helpful for various other digestive issues. The diet is based on the premise that specific types of carbohydrates can be hard to digest (hence the name) and can lead to gut inflammation and symptoms.

It primarily allows monosaccharides (simple sugars found in fruits, vegetables, and honey) while excluding disaccharides (found in dairy and grains) and most polysaccharides (like starches from grains). The diet follows a phased approach, starting with a restrictive introduction phase that includes bone broth, non-processed meats, vegetables, certain fruits, and homemade yogurt (if tolerated). Foods like grains, potatoes, milk, canned beans, and added sugars are avoided. Over time, many people are able to reintroduce previously excluded foods. The book *Breaking the Vicious Cycle* by Elaine Gottschall is a helpful resource for SCD, written by a mother who healed her daughter's ulcerative colitis with the SCD. It is a temporary diet to reduce pathogenic bacteria, inflammation, and promote gut healing.

Low Sulfur Diet

The low-sulfur diet can help reduce levels of hydrogen sulfide, which may be a source of inflammation in IBD. Additionally, a diet low in sulfur-containing foods may help eliminate SIBO, which can cause symptoms similar to IBD (and may be a trigger for IBS). The diet includes limiting the intake of sulfur-rich foods like red meat and other animal proteins, eggs, dairy, certain vegetables like broccoli and cabbage, and certain dried fruits.

Mediterranean Diet

The Mediterranean diet is another popular choice that may help reduce inflammation and even improve bacterial diversity in the gut. Several studies have been carried out that highlight the benefits of the

Mediterranean diet that excludes foods that can cause inflammation and incorporates foods like salmon, avocado, sweet potatoes, a variety of fresh vegetables, olive oil, green tea, and honey. Some of the studies even found that this pattern of eating improved nutritional status, improved body composition, and reduced inflammatory markers like C-reactive protein (CRP) and fecal calprotectin, markers often elevated in IBD.

Autoimmune Paleo Diet

The Autoimmune Paleo (AIP) Diet is often recommended for those with autoimmune disease. By removing potentially inflammatory foods, the goal of the AIP diet is to bring the inflammatory response in the body down, and help pinpoint any individual food sensitivities. It has been used in the treatment and management of IBD. A small study in patients with UC and CD had participants complete a six-week elimination phase, where they removed potentially inflammatory foods such as grains, legumes, nightshades, dairy, eggs, and other foods, followed by a five-week maintenance phase, where they eliminated all of the suspecting foods. At the end of six weeks, 73 percent achieved clinical remission, and all of them stayed in remission during the maintenance phase. The patients reported an improvement in symptoms and quality of life, and fecal calprotectin levels were reduced. However, levels of CRP did not change significantly, and two patients with CD developed increased symptoms or partial bowel obstruction. The AIP diet is promising for IBD, but may not be appropriate for all cases.

Semi-Vegetarian Diet

In a case report, the semi-vegetarian diet was found to induce remission without medication in a patient with UC that developed after a low-carbohydrate weight-loss diet. Another study on 22 patients with CD found that the semi-vegetarian diet led to remission in 94 percent of patients, versus 33 percent in the control group. It was effective in maintaining remission, with none of the patients relapsing at the one-year mark, and only 8 percent relapsing at the two-year mark. In the control group, these numbers were 33 percent at year one and 75 percent at year two. More than half of the patients with CD also achieved normal CRP levels. In this particular study, the semi-vegetarian diet group was given fish once per week, and meat every two weeks. The rest of their diet was filled with brown rice, eggs, milk, miso soup, vegetables, fruits, legumes, potatoes, pickled vegetables, and plain yogurt. The semi-vegetarian diet may be effective because it removes a considerable amount of animal protein, which is rich in sulfur. (see, the low-sulfur diet above).

Additive-Free Diet

Of all of the diets, I think the most compelling one for IBD is the additive-free diet. Research suggests that additives are an environmental factor in triggering IBD, and many food emulsifiers such as carrageenan, artificial sweeteners such as sucralose and saccharin, colorants, and preservatives have been implicated in the development of IBD. The artificial sweetener erythritol, found to exacerbate colitis was a particularly important trigger for my husband.

Supplement Recommendations

The following supplements can be used to reduce inflammation in the body, as well as the gut. Most of these supplements work systemically and have been shown to induce remission in inflammatory bowel disease, some of them have been shown to maintain remission, and some of them have been shown to do both. In addition to normalizing gut inflammation, people also report pain and puffiness in the body resolving as well.

Aloe Vera

Known to help lower inflammation, supplementation with aloe vera gel at 100 mL for four weeks in one study induced remission in 30 percent of UC patients and 37 percent of patients taking aloe vera experienced symptom improvement. Nature's Way Organic Aloe Vera Whole Leaf Juice is a liquid option and capsule options include Rootcology Aloe (1 capsule at breakfast) and Designs for Health Aloe/200x.

Andrographis paniculata

Andrographolide, the main active component of *Andrographis paniculata,* is known for its anti-inflammatory properties. Studies have shown it can inhibit levels of multiple proinflammatory factors including certain immune cells and the expression of certain proteins in patients with UC, relieving digestive symptoms. One study of UC patients found 34 percent of those who received 1,200 mg and 38 percent of those who received 1,800 mg per day of *Andrographis paniculata* daily were in clinical remission of UC at the end of eight weeks.

Boswellia/Frankincense

A valued herb in Ayurvedic medicine, Boswellia (common name frankincense) has been shown to have potent anti-inflammatory properties that can help improve markers of IBD, and it can help induce remission in UC. In one small trial, 350 mg of boswellia, three times a day, had a remission rate of 82 percent, which was higher than 75 percent remission rate of sulfasalazine, a commonly prescribed drug for IBD. Additionally, a randomized, double-blind study found boswellia to be non-inferior to mesalamine for initiating and maintaining remission. Consider Pure Encapsulation Boswellia (AKBA).

Omega-3 fish oils

Anti-inflammatory and supportive of intestinal barrier integrity, fish oil has been shown to induce and maintain clinical remission of UC and decrease disease activity and increase quality of life in those with Crohn's disease. These fatty acids may also play a role in preventing IBD. 1 to 4 grams per day of EPA/DHA is generally a therapeutic dose of fish oil for IBD. For more on omega-3s, see chapter 6.

Serum-based Immunoglobulin

This animal-derived protein isolate contains IgG molecules that reduce inflammation, bind harmful gut bacteria, and support the intestinal barrier. It's been studied in IBS and IBD; in one study, 49 percent of people with IBD reported improvement after one week of taking 5 grams daily, with 9 percent seeing significant symptom relief. At the end of twelve weeks, these numbers increased to 76 percent and 20 percent respectively. Serum-based immunoglobulins are available as the prescription medical food EnteraGam, as well as Ortho Molecular Products SBI and Microbiome Labs Mega IGG2000.

Butyrate

A beneficial short chain fatty acid produced by the "good" bacteria in the gut, butyrate can increase the tight junctions of the gut lining, reduce food reactions, balance the microbiome, and modulate the immune system. Some studies suggest butyrate may reduce inflammation through a prebiotic effect. A 2019 study found people with IBD have fewer bacteria that produce butyrate and thus lower butyrate levels. While you can supplement with butyrate directly, one study found consuming 60 grams of oat bran daily can increase butyrate levels by as much as 36 percent, and at the end of twelve weeks UC patients reported significant improvement in abdominal pain and reflux symptoms. High-quality supplement options include: Rootcology Butyrate Balance, Designs for Health Tri-Butyrin Supreme, Healthy Gut TriButyrin, and Pure Encapsulations Butyrate.

P5P (the most bioavailable form of vitamin B_6)

Inflammation increases the uptake of P5P into tissues, limiting its availability in the bloodstream, and low levels are associated with IBD. Supplementing has been shown to lower inflammation of the colon. Additionally, supplementing with P5P may help produce neurotransmitters and help resolve the anxiety, insomnia, and depression which sometimes co-occur with IBD. Consider 50–200 mg/day of Rootcology P5P, Designs for Health P-5-P, Pure Encapsulations P5P 50, or SFI Health P-5-P. Do not use more than 300 mg/day of B_6 in the pyridoxine form.

> ### The Mood and Inflammatory Bowel Connection
>
> IBD often overlaps with depression and anxiety, likely due to shared pathways involving inflammation, vagus nerve signaling, and gut dysbiosis. In one study, 58 percent of people with active ulcerative colitis had depression and 50 percent had anxiety. Those with both UC and mood issues had lower microbial diversity compared to healthy controls, with more Lactobacillales, Sellimonas, Streptococcus, and Enterococcus, and less Prevotella and Lachnospira.
>
> Neurotransmitters like serotonin, dopamine, and GABA—which are involved in both gut and brain function—are produced in part by gut bacteria. This might be why SSRIs, which act on serotonin receptors, can be helpful for some people in alleviating symptoms of IBD, and why the dopamine agonist antidepressant bupropion (Wellbutrin) has resulted in numerous cases of IBD remission. As a pharmacist, I don't love SSRIs due to their side effects, but I do find bupropion to be generally well tolerated.
>
> Natural support options include 5-HTP (for serotonin), L-tyrosine (for dopamine), and P5P, the active form of vitamin B_6, which is often low in IBD and crucial for neurotransmitter production.

Vitamin D

Vitamin D plays a large role in immunity and in modulating inflammation, and I generally recommend levels between 60 and 80 ng/mL for optimal immune system function. Studies have found vitamin D can have both a preventative and therapeutic effect on mice with UC because of its antibacterial and anti-inflammatory action, and its role in the repair of the intestinal barrier.

I always recommend testing vitamin D levels before supplementing, as it is possible to get too much. Please note a recent review has suggested doses of 1,800–10,000 IU daily may be required for therapeutic effects in IBD, which is higher than typical Vitamin D dosing. For more on vitamin D, see chapter 6.

Mucilaginous herbs

These botanicals, which include DGL (deglycyrrhizinated licorice), slippery elm, marshmallow, chamomile, okra extract, and cat's claw, can provide support for healthy intestinal function by coating and soothing the intestinal lining, promoting the healing of ulcers and inflamed tissue, and reducing cramping by relaxing the intestines. Rootcology Gut R&R (1 scoop in 6 to 8 ounces of water, daily at bedtime), Designs for Health GI Revive, Biosense Clinic Mucosa-Heal, XYMOGEN GI Balance Powder, DaVinci Laboratories G.I. Benefits, Pure Encapsulations G.I. Fortify, and ReLeaf MucosaCalm are high-quality options.

Curcumin

Curcumin, the active ingredient in turmeric, has established anti-inflammatory properties and a recent study found it improved the odds of maintaining ulcerative colitis remission by a factor of three compared to placebo (the study used it in combination with mesalamine, a nonsteroidal anti-inflammatory drug used to treat ulcerative colitis, but when I consulted my friend Steve Wright, founder of the Healthy

Gut Project, about my husband's UC, he had experience using it as a stand-alone for inducing remission). Consider 500–2,000 mg per day of Rootcology Curcumin Absorb or Thorne Curcumin Phytosome.

Beneficial *E. coli* Nissle

Isolated by Alfred Nissle in 1917, this beneficial strain of the bacteria *E. coli* has been found to be as effective in maintaining remission of ulcerative colitis as mesalazine, a first-line anti-inflammatory prescription drug used to treat IBD, and may also help relieve anxiety (frequently co-occurring with IBD) by increasing the bioavailability of serotonin in the gut. This probiotic is currently manufactured and available in Germany as Mutaflor. Some importers will ship it to the U.S., and while it does require refrigeration to stay stable, keeping it out of the fridge for several days will normally have no effect on bacterial availability. That said, prolonged heat exposure can cause the bacteria to lose some of their viability. Keep this in mind when ordering.

Milk thistle

The antioxidant and anti-inflammatory properties of this liver- and gut-supporting herb support healthy bile flow and digestion and milk thistle has been found to promote healing and maintain remission in people with UC. In one study, 35 out of 38 people with UC who were given 140 mg of milk thistle daily were in complete remission with no flare-ups after six months, compared to 21 out of 32 people given a placebo. Designs for Health Milk Thistle is a high-quality option.

Psyllium

This prebiotic has been found to suppress inflammation and be particularly helpful in easing UC. In one study, 10 grams twice daily was found to significantly reduce symptoms while in another study, the same dose was as effective as mesalazine in maintaining remission. It is a main ingredient in Metamucil, Citracel, FiberCon, and other OTC fiber supplements.

Lactobacillus rhamnosus GG

This probiotic has strong anti-inflammatory properties and has been found to be as effective as mesalazine in maintaining remission of UC. Pure Encapsulations Pure GG 25B and Culturelle are two potential options.

Resveratrol

A type of polyphenol found in the skin of red grapes, peanuts, and berries, resveratrol has prebiotic, immune-modulating, anti-inflammatory, and antioxidant benefits with studies supporting its effectiveness against several autoimmune diseases, including IBD. In one study of people with active UC, supplementing with 500 mg of resveratrol for six weeks significantly improved symptoms and reduced inflammation. High-quality options are available from various companies.

Thiamine

Thiamine deficiency has been found in people with IBD and one study on the effect of thiamine on patients with Crohn's disease and ulcerative colitis published in the *Journal of Alternative and Complementary Medicine* found dosages ranging from 600 to 1,500 mg per day, depending on the body size of the individual, were effective at completely reversing symptoms associated with fatigue, one of the most common and debilitating symptoms associated with IBD, and overall intestinal functionality. I encourage you to work with a practitioner to determine the proper dosage for your needs. For more on thiamine, see chapter 6.

Seacure

Made from deep-ocean whitefish, this whole-food supplement contains naturally occurring nutrients from the fish, including omega-3 fatty acids and high concentrations of glutamine and glutamine-containing peptides. I have personally used this supplement in people with IBS and IBD with good results, and many other practitioners report Seacure reduces symptoms and restores gut integrity in their patients with Crohn's disease, UC, and IBS.

Research Corner: Emerging Treatments for IBD

Wormwood (*Artemisia absinthium*)

This herb has shown promise in inducing remission in Crohn's disease. In one study, 65 percent of participants taking 500 mg three times daily achieved near-complete remission after 8 weeks; another trial found 80 percent remission with 750 mg doses over 6 weeks (vs. 20 percent in placebo). However, wormwood contains thujone, a potentially toxic compound that can cause seizures, kidney failure, and hallucinations, so it must be used with extreme caution under medical supervision.

Please Note: Artemisia annua (sweet wormwood), a similar sounding, yet different herb, is often used in integrative GI protocols and has a better safety profile, but hasn't been specifically studied for IBD.

Hyperbaric Oxygen Therapy (HBOT)

Hypoxia, or low oxygen levels in tissues, plays a significant role in the inflammation seen in inflammatory bowel disease (IBD). When the gut lining is deprived of oxygen, it can lead to increased inflammation and damage, worsening symptoms. HBOT delivers concentrated oxygen under pressure to oxygen-deprived tissues, reducing inflammation, promoting healing, and supporting immune function. It's a promising option for IBD patients not fully helped by conventional treatments.

> **Fecal Microbiota Transplant (FMT)**
>
> FMT has demonstrated increased remission rates in both ulcerative colitis and Crohn's. One meta-analysis showed a 50 percent remission rate in UC patients receiving FMT, and a Crohn's trial found 87.5 percent stayed in remission after 10 weeks post-FMT, compared to 44.4 percent in the control group.

Things to Avoid with IBD

While the research I studied and my functional medicine training suggested high-dose probiotics and berberine could be helpful for IBD (they're often safe and very helpful in IBS), my experience with my husband and clients has revealed they can actually be triggering. Colleagues, including Debbie Steinbock, have seen the same.

I decided to create a list of things to avoid with IBD when trying to get into remission and even when staying in remission. Please note, some of these may be very helpful for other causes of IBS (and this is reason #124523 why I recommend knowing what you're dealing with)!

High-dose probiotics, such as VSL#3

VSL#3, this high-potency probiotic containing 8 strains (4 Lactobacillus, 3 Bifidobacterium, and 1 Streptococcus salivarius) is classified as a medical food and studied to help ulcerative colitis, yet in recent years, some clinicians report it can trigger IBD flares. This could be because the original formulator, Dr. Claudio De Simone, left the company that produces VSL#3 and took his proprietary formula with him. According to the Dr. De Simone the current VSL#3 formula is different from the one used in clinical trials. Dr. De Simone has sued for false advertising and unpaid royalties and taken the original formula to a new company, called Visbiome. While some clinicians are now using Visbiome instead, I have not used it personally and do not recommend VSL #3.

Berberine
Berberine has been shown to inhibit proinflammatory responses in epithelial cells, support gut barrier function, and promote recovery of colitis. Although some research and clinicians suggest this supplement may help with IBD, my experience has been that it can cause flare-ups, including GI bleeding. I personally believe berberine should be avoided, especially in the early stages of healing.

Oil of Oregano
While oil of oregano has a number of benefits for gut health, it may be too strong to use initially in those with IBD. This could be due to major changes in the gut microbiome.

Food Additives, Especially Carrageenan and Erythritol
Carrageenan
Carrageenan has been linked to increased inflammation and the development of IBD. In one small study, people with UC in remission who were given carrageenan-containing capsules relapsed while controls on a carrageenan-free diet did not! Lab tests indicated higher inflammatory markers and fecal calprotectin (a protein that may indicate inflammation) in the group exposed to carrageenan!

Erythritol
This sugar alcohol may feed *Clostridia,* a bacteria that can cause serious inflammation of the colon and is a potential UC trigger. That seemed to be the case with my husband. While healthy people may be able to tolerate this additive (I have not had issues with it personally), it can exacerbate inflammation and colitis in those who already have gut inflammation.

Other Additives

In addition to erythritol, many food additives have been linked to the development of autoimmune disease, including IBD: other sugar alcohols (including maltitol, mannitol, sorbitol, xylitol), maltodextrin, titanium dioxide, guar gum, xanthan gum, polysorbate-80, carboxymethylcellulose, soy lecithin, carrageenan, MCT oil, noncaloric artificial sweeteners such as sucralose and saccharin, ethylenediaminetetraacetate (EDTA), and microbial transglutaminases.

Systemic Enzymes

Proteolytic enzymes, especially when taken in doses higher than recommended, may lead to intestinal inflammation in people with IBD.

Fibrous Foods

These are hard to digest for anyone and may irritate the digestive tract in those with IBD and aggravate symptoms. High-fiber fruits and vegetables (avocado, artichokes, pears) as well as nuts, seeds (chia, flax, pumpkin seeds with shells), and beans are best avoided while getting into remission and perhaps a few months after.

Resistant Starch

This last one is not a definite no-no, but this type of prebiotic may fuel pathogenic bacteria such as *Klebsiella*, which may induce inflammatory bowel diseases.

My Husband's Story

I'm grateful to say that thanks to my functional medicine training and the help of some great friends and practitioners, we were able to get my husband into remission within a month of his UC diagnosis.

He's back to waking up earlier than me, going to the gym, and feeling well overall.

He does not have any remaining UC symptoms and his calprotectin level has remained at 0, though it was in the 900 range at the time of diagnosis!

He has only had two, short-lived flare-ups of UC in the last seven years, and both were due to consuming products made with erythritol! He eats everything without any digestive issues, though we do eat a mostly clean, home-cooked and gluten-free diet and avoid erythritol like the plague, he often likes to eat out and has no issues in doing so.

While protocols and causes will vary for each person, I feel these were the most helpful for him: Canasa suppositories, the semi-elemental diet, soft and mushy foods, SBI, boswellia, high-dose turmeric (curcumin), high-quality fish oil, milk thistle, mucilaginous herbs (we used Biosense Clinic Mucosaeal), and LDN. He used the suppositories, semi-elemental diet, and soft-mushy foods for approximately one month, while all of the other interventions were continued for approximately six months. He continues to take LDN, the only medication/supplement he takes regularly.

His potential causes included: hemochromatosis (iron overload, phlebotomies helped reduce inflammation while we lived in Boulder, and it actually resolved when we moved to sea level), Shiga-like toxin-producing *E. coli* (found on a GI-MAP test), and reactivated EBV (he used the herb lomatium to get the virus back into a dormant state). Stress was also a likely factor and getting it under control is a work in progress.

Inducing Remission vs. Keeping IBD in Remission

In the following chart, I have done my best to summarize the research-backed support for supplements and diets that can get IBD into remission and maintain remission. I've divided the chart by UC and Crohns', but in my experience, many of the supplements that help Crohn's disease will help UC and vice versa, even in the absence of specific studies. Please note that while there aren't many compelling studies connecting mucilaginous herbs to UC or Crohn's disease remission, they do have evidence of healing ulcers and anecdotally, they do seem to be helpful in inducing remission. Furthermore, while there are fewer studies on microscopic colitis, many of the strategies for both UC and Crohn's disease are likely to be effective for microscopic colitis.

Supplement or Diet Name	Induce Remission UC	Maintain Remission UC	Induce Remission Crohn's disease	Maintain Remission Crohn's disease
AIP Diet	X	X	X	X
Aloe vera	X	X		
Andrographis paniculata	X 1,200 mg, equal to mesalazine			
Artemisia (wormwood)			X	
Boswellia	X	X	X	X
Butyrate oral	X (adding oat bran to increase butyrate has been found to help)	X	X	
Butyrate suppositories	X			
Curcumin oral (Thorne Meriva)	X	X		
Curcumin enema	X			
Elemental Diet	X		X	
Lactobacillus rhamnosus CG		X		

Supplement or Diet Name	Induce Remission UC	Maintain Remission UC	Induce Remission Crohn's disease	Maintain Remission Crohn's disease
LDN	X	X	X	X
Milk thistle		X		
Mucilaginous herbs: slippery elm, DGL, and others	X			
Beneficial *E. coli* Nissle		X		
Omega-3 fatty acids	X	X	X	X
Psyllium		X		
Semi-Vegetarian Diet	X	X		
SBI	X			
SCD Diet	X		X	
Soft and Mushy Diet	X		X	
Vitamin B$_6$ (P5P)	X			
Vitamin D	X	X		X

Chapter Summary

- Up to 10 percent of people with IBS may actually have ulcerative colitis (UC) or Crohn's disease and 10-23 percent may have microscopic colitis, autoimmune conditions commonly referred to as inflammatory bowel disease (IBD).

- Ulcerative colitis is characterized by inflammation and ulcers (sores) along the lining of the colon and rectum, Crohn's disease involves inflammation throughout the digestive tract, and microscopic colitis refers to inflammation of the colon and rectum that is only visible under a microscope.

- Various potential causes of IBD have been proposed including immune system triggers, chronic stress, mold exposure, reactivated EBV, food additives, pathogenic *E. coli,* and certain medications.

- Prescription drugs, such as anti-inflammatories, corticosteroids, immunosuppressants, and biologics, can be helpful in lowering systemic inflammation, allowing the intestines to heal, and getting IBD into remission.

- Low dose naltrexone (LDN) can be incredibly helpful with IBD.

- Several diets, including the Soft and Mushy Diet, semi-elemental diet, semi-vegetarian, and additive-free diet, can be effective tools for inducing remission.

- Supplements to help reduce inflammation in the body include aloe vera, *andrographis paniculata,* boswellia, SBI, and butyrate.

Visit https://ibsrootcause.com/bonus for notes on this chapter.

CHAPTER 14

Toxins and Chemical Triggers

Toxins in our environment can be a hidden trigger for IBS, affecting everything from gut health to immune function. While we can't completely avoid them, awareness and small changes can make a big difference. Studies have linked IBS to certain medications, pesticides, air pollution, and contaminants in drinking water, but the list doesn't stop there. Mold toxins, heavy metals (with nickel being the most widely studied), breast implants, and toxic estrogen metabolites as well estrogen-mimicking substances like xenoestrogens can all influence gut health.

All of these toxins can disrupt the gut microbiome, lead to inflammation, and aggravate IBS symptoms, making detoxification one of the essential strategies for managing IBS.

The gut, liver, and skin are the primary organs that process toxins, and when a person has digestive issues, this puts an undue burden on the liver and skin. Normally, the liver processes toxins and waste products, sending them to the gut for elimination. If they're not properly eliminated due to constipation, they can recirculate. If a person has diarrhea, they will often lack the ability to absorb the required nutrients that act as cofactors for liver detoxification pathways.

When the liver is overwhelmed, it struggles to clear out hormones, toxins, and other waste, leading to symptoms such as fatigue, mood issues, hormonal imbalances, skin issues, and a sluggish metabolism.

Signs and symptoms of toxic exposure, liver congestion, or chemical sensitivity may include digestive problems such as gas, diarrhea, and constipation, bad breath, fatigue, weakness, headaches, skin issues like breakouts, rashes, and itchiness, joint pain, brain fog, weight loss resistance, and hormonal imbalances.

If you have multiple chemical sensitivities and/or skin reactions, in addition to digestive symptoms, this is a red flag to me that toxins may be a part of what's triggering (or worsening) your IBS or leading to co-occurring symptoms like anxiety and hormonal issues.

This chapter will focus on the most impactful toxins that can trigger IBS symptoms and strategies for mitigation. I will also share some foundational methods supporting detox pathways that I've used with my clients over the last decade. Supporting detox pathways can be an integral part of healing residual IBS symptoms and staying in balance.

Medications

Medications are an incredibly powerful healing tool, but when used inappropriately or in excess, they can cause more problems than they solve. As a pharmacist, I have unfortunately seen the dire consequences of a prescription cascade, a situation in which a person takes a medication for one symptom, only for the medication to cause additional symptoms that are then addressed with additional medications!

Often time medications used for other conditions can produce GI side effects that mimic IBS symptoms. GI distress is such a common symptom of various medications that during my years of "cramming" for pharmacy school exams that tested my knowledge of medication side effects, I chose to say "digestive disturbances" when in doubt, because most of the medications do cause digestive problems!

Opiates, for instance, are notorious for causing constipation—there's even a medication specifically designed to treat opiate-induced constipation! But there are plenty of other medications, less commonly recognized, that can quietly wreak havoc on digestion.

Could Your Medication Be Causing Your IBS Symptoms?

GI side effects from medications are so common that back in pharmacy school, if I didn't know a drug's side effects on a quiz, "digestive issues" was usually a safe guess.

If you're taking one of these medications and dealing with constipation, diarrhea, or IBD symptoms, I strongly encourage you to talk to your doctor or pharmacist about possible alternatives.

Medications That Can Cause Constipation

These can reduce gut motility, dry the stool, or block neurotransmitters needed for digestion:

- **NSAIDs (e.g., ibuprofen, naproxen):** Cause hard stools, GI damage, and have also been linked to IBD and microscopic colitis.
- **Tricyclic antidepressants (e.g., Elavil, Pamelor):** Have anticholinergic properties that slow peristalsis.
- **Antipsychotics (e.g., clozapine, olanzapine):** Block dopamine receptors, leading to sluggish digestion.
- **Opioids (e.g., oxycodone, morphine, codeine):** Activate gut opioid receptors, causing delayed transit and hard stools (opioid-induced constipation).
- **Diuretics:** Cause dehydration by flushing fluids, a major cause of constipation.
- **Antihistamines (e.g., diphenhydramine/Benadryl, cetirizine/Zyrtec):** Dehydrate and disrupt gut histamine signaling; Claritin and Allegra may have a gentler effect.

- **H2 blockers (e.g., famotidine/Pepcid, cimetidine/Tagamet):** Block histamine in the GI tract, impairing digestion.
- **Anticholinergics (e.g., tiotropium/Spiriva, benztropine/Cogentin, hyoscyamine/Levsin, diphenhydramine):** Inhibit acetylcholine, reducing gut muscle contractions. Found in meds for allergies, Parkinson's, COPD, and overactive bladder.
- **Antihypertensives (e.g., clonidine, verapamil):** Reduce smooth muscle action in the intestines, slowing motility.
- **Calcium channel blockers (e.g., verapamil, diltiazem):** Relax intestinal muscles, slowing digestion.
- **Antispasmodics (e.g., dicyclomine/Bentyl):** Reduce gut contractions, relieving cramps but potentially worsening constipation.
- **Supplements:**
  - **Calcium (especially calcium carbonate):** Contracts intestinal muscles.
  - **Iron:** Hard to digest; often causes slow, dry stools.
  - **Activated charcoal:** Binds toxins but may worsen constipation.
- **Hormones and birth control (especially those containing drospirenone):** Can alter gut motility, causing constipation in some. (Please see box for more information.)

Did Your Birth Control Trigger Your IBS?

A 2012 large-scale study found that women who used oral contraceptives containing the progestin drospirenone had a higher risk of being diagnosed with IBS compared to those taking contraceptives with levonorgestrel.

Drospirenone-based birth control pills entered the US market in 2001 with the launch of Yasmin. They quickly gained popularity due to their diuretic effect, which caused water loss, a desirable alternative to the water retention and weight gain often associated with other progestins.

However, this same diuretic action can come with trade-offs. Drospirenone, like other diuretics, blocks mineralocorticoid receptors, which are important for tissue repair. In the GI tract, this receptor blocking has been linked to a range of digestive side effects, including nausea, cramping, vomiting, diarrhea, gastritis, abdominal pain, dyspepsia, gastric bleeding, gastroenteritis, and even ulceration.

Research suggests that long-term use of drospirenone-containing contraceptives may be a trigger or exacerbating factor for IBS in some individuals.

Common drospirenone-containing birth control options include: Gianvi, Loryna, Nikki, Ocella, Syeda, Vestura, Yasmin, YAZ, Yaz 28, and Zarah.

Medications That Can Cause Diarrhea and/or IBD

Several drugs and supplements can disrupt digestion, stimulate gut motility, or alter the microbiome, leading to diarrhea and, in some cases, triggering inflammatory conditions:

- **NSAIDs (e.g., ibuprofen, naproxen):** Can irritate the GI lining, causing ulcers, diarrhea or constipation.
- **Aspirin:** has been linked to gastrointestinal irritation, may cause ulceration and diarrhea in some individuals, studies suggest long-term use may increase the risk of developing inflammatory bowel disease, particularly Crohn's disease.
- **Metformin (antidiabetic):** Alters the gut microbiome, increases bile acids, and draws excess glucose into the intestines, leading to loose stools.

- **Antibiotics:** Disrupt beneficial bacteria and may trigger overgrowth of pathogens or infections like *C. difficile*. Repeated use is linked to higher IBD risk in both children and adults.
- **SSRIs (e.g., sertraline, fluoxetine):** Stimulate gut serotonin receptors, increasing motility and cramping; sertraline in particular is linked to microscopic colitis.
- **Magnesium (supplements/antacids):** Unabsorbed magnesium pulls water into the intestines and stimulates contractions, often causing diarrhea.
- **Hormones and birth control (especially drospirenone):** Can trigger diarrhea in some, and have been linked to IBS and IBD.
- **Mycophenolic acid:** An immunosuppressant used post-transplant and in autoimmune conditions; associated with diarrhea, abdominal pain, and, in some cases, severe GI inflammation and bleeding ulcers.

Estrogen Dominance

Hormones, especially estrogen, play a key role in gut motility and imbalances can significantly worsen IBS symptoms. Estrogen dominance—where estrogen levels are too high compared to progesterone—is particularly troublesome for women with IBS-C, as excess estrogen slows down gut motility, leading to constipation, bloating, and discomfort.

Estrogen dominance can occur from using oral contraceptives, hormone replacement therapy and sometimes naturally during perimenopause, though not everyone with perimenopause experiences it.

Estrogen dominance can also occur due to certain environmental toxins, such as xenoestrogens (chemicals that mimic estrogen), found in plastics, personal care products, pesticides, and mold mycotoxins, which impair estrogen metabolism. Chronic stress and excess fat (fat cells can produce estrogen) are additional factors that can exacerbate estrogen dominance, regardless of perimenopausal status. Poor liver function and certain genetic factors, like a slow COMT enzyme, can also contribute.

How Do You Know You Have Estrogen Dominance?

Symptoms

Estrogen dominance is linked to symptoms such as:

- Anxiety, irritability, and mood swings
- Fibroids (growths in or on the wall of the uterus)
- Hot flashes
- Breast lumps and fibrocystic breasts
- Heavy periods or postmenopausal bleeding
- Irregular, frequent, sporadic, or absent periods
- Worsening symptoms of PMS or PMDD
- Thyroid nodules
- Elevated anti-thyroglobulin antibodies
- Hair loss
- Brain fog
- Autoimmunity

Testing

- A blood test can assess estrogen (estrone, E1; estradiol, E2; and estriol, E3) and progesterone levels. However, these tests often reflect highs and lows based on conventional standards and may not fully capture estrogen dominance. They don't account for the estrogen-progesterone ratio, meaning levels can appear normal while symptoms persist if estrogen is high relative to progesterone. Normal estrogen levels for menstruating women range from 15 to 350 picograms per milliliter (pg/mL), while for postmenopausal women, levels should be below 10 pg/mL.

- Precision Analytical DUTCH Complete, a dried urine test that gives a much bigger picture of what is going on with hormone levels, including estrogen metabolism, testosterone, adrenal hormones, and other markers that can be useful for uncovering the root cause of your hormone imbalance. This test is also helpful for creating a personalized treatment plan with your practitioner. While I am a big proponent of patient self-management and often recommend people self-order and interpret their own labs, I recommend working with a practitioner for interpretation of this particular test. This is because, while the test is easy to do, it's a bit complicated to interpret.

Mitigation Options
Balancing Female Hormones

There are three hormonal patterns that can be considered estrogen dominance:

1. Normal estrogen with low progesterone
2. High estrogen with normal progesterone
3. High estrogen with low progesterone

Some women may need to focus on lowering estrogen, others on increasing progesterone, while some women will need to focus on both strategies!

To balance hormones, consider the following:

- Stress less: Stress can lead to the "pregnenolone steal," which forces our adrenals to decline the production of progesterone in favor of making more cortisol. The strategies in chapter 11 can help.

- Review your hormonal therapies: Work with your doctor to adjust your hormonal medications to ensure you're dosed properly.

You may wish to consider birth control pills without drospirenone or hormone-free alternatives such as fertility tracking apps including Natural Cycles or the Lady-Comp device.

- Clean up your personal care and cleaning products in order to avoid exposure to xenoestrogens: Women, on average, use 12 personal care and cosmetic products per day, which amounts to 168 different chemical ingredients! Environmental Working Group's Guide to Healthy Cleaning and Skin Deep Database (ewg.org) can help you find cleaner alternatives to conventional personal care and cleaning products.

- Filter your water: Remove xenoestrogens, chlorine, fluoride and hormones from drinking and cooking water with a high-quality filter.

- Include brassica/cruciferous vegetables: broccoli sprouts, turnips, cauliflower, cabbage, and collard greens contain indole-3-carbinol and (I3C) and diindolylmethane (DIM), compounds that support estrogen metabolism and detoxification.

- Add high-fiber produce: Fiber binds excess estrogen it in the digestive tract allowing for its excretion through the stool. Aim for at least 25 to 35 grams of fiber per day from sources like vegetables, fruits, and whole grains. Soluble fiber found in foods such as flaxseeds and oats can be particularly effective in supporting healthy estrogen metabolism. Aim for 1 to 2 tablespoons of flaxseeds per day. For additional support, consider Pure Encapsulations PureLean Fiber, a blend of fibers and prebiotics.

- Reduce or eliminate coffee and caffeine: Caffeine intake, especially in high doses has been associated with higher levels of estrogen and may cause a decline in progesterone by contributing to the "pregnenolone steal."

- Incorporate seed cycling to support hormones throughout your menstrual cycle.
    - During the first half of your cycle (days 1 to 14), eat 2 tablespoons of fresh (not roasted) ground flax or pumpkin seeds per day to help the body produce estrogen.
    - During the second half of the cycle (days 15–28), eat 2 tablespoons of fresh (not roasted) ground sunflower seeds or sesame seeds per day to support progesterone production through zinc and vitamin E. Seed cycling has been studied in women ages 18 to 45 to support hormone balance.
    - You can prepare your own seeds, and I also like using the Beeya blend of nutrient- dense seeds in my salads and smoothies.

- DIM (diindolylmethane): A natural substance found in many cruciferous vegetables that can also be taken in capsule form, DIM is helpful for estrogen dominance, specifically in the case of excess estrogen with normal levels of progesterone. The therapeutic dose is 200 mg per day and high-quality options are Wellena DIM and Pure Encapsulations DIMPRO 100.

- Vitamin C: Research shows women who take vitamin C have significantly increased levels of progesterone. One study showed women who took 750 mg of vitamin C daily increased their progesterone levels by 77 percent. For more on vitamin C, see chapter 6.

- Zinc: Zinc helps the pituitary gland to release follicle-stimulating hormone (FSH). FSH is needed for ovulation and it also signals to your ovaries to produce more progesterone. For more on zinc, see chapter 6.

- Magnesium: This important mineral can help support progesterone levels by supporting stress and helping you feel calmer. It also assists in the breakdown of the antagonistic estrogen metabolites, which helps to reduce estrogen dominance. For more on magnesium, see chapter 6.

- Vitamin E: Research shows vitamin E can help to improve luteal blood flow and raise progesterone levels in some women. NOW Foods Sun-E 400 is a high-quality supplement option for additional support.

- Vitamin B_6 (as the most bioavailable form, P5P): B vitamins help combat stress and assist the liver in breaking down estrogen byproducts, which can help reduce estrogen dominance. Studies have shown 200–800 mg per day of vitamin B_6 can raise progesterone levels and reduce estrogen, with noticeable improvements in PMS symptoms. Please note the pyridoxine form of B_6 in doses above 300 mg has the potential to cause peripheral neuropathy, due to buildup from a toxic pyridoxine metabolite. Using the P5P version of B_6 prevents this potential side effect. High-quality options of P5P in therapeutic doses include: Rootcology P5P, Designs for Health P-5-P, Pure Encapsulations P5P 50, and SFI Health P-5-P.

- Bio-identical, or natural, progesterone: Using a bioidentical oral or topical progesterone may help balance female hormones. Prescriptions for oral progesterone include Prometrium (and generics), as well as compounded options. Topical preparations can be made by compounding pharmacies and supplement companies including my friend's company Wellena (Wellena ProgestPure Cream). I generally recommend working with a practitioner for proper dosing.

Mycotoxins (Mold)

Mold toxicity is an often-overlooked trigger for various health issues, including IBS and IBD. While mold is all around us, indoor exposure in water-damaged buildings poses the greatest risk. Mold thrives in damp, poorly ventilated spaces like basements, bathrooms, or areas previously flooded. While mold can sometimes be detected visually or by its musty smell, not all mold is visible. We also encounter mycotoxins through food, though this impact is typically low unless we're already dealing with a high mold burden. Our liver can detoxify mycotoxins, but if exposure is high or detox pathways are impaired—due to factors like nutrient deficiencies, overloaded detox systems, or MTHFR gene mutations—mycotoxins can build up and lead to illness.

The most common molds—*Cladosporium, Penicillium, Alternaria,* and *Aspergillus*—can produce toxic compounds called mycotoxins. These harmful substances can enter the body through inhalation, skin contact, or ingestion, and impair health in the following ways:

- Promoting dysbiosis: Mycotoxins kill beneficial bacteria and allow harmful microbes to flourish. For example, the mycotoxin deoxynivalenol (DON), found in cereals, increases *Bacteroides* levels, which are linked to Crohn's disease and celiac disease. Mycophenolic acid, an immune-suppressing mycotoxin produced by multiple strains of *Penicillium,* decreases beneficial *Firmicutes* and *Bacteroidetes* and the production of butyrate. Interestingly, mycophenolic acid has been turned into an immune suppressing medication and 30 percent of people taking it experience GI symptoms, ranging from abdominal pain and diarrhea to life-threatening bleeding ulcers!

- Increasing intestinal permeability and vulnerability to gut infections: mycotoxins, including DON, can weaken the gut lining, contributing to intestinal permeability and food allergies. Ochratoxin reduces gut-protective SCFAs such as butyrate. This leaves individuals vulnerable to gut infections such as *Candida* overgrowth, *Clostridia, H. pylori,* and parasitic infections.

- Impacting bile flow: Bile is thought to be reduced in the presence of mycotoxins, and this may create a vicious cycle where mold reduces bile, which is needed to excrete mold from the body.

- Cntributing to histamine intolerance: Mold exposure can trigger mast cell activation and excess histamine production.

- Compromising nutrient absorption: Mycotoxins damage intestinal villi, leading to nutrient deficiencies.

- Disrupting hormone balance: Mycotoxins can mimic estrogen and interfere with the body's ability to detox excess hormones, resulting in estrogen dominance.

How Do You Know You Have Mycotoxin Toxicity?
Symptoms

When it comes to mold exposure, not everyone is affected in the same way. Even those living in the same home may develop different symptoms—or no symptoms at all—depending on their genes. That said, common symptoms of mold exposure include:

- Brain issues: such as brain fog, anxiety, depression, tremors, vertigo, trouble focusing, cognitive impairment, insomnia, fatigue, potentially due to mitochondrial damage

- Digestive problems: abdominal pain, gas, bloating, diarrhea

- Respiratory and Sinus Issues: difficulty breathing, cough, sinus congestion, nasal blockages, sneezing, watery eyes

- Inflammation and Pain: Arthritis, joint pain, inflammation, headaches, migraines, muscle weakness

- Additional: urinary frequency, eczema, rashes, immune suppression, developmental delays in children, chemical sensitivity, autoimmune flare-ups

Testing

These tests will help you determine if your body has been colonized by mold and if you are currently being exposed to mycotoxins—and if so, which ones. Knowing exactly which molds and mycotoxins are in your body can help you identify the specific binders, nutrients, herbs, and medications most effective at targeting and clearing them.

To determine whether mold has colonized your body:

- Organic Acids Test (OAT), a urine test which checks for mold metabolites and oxalate metabolites that may indicate mold colonization in the body. This test is especially relevant to people who may have gotten out of a moldy situation but are still symptomatic, as well as those who are currently exposed.

- Mycotoxin Testing: Urine testing such as Mosaic Diagnostics MycoTOX Profile, Vibrant Wellness Mycotoxins Test, and Real-Time Laboratories MycoToxin Panel can help reveal which types of mold mycotoxins are present. Knowing which mycotoxin is present can help us tailor the treatment approach.

- Comprehensive stool analysis, to reveal if you have additional mold-induced dysbiosis necessary to address. Some common patterns I see in people with mold exposure are *H. pylori,* high beta-glucuronidase (an enzyme produced by pathogenic gut bacteria that can interfere with the body's detoxification process and estrogen levels), low secretory IgA (a gut-protective antibody) due to immune suppression from mold, low beneficial flora, and a higher susceptibility to parasites.

To determine whether mold has colonized your home, mold testing can be conducted by a professional service or you can do it yourself with a home kit. Some individuals have found using ImmunoLytics in-home testing or the ERMI test helpful.

What To Do About Mold Toxicity

Recovering from mold toxicity often requires a comprehensive approach. First, it's essential to limit further exposure by addressing mold in your environment. Additionally, supporting detoxification pathways, especially the liver and bile flow, is crucial, as mold produces various toxins that may build up in the body. Taking binders can help move mold out of the body, while antifungals are necessary to kill the mold if it has colonized your gut or sinuses. In some cases, working with a practitioner who specializes in mold and mycotoxin illness is necessary. Additionally, it may involve moving out of your home or workplace and hiring a qualified inspector and remediation company to remove mold from your environment.

Limiting Mold Exposure
Eliminate your exposure
Depending on the circumstances, this can be as easy as finding a leak in a bathroom, cutting off the wet baseboards, replacing them, and running an air filter, or as complicated as hiring specially trained inspectors

and a professional mold remediation service to safely remove the contaminated parts of your home and prevent additional mold exposure.

Air filter

A quality air filter, such as the Air Doctor and JASPR, can help purify your living environment of airborne molds and other allergens. Air filters are best for maintenance and prevention of mold-related issues.

Supporting Detox Pathways

Supporting liver detox pathways is essential in mold toxicity, as the liver can become overwhelmed and allow toxins to recirculate. It relies on processes like glucuronidation, sulfation, methylation, and glutathione conjugation to neutralize mycotoxins for elimination via bile or urine. Each mold toxin is cleared through different pathways and responds to specific binders and nutrients.

If you don't know which mycotoxins you're dealing with, begin with a broad-spectrum liver support and binder protocol. Once identified, you can tailor support accordingly:

- Glutathione pathway clears aflatoxin B-1 and ochratoxin A; supported by alpha lipoic acid, selenium, and magnesium.
- Methylation pathway clears *fusarium* and *zearalenone*; supported by B vitamins, zinc, and SAMe.
- Sulfation pathway clears *deoxynivalenol* and *trichothecene*; supported by sulfur-rich foods and retinoic acid.
- Glucuronidation clears multiple mycotoxins and is enhanced by calcium D-glucarate, dandelion root, and astaxanthin.

Starting broad ensures you're covering all bases before customizing your detox to match specific mycotoxin test results. See page 75 for the protocol I use with clients.

Binders

Binders are compounds that help remove toxins from the body, preventing their reabsorption before they're eliminated. They can be particularly helpful for clearing mycotoxins from mold exposure. Here are some commonly used binders:

- Cholestyramine powder: A prescription binder often used for thirty to ninety days to help bind and remove mold toxins from the body.

- *S. boulardii*: A beneficial yeast that can assist in reducing mycotoxins in the gut while supporting overall gut health. High-quality options include Rootcology *S. Boulardii*, Pure Encapsulations *Saccharomyces boulardii*, Designs for Health Floramyces, and XYMOGEN Saccharomycin DF.

- Glucomannan: This soluble fiber binds with mold toxins in the gut and can also help with constipation. Take ½ teaspoon 1-2 times daily with water, 30-45 minutes before meals. NOW Glucomannan is a good option.

- ION Gut Support*: A humic acid-based product that helps the body clear out mold toxins and glyphosate, while also supporting mineral balance.

- Activated charcoal: Known for binding toxins and supporting loose stools, activated charcoal is popular for mold detox. However, it may cause constipation, so avoid it if you're prone to constipation. Take 1-3 capsules once per day, at least an hour away from food or supplements. Integrative Therapeutics Activated Charcoal is an option to consider.

Each binder has a unique affinity for various mycotoxins, and the right one for you may depend on your individual mycotoxin exposure and symptoms. Some companies offer combination products that target multiple mycotoxins, such as Biocidin Botanicals GI Detox, which includes zeolite clay, activated charcoal, aloe vera, pectin, silica, and humic powder.

Antifungals

Antifungals are often a forgotten, but important step for removing the mold from the body. Even if we are out of a moldy environment, our bodies can become "mold factories" if we are colonized. Most people will benefit from a sinus protocol, as well as a gut protocol.

Please note, taking antifungals without supporting detox pathways and using binders can result in worsening symptoms, so please consider using both for at least one to two weeks before considering antifungals.

For gut colonization:
- Antifungal medication such as amphotericin B, nystatin, fluconazole, or itraconazole: for thirty to ninety days for killing mold in the body
- Antifungal supplements may include: oil of oregano, berberine, and various botanical blends such as Biocidin Botanicals GI Detox

For sinus colonization:
- Propolis nasal spray (consider Beekeeper's Naturals Nasal Spray)
- Xlear nasal spray
- Itraconazole nasal spray compounds (available with a prescription through a compounding pharmacy)

As much as I wanted to, I couldn't fit my detailed, 60-page mold protocol that identifies the best treatments for specific mold symptoms and toxins in this book. If you're dealing with mold toxicity, please go to ibsrootcause.com/bonus to get my full protocol.

> ### Preventing Mold Growth
>
> An ounce of prevention is worth a pound of cure! A few steps to inhibit mold growth include the following.
>
> - All sources of uncontrolled moisture should be eliminated (e.g., roof leaks, pipe leaks, flooding).
>
> - All heat/air ductwork systems should be cleaned every two years, and all of the seals on the ductwork should be inspected and repaired, if necessary.
>
> - Leave your washer and dryer doors open while not in use, and spray with a non-toxic bio-balancing spray after each use.
>
> - Increase ventilation in bathrooms (open windows, turn on fan) to help remove moisture during and after use.

Cleaning Up Your Home Environment

Reducing toxic exposure can be a helpful tool for IBS symptoms, and small changes can make a big difference. I always say that healing starts at home, and a big part of what I have recommended to my clients is to focus on making your home a safe space.

I generally recommend starting in the kitchen, opting for non-toxic cookware like glass, ceramic, or cast iron, and swapping out plastic food storage for glass or BPA-free options. Using chlorine-free parchment paper in place of aluminum foil, and replacing plastic cutting boards and cooking utensils with wood can limit the microplastics that get into our circulation.

Water is an important source of toxins (and in some cases parasites!), so installing a reverse osmosis filter to remove contaminants can be a game changer for getting well and staying well.

To reduce exposure to airborne toxins:

- Invest in an Air Purifier: Using a high-efficiency particulate air (HEPA) filter in your home, especially in bedrooms, can significantly reduce indoor air pollution. Consider the JASPR and AirDoctor as potential options.

- Houseplants: Plants such as Golden Pothos and snake plants can naturally help filter toxins from the air.

- Limit Outdoor Activity on High-Pollution Days: Check air quality reports and try to avoid strenuous outdoor activities during periods of high pollution.

Do Airborne Toxins Impact the Gut?

Airborne toxins, especially fine particulate matter from industrial activities and traffic, are known to affect lung health, but they also have a significant impact on the gut. Studies have demonstrated that air pollution can alter the gut microbiome, leading to an increased risk of IBS and other gastrointestinal issues.

Fine particulate matter can enter the body through inhalation, accumulate in the digestive system, and cause oxidative stress, inflammation, and alterations in gut motility. Research has shown that exposure to air pollution can lead to an increase in harmful bacteria in the gut, while reducing beneficial bacteria like *Akkermansia*, which are essential for maintaining a healthy gut barrier.

Implant Illness

There is increasing awareness about something called implant illness that can occur due to various types of implants. The two types of implants that seem to be most relevant with regard to IBS include mesh implants for hernias as well as various types of breast implants.

A "Mesh" of a Situation

Mesh implantation is commonly used for hernia repair, but some patients experience complications that start with insertion and resolve after mesh removal, a condition known as mesh implant illness (MII). Symptoms may include chronic inflammation, fatigue, pain, rashes, bloating, autoimmune issues, and signs of chronic infection. While the exact cause is unclear, MII is thought to be a systemic immune reaction to the mesh as a foreign body.

In one study of 28 symptomatic patients, 68 percent saw symptom improvement within a month of mesh removal. A case study of a fifty-year-old woman diagnosed with IBS after hernia mesh placement reported complete resolution of symptoms after surgical removal, which revealed the mesh had eroded into her small bowel. Since many mesh materials contain nickel, systemic nickel sensitivity may also play a role (see chapter 4).

Breast Implant Illness

Breast implant illness (BII) is a condition where women develop systemic symptoms after receiving implants, including inflammation, fatigue, brain fog, joint pain, anxiety, loss of sight and hearing, and weight loss. Gastrointestinal symptoms are also common, with many women reporting IBS-like issues such as abdominal pain and alternating constipation and diarrhea. In some cases, symptom resolution occurs only after implant removal, suggesting a possible immune or inflammatory reaction to the implants.

Glyphosate

Glyphosate, the active ingredient in Roundup, is a controversial herbicide. Although the EPA stated in 2020 it's "unlikely to be a human carcinogen," over 20 countries, including France, Italy, and Thailand, have banned or restricted its use due to health concerns.

Research suggests glyphosate may disrupt the gut microbiome. One study found it harmed 54 percent of common gut bacteria, including beneficial species like *Bifidobacterium*, while more harmful bacteria like *Clostridium* were resistant and could flourish, potentially weakening the gut lining and increasing infection risk.

Some experts believe glyphosate use on wheat may contribute to rising rates of celiac disease and gluten sensitivity, as it mimics celiac-like effects and impairs vitamin D metabolism. It's also been linked to increases in rod-shaped bacteria (*Prevotella* and *Actinomyces*) associated with celiac risk.

Glyphosate enters the body through contaminated food, water, soil, and air. While eating organic helps, exposure can still occur through herbicide drift. If you live in a country where glyphosate is still used and have digestive issues, consider testing your levels. I recommend the Glyphosate Test from Mosaic Diagnostics (urine-based).

What To Do About Glyphosate Toxicity
Avoidance
It can be difficult to avoid glyphosate exposure completely, even on a one hundred percent organic diet, but prioritizing a mostly organic diet may still help reduce exposure. Studies have shown organic fruits and vegetables have lower levels of pesticide residue—and glyphosate is not allowed to be used on organic products—and higher levels of antioxidants, which have anti-inflammatory benefits. If you cannot buy organic all the time, use the Environmental Working Group's (EWG)

Clean Fifteen (the least contaminated fruits and veggies) and Dirty Dozen (most pesticide-contaminated produce) lists to help prioritize which produce to buy organic. (Access the most up-to-date versions of these lists at ewg.org.)

Filter air and water
The glyphosate used in agriculture tends to end up in our air and our water supply. To help reduce your exposure, use an air filter and a water filter in your home. For countertop water filters, I recommend the AquaTru or Clearly Filtered. For air filters, consider the JASPR or Air-Doctor.

Support detox pathways
While the research on how to accelerate glyphosate elimination from the body is lacking, I have seen some people lower levels by using my two-week Liver Support Protocol in my book *Hashimoto's Protocol* and sauna. Additionally, current research suggests it is excreted primarily through the urine and feces, largely unchanged, thus proper hydration and adequate bowel movements are important. See the box on page 446 for more.

Supplement Recommendations
Glycine
Glycine is an amino acid that may help remove glyphosate from the body. Experts suggest starting with 1 teaspoon (4 grams) of glycine powder twice a day for a few weeks, then reducing to ¼ teaspoon (1 gram) twice daily. This process helps flush glyphosate through urine. High-quality brands include Pure Encapsulations and Designs for Health. If you're low in vitamin B_6/P5P, glycine may cause restlessness, so consider adding Rootcology P5P to your routine.

ION* Gut Support

The humic acid in this liquid supplement improves the gut lining's ability to keep glyphosate out, promotes the production of beneficial enzymes, and repairs intestinal permeability.

Chlorella

This blue-green algae is known for its ability to help bind to and pull heavy metals from the body, and it can act similarly in removing glyphosate from the digestive tract. NOW Foods Chlorella is a high-quality option. Please note that I don't recommend high iodine foods or supplements like chlorella for those with Hashimoto's, as excess levels can actually trigger and worsen Hashimoto's symptoms.

Additional Interventions to Consider

Avoid gluten

Some experts believe the real reason for gluten sensitivity may be due to glyphosate contamination, as conventional wheat in the U.S. is often sprayed with this chemical. Studies have noted the similarities between the effects of glyphosate on our health and the symptoms of celiac disease, suggesting glyphosate may be a causal factor in the increasing rates of celiac disease in the US.

> ## Supporting Detox Pathways
>
> When I realized that a lot of my clients were dealing with chemical sensitivities, I developed a two-week-long program that focuses on removing toxic backlogs. Participants in this program find that digestive symptoms, fatigue, pain and chemical sensitivities greatly improve after completion. We focus on removing common reactive foods (gluten, dairy and soy), while adding liver supportive foods, lifestyle changes, dietary adjustments and sweating.

Here are the key elements of the program:

Liver-Supportive Foods

- Hot lemon water: Drink first thing in the morning to support liver detox.
- Beets: Rich in phytonutrients for detoxification.
- Cruciferous vegetables: Support estrogen metabolism.
- Cilantro: Acts as a natural chelator.
- Fiber: Helps excrete toxins and excess hormones, especially when addressing constipation.
- Sprouts: Natural enzymes in sprouts aid detoxification.
- Green juices and chlorophyll: These support detox and reduce inflammation.
- Fermented foods: Probiotics aid detox but should be avoided if dealing with overgrowth.
- Turmeric: Curcumin detoxifies metals and toxins.
- Berries: High in antioxidants to support detox.

Hydrotherapy and Sweating

- Hot baths: Stimulate circulation and detoxification, especially with Epsom salts to promote magnesium absorption.
- Saunas: Infrared saunas are gentle and help detox through sweat. Aim for 30-minute sessions, four times a week.
- Exercise: Regular movement boosts lymphatic flow and sweat, aiding detoxification. Choose the intensity that suits your health journey.
- Hot yoga: Combines heat and movement to enhance detox.

Supplements for Detox Pathways

- Liver supportive herbs: (milk thistle, quercetin, green tea extract): Support liver detoxification. Options include Rootcology Liver Reset Powder, and Designs for Health VegeCleanse or PaleoCleanse.
- Gallbladder supportive supplements: (dandelion, taurine, methionine, ox bile): Help bile flow, which is essential for detox. Options include Rootcology Liver and Gallbladder Support, Designs for Health LV-GB, or Pure Encapsulations Digestion GB.
- Methylated B vitamins and methylfolate: Support methylation pathways for detox, especially for estrogen dominance and mold toxicity. Consider Rootcology MTHFR Pathways, XYMOGEN Methyl Protect, Ortho Molecular Methyl CpG, or Pure Encapsulations Homocysteine Factors.
- Amino acids (glycine, taurine, cysteine, methionine, glutamine): Aid in toxin elimination. Rootcology Amino Support or Designs for Health Amino-D-Tox.
- NAC (N-acetyl cysteine): Supports detox by boosting glutathione levels. Consider Rootcology Pure N Acetyl Cysteine, Pure Encapsulations NAC, or Designs for Health N Acetyl-Cysteine.
- Magnesium citrate: Supports regular bowel movements, essential for toxin elimination. For ways to replenish magnesium, see chapter 6.

I have outlined the details of this program in my book *Hashimoto's Protocol* and in a guided two-week course called the Root Cause Reset. I also created a detailed supplement guide for readers of this book that can be found at ibsrootcause.com/bonus.

Chapter Summary

- Certain medications (NSAIDs, opioid pain medications, antidepressants, allergy medications, and antispasmodics, among others), the weed killer glyphosate, breast implants, and mold mycotoxins can cause IBS symptoms.

- Sweating (hot yoga, sauna) and supplements including liver supportive herbs, amino acids, NAC, and magnesium citrate support the liver's detoxification pathways.

- Targeted interventions may be necessary depending on the toxin you have been exposed to.

- Testing can be helpful in tailoring your detoxification protocol.

Visit https://ibsrootcause.com/bonus for notes on this chapter.

PART III

Creating Your Healing Plan

CHAPTER 15

Where to Start

I know I've shared a lot of potential IBS triggers with you, and if you're feeling a bit overwhelmed, that's completely understandable. It can seem like there's a mountain of things to address, but take a deep breath, you're not alone on this journey, and healing doesn't have to happen all at once. The good news is that every small step you take is a step toward feeling better. Together, we'll break this down into manageable pieces, and with each change, you'll be one step closer to reclaiming your health. You've already made it this far, and I have every confidence that you can do this! Let's take it one step at a time, and I'll be here to guide you along the way.

While there's always more than one way to peel a potato, I generally take a streamlined, stepwise approach to help guide people through gut healing. Doing everything at once can be overwhelming, and some steps, while necessary, if done too soon may produce less than desirable outcomes.

If I were working with you as a health consultant, I would review a list of your symptoms and your medical records and recommend relevant testing, as well as some dietary approaches to kick off your healing process. I may also recommend some helpful strategies to manage symptoms while healing.

As you start making changes, I would recommend that you observe and track your symptoms and bowel movements. These will help to determine next steps.

Step 1 Fundamental Protocols
Remove Reactive Foods

Diet is often the very first intervention I would recommend for someone with digestive symptoms, as it's a quick path to feeling better, and doesn't necessarily require testing right away, but can be adjusted based on test results.

Multiple diets have been reported to relieve IBS-related symptoms but the right healing diet for you will depend on your unique health history, food sensitivities, microbiome health, infections, and many other individualized factors.

In some cases, the diets are a temporary measure to reduce symptoms, while working on underlying causes, in other cases, the diets may be lifelong.

A great place to start for most people with IBS symptoms is the gluten-free, dairy-free, soy-free, and additive-free diets, with many people reporting symptom relief with the elimination of the aforementioned foods. For people who have already tried this approach, I may recommend a more comprehensive elimination diet, while awaiting test results. See appendix, How to Do an Elimination Diet.

Support Good Digestion

As you embark on a healing diet, I would also encourage you to focus on calming your "fight-or-flight" response and getting your body into a parasympathetic ("rest and digest") state for optimal healing through many of the strategies shared in chapter 11 and focusing on the best practices for digestion. Digestive enzymes may be helpful here, though avoid Betaine with Pepsin until testing confirms you are negative for *H. pylori* or have cleared the infection as it can potentially worsen *H. pylori* infections.

Address Motility Issues and Add Probiotics

As we focus on good digestion, we also address any motility-related issues and support your body's microbiome. I often find that using *bifido*-based and spore-based probiotics and motility support such as P5P, magnesium citrate, and carnitine can be a great way to start resolving slow motility and constipation, while using the SIBO-safe beneficial yeast *S. boulardii* can help with resolving diarrhea as well as help with overcoming infections.

Step 2 Testing

In some cases, a few weeks of dietary changes, digestion best practices, motility support, and probiotics will resolve IBS. In other cases, individuals may have additional causes contributing to IBS symptoms that may need to be addressed. Think of the various IBS triggers as tacks stuck on the bottom of your heel. If you only have one tack and remove it, you'll feel a lot better. If you have multiple tacks and remove just one, you might feel somewhat better, but not all the way!

Root cause testing allows us to uncover the additional tacks!

Once a person receives the results of root cause testing, I would recommend a targeted protocol that's described in detail in each of the chapters in this book. In some cases, the protocol may be based on medications or supplements, in other cases, lifestyle changes.

IBS

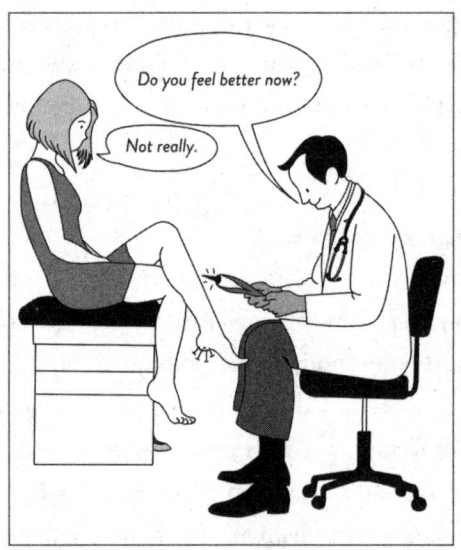

Testing to Consider

In addition to red flag testing done with a gastroenterologist to rule out differential diagnoses for IBS such as celiac disease, IBD, and stomach cancer (see page 304), I would also often suggest the following tests for most people with IBS.

- An IgG food sensitivity test, specifically Alletess Lab 96 Food Sensitivity Panel or Alletess Lab 184 Food Sensitivity Panel to find trigger foods
- A comprehensive stool analysis test such as Diagnostic Solutions GI-MAP, Vibrant Wellness Gut Zoomer 3.0, Genova Diagnostics GI Effects, Mosaic Diagnostics Comprehensive Stool Analysis, Doctor's Data GI 360
- An additional parasite test, either Parawellness Research Comprehensive Parasite Test or Vibrant Wellness Gut Zoomer 3.0
- An Organic Acids Test (OAT) from Mosaic Diagnostics to test for yeast, mold, *Candida,* and *Clostridia* metabolites, elevated

ammonia, neurotransmitter metabolites, oxalates, salicylates, and many other root causes.
- A SIBO test such as the Genova Diagnostics 3-Hour Lactulose Kit, Gemelli Biotech Trio-smart SIBO breath test, or Commonwealth Diagnostics SIBO and IMO tests
- A full thyroid panel, which includes not only TSH and T4, but also T3, and the two most common Hashimoto's antibodies, TPO and TG antibodies, to determine if thyroid hormones were playing a role in IBS symptoms

I may consider additional tests, such as adrenal, hormone, or toxins tests, depending on the person's symptoms or test results.

Step 3 Advanced Protocols Based on Test Results
Adjusting Your Diet

Based on your test results, you may wish to change your diet accordingly.

1. If you have atopy and have pursued IgE testing, you may wish to avoid the foods that came up on the test and to follow the IgE guided elimination diet.
2. If you have celiac disease, you may require a lifelong gluten-free diet and you may also need to avoid dairy and gluten cross reactive foods.
3. If testing has confirmed systemic nickel sensitivity, follow the low-nickel diet.
4. If you have done IgG testing, you will want to consider an IgG guided elimination diet.
5. If testing shows that you have SIBO, consider the low FODMAP diet.
6. If you have *Candida*, mold, and/or oxalate issues, consider the anti-*Candida* diet, the low-histamine diet, and/or low-oxalate diet.

7. The low-salicylate diet can be helpful if you have elevated salicylates and allergic symptoms.
8. If you have Hashimoto's, you may wish to start with a gluten-, dairy-, and soy-free diet, and perhaps consider a Paleo diet and an autoimmune Paleo diet. The low-iodine diet may also help.
9. If testing reveals you have a parasitic infection, you may wish to consider a polyphenol-rich diet to support healing in addition to a parasite clearing protocol.
10. If testing reveals you have inflammatory bowel disease, you may wish to consider the Elemental Diet, Soft and Mushy Diet, the Additive-Free Diet, and the Specific Carbohydrate Diet.

Go to ibsrootcause.com/bonus to download various IBS Dietary Plans, including a FODMAP plan, a simple elimination diet plan, and a comprehensive elimination diet that includes food lists and twenty-one days' worth of recipes and a symptom journal.

Resolve Infections with Antimicrobial Therapies

In my experience with complex clients, they often have more than one thing going on. It's not uncommon for tests to find SIBO, fungal overgrowth, protozoa, and *H. pylori* in one person with digestive issues.

The functional medicine approach for treating these infections and overgrowths is a top-down one, starting with the stomach (*H. pylori*), then small intestine (SIBO), and lastly the colon (protozoa). Many times, treating *H. pylori* can resolve SIBO, and treating protozoa can resolve yeast issues, so *Candida* is treated last.

Generally speaking, both medications and herbal remedies have pros and cons for treating infections and overgrowths, and so I always take into consideration the client's test results, sensitivities and preferences when choosing a protocol.

If my clients aren't able to do testing, I may instead recommend broad-spectrum herbal protocols for *H. pylori*, SIBO, and protozoa, keeping the same order in mind to cover all of our bases. The beauty of herbal protocols is that many of the herbs have activity against multiple infections. For example, Berberine works for *H. pylori*, SIBO, and certain protozoa, while oil of oregano has anti-SIBO, antiparasitic, and antifungal properties!

A sample broad-spectrum infection protocol may look like this . . .

H. pylori *Protocol*
- Mastic Gum: three times per day for thirty to sixty days
- DGL: three times per day for thirty to sixty days
- S. boulardii: once per day for thirty to sixty days

After that point, we would focus on the SIBO, protozoa, and yeast . . .

- Oil of Oregano: three times per day for sixty days
- Berberine: three times per day for sixty days
- S. boulardii: twice per day for sixty days

Antimicrobial Herbs and Supplements

Berberine

Berberine reduces intestinal permeability and increases the thickness of the mucus layer in the gut. It helps clear hydrogen and methane SIBO and its anti-yeast and antifungal properties help clear Candida. It contains powerful antimicrobial properties that can help clear a variety of infections, including *H. pylori* strains resistant to antibiotics. It can help clear out protozoa such as *Blastocystis hominis, Dientamoeba, Giardia, Pentatrichomonas,* and *Entamoeba histolytica*. Its antifungal properties help clear mold from the body. Therapeutic doses are about 1,200 mg per day, divided in three doses and taken for about sixty days. In certain cases of *B. hominis* infections, I pair berberine with oil of oregano and *S. boulardii*.

Brand options include Rootcology Berberine, Candibactin-BR, Integrative Therapeutics Berberine, NOW Foods Berberine, and Pure Encapsulations Berberine UltraSorb.

Biocidin Botanicals Biocidin Liquid

This broad-spectrum formula removes pathogens including Clostridia. Begin with 1 drop and gradually increase up to 5 drops 3 times per day, or as directed by your health care professional.

Black seed oil (*Nigella sativa*)

Black seed oil exhibits anti-microbial properties against *Candida*, *H. pylori*, *Blasto*, *Giardia*, *Entamoeba histolytica*, and *Pentatrichomonas* infections.

Therapeutic doses range from 2-4 g per day, divided in 2-3 doses and taken for 15 days.

Brand options include Rootcology Black Cumin Seed Extract and Organika Black Cumin Seed Oil Capsules.

Cat's claw

Cat's claw supports the clearance of multiple pathogenic infections and is effective against a variety of protozoa such as *Plasmodium* and *Babesia*. It works in synergy with monolaurin, which has antiparasitic properties against *Blastocystis hominis*, *Giardia*, and *Entamoeba histolytica* and activity against *H. pylori*. Quicksilver Scientific Cat's Claw Elite contains both cat's claw and monolaurin.

Deglycyrrhizinated licorice (DGL)

DGL promotes the healing of ulcers, a common complication attributed to *H. pylori*, and may also help with clearing *H. pylori*, infections, and acid reflux. It's typically taken three times per day for sixty days. Consider Pure Encapsulations DGL Plus.

Garlic oil

Garlic oil helps clear methane SIBO and antifungal properties can help treat *Candida*, helps clear rotavirus and has antiparasitic properties against protozoa such as *Blastocystis hominis, Babesia, Dientamoeba, Giardia, Endolimax nana,* and *Entamoeba histolytica* and antimicrobial activity against *H. pylori*. Typically taken three times per day for sixty days. Brand options include NOW Foods Garlic Oil and Designs for Health Allicillin.

Grapefruit seed extract

Help inhibits the growth of fungal cells. Follow package instructions. Consider Pure Encapsulations Grapefruit Seed Extract and Nutribiotic GSE.

Mastic gum

Effective against multiple strains of *H. pylori*. Usually taken three times per day for sixty days. Consider Allergy Research Group Mastica.

Oil of oregano

It helps clear hydrogen and methane SIBO, Candida, and norovirus. It has powerful antibacterial and antiprotozoal properties, and is particularly effective for treating *Blastocystis hominis, Cyclospora, Dientoamoeba, Entamoeba histolytica,* and *Endolimax nana* infections. It also helps clear mold from the body. Typically taken three times per day for sixty days. Brand options include Rootcology Oil of Oregano, Designs for Health Oil of Oregano, Candibactin-AR.

Olive leaf

Its antifungal properties can help reduce *Candida*. Consider Pure Encapsulations Olive Leaf Extract, follow package instructions.

Pau d'arco

Its antifungal properties can help reduce *Candida*. NOW Foods Pau d'arco, is one option. Follow package instructions.

Saccharmyces boulardii

S. boulardii helps restore a healthy microbiome, can resolve diarrhea, clear many gut infections, and may help crowd out pathogenic yeast. It has activity against *C. diff.*, rotavirus, and norovirus and supports the immune system to help clear *H. pylori*. It helps raise secretory IgA levels and helps the body overcome many protozoan infections, including *Blastocystis hominis, Giardia, Chilomastix, Entamoeba histolytica,* and mold mycotoxins. It should be avoided by those who have Crohn's disease. Therapeutic dosing is usually 5 billion-15 billion CFUs, 2-4 times per day. Start low and go slow to build up to a therapeutic dosage. Consider Rootcology *S. Boulardii,* Pure Encapsulations *Saccharomyces boulardii,* Designs for Health Floramyces, XYMOGEN Saccharomycin DF or Florastor.

For additional supplement and medication protocols, visit ibsrootcause/bonus.

Support Probiotic Growth

Once SIBO and pathogenic microbes are cleared and we have seeded with probiotics, we can add prebiotics, which can help the beneficial microbes grow. I sometimes may add butyrate and aloe earlier in the game as they can help with microbial balance and symptom relief without feeding potentially pathogenic microbes.

Heal Intestinal Permeability

While for most people L-glutamine and bone broth can be added at anytime during the healing journey, I have learned that people who have a B_6/P5P deficiency and histamine-producing gut infections may present with histamine reactions to gut-healing protocols, such as L-glutamine and bone broth, so in some cases I add in the healing foods after a person has been on a P5P supplement and has cleared the histamine producers. An intestinal permeability support blend such as Rootcology Gut R&R, Biosense Clinic MucosaHeal, Designs for Health GI Revive, XYMOGEN GI Balance Powder, DaVinci Laboratories G.I. Benefits, Pure Encapsulations G.I. Fortify, and ReLeaf MucosaCalm can help seal and repair the gut lining, promoting long-term healing.

Chapter Summary

- Healing is not always a straight path, and setbacks are part of the process, but every small change you make brings you one step closer to feeling your best. Whether it's discovering the right diet, finding balance with probiotics, or simply learning to listen to your body's signals, there is always an opportunity to improve your quality of life.

- You deserve to feel good in your own skin, and I believe that with the right approach, you can. Take this information, apply it at your own pace, and trust in the power of your body's ability to heal. This journey is about progress, not perfection, and I'm honored to have been part of it with you.

Visit https://ibsrootcause.com/bonus for notes on this chapter.

CHAPTER 16

Symptom Solutions While You Heal

In developing a plan for a client, I do take into consideration symptoms to adjust dietary, testing, and supplement recommendations. I may also recommend some helpful strategies to manage symptoms while healing. I would recommend that you observe and track your symptoms and bowel movements.

As you're diving into a healing diet and perhaps waiting for test results, consider these strategies to address specific symptoms. I've listed them in order of relevance as I have seen these symptoms in my experience.

Acid Reflux

In my experience, acid reflux is commonly caused by IgG food sensitivities (especially dairy), *H. pylori,* low stomach acid, slowed motility, SIBO, and occasionally suppressed emotions.

If gluten and dairy elimination doesn't help, I may recommend an IgG food sensitivity test and eliminating foods based on the results.

Subsequently, I would suggest a comprehensive stool analysis to test for *H. pylori* and working on supporting stomach acid levels.

I would consider looking into SIBO and slowed motility next.

Of course if you have suppressed emotions, that would be a high priority.

To find resolution from acid reflux symptoms while you heal, consider the following:

Helpful Dietary Recommendations
- Eliminate dairy/gluten
- Eliminate based on IgG food sensitivities
- Try bone broth: Bone broth can soothe the intestinal lining and stimulates the production of stomach acid.
- Try a soothing and digestion-supporting tea: Ginger tea is particularly helpful for acid reflux, as ginger has soothing, digestive and prokinetic properties. Of course, if your food sensitivity test results show you're sensitive to ginger (like I was), don't drink it! Other herbal teas that can help soothe acid reflux symptoms include chamomile, slippery elm, anise seed, fennel seed, peppermint, slippery elm, marshmallow, lemon balm, and licorice.
- Don't overeat. Putting too much food in the stomach at one time can put pressure on the LES, causing reflux symptoms. Instead, eat until you are comfortably full or consider smaller, more frequent meals to help manage symptoms.
- Stop eating two to three hours before bed. Allowing your last meal to fully digest before lying down can help with nighttime reflux symptoms.
- Chew gum. Chewing gum (not flavored with spearmint or peppermint) increases saliva production, thus reducing the amount of acid in the esophagus.

OTC Medications

For occasional acid reflux, H2 receptor blockers such as famotidine (Pepcid) and calcium carbonate (Tums) may be helpful. I do caution against the use of Proton Pump Inhibitors as they can produce rebound acid reflux.

Helpful supplements may include:

1. DGL and mastic gum: Taking a supplement that contains deglycyrrhizinated licorice extract (DGL) and mastic gum can help support and soothe your digestive tract while healing damaged mucous membranes. This supplement may also help for combating *H. pylori,* the bacteria that may lead to ulcers, bloating, reflux, and upset stomach. Generally, people see symptom resolution of reflux in days, but a full sixty-day course is used to clear out non-resistant *H. pylori* infections.

2. D-limonene: A major constituent in several citrus oils (orange, lemon, mandarin, lime, and grapefruit), it is used for relief of heartburn and GERD. Integrative Therapeutics and Jarrow make high quality D-limonene supplements.

3. Melatonin: If acid reflux wakes you up at night, you may wish to try melatonin, as research suggests it offers gastroesophageal protective effects. Consider taking 1 capsule of Pure Encapsulations Melatonin about an hour before bedtime.

Some lifestyle strategies I would recommend:
1. Sleeping on a wedge pillow if reflux occurs at night.
2. Speaking your truth and working on repressed feelings, such as EMDR therapy.

3. Stress reduction and management. Activities such as yoga, meditation, walking, acupuncture, and reading, can help you to manage stress and improve the body's ability to digest. To put your body in a relaxed mode before eating, try taking five deep breaths before your meal and eating mindfully instead of multitasking.

Bloating, Cramping, and Stomach Pain

Bloating, cramping, and stomach pain often go hand in hand and are common symptoms of IBS. They can be caused by a plethora of issues, such as dietary triggers, SIBO, stress, and parasitic infections.

If you are dealing with bloating and stomach pain, consider getting an IgG food sensitivity test next and eliminating foods based on that.

Subsequently, I would suggest a comprehensive stool analysis, a test for SIBO, and a test for parasitic infections.

To find resolution from bloating and stomach pain symptoms while you heal, consider the following:

Helpful Dietary Recommendations

- Eliminate dairy/gluten
- Eliminate based on IgG food sensitivities
- Try bone broth: Promotes healthy digestion.
- Try a soothing and digestion-supporting tea: fennel tea is particularly helpful for bloating. Ginger tea, chamomile, and peppermint tea may also help.
- To put your body in a relaxed mode before eating, try taking five deep breaths before your meal and eating mindfully instead of multitasking.

OTC Medications

The medications Simethicone, marketed as GasX, can work well for deflating the bloat.

Helpful supplements may include

1. Lycopodium: Derived from the spores of the club moss, *Lycopodium clavatum* is a homeopathic remedy believed to help with various digestive symptoms, including gas and bloating. My clients and my baby seem to respond well to this.
2. Digestive enzymes: Enzyme supplements, such as amylase, protease, and lipase, can aid in the digestion of specific nutrients, potentially reducing bloating caused by poor digestion.
3. Multi-ingredient enzymes: These contain a variety of enzymes to provide broad-spectrum digestive support for the digestion of fat, protein, carbs, and dairy (lactase enzyme). Each company has a unique formulation and you may need to try different ones to find the combination of enzymes that works best for you. As a starting point, consider Rootcology Broad Spectrum Enzymes, SFI Health Ther-Biotic SIBB-Zymes, SFI Health Ther-Biotic Vital-Zymes Complete, Pure Encapsulations Digestive Enzymes Ultra, and Transformation Enzymes Digest.
4. Probiotics: Probiotic supplements can help improve the balance of beneficial bacteria in the gut, potentially reducing gas and bloating and promoting healthy digestion. Probiotics such as *Lactobacillus* and *Bifidobacterium*, which can help with digestion and motility, potentially reducing gas and bloating. Rootcology ProB50 is a blend that may help.
5. *Saccharomyces boulardii (S. boulardii):* S. boulardii is a beneficial probiotic yeast that can help ease stomach pain and bloating by restoring microbial balance, preventing infections

and reinfection of the gut, and supporting gut barrier integrity. Additionally, unlike most probiotics that can make a SIBO infection worse, *S. boulardii* is well-tolerated and helpful for SIBO. Consider a dose of 250 mg to 2,000 mg per day of Rootcology *S. Boulardii*, Pure Encapsulations *Saccharomyces boulardii*, Designs for Health FloraMyces, or XYMOGEN Saccharomycin DF.
6. Activated charcoal: Activated charcoal may help absorb gas and toxins in the digestive tract, providing short-term relief from bloating. It may be constipating, which can be helpful if you tend toward diarrhea, but please avoid it if you're already constipated. Consider taking 1 to 3 capsules once per day, at least 1 hour away from food and supplements. Integrative Therapeutics Activated Charcoal is a high-quality option.

Some lifestyle strategies I would recommend
1. Use heat therapy to relieve pain, cramping, and bloating. I love to soak in a warm Epsom salt bath to help relieve cramping as well as heated rice bags or heat packs.
2. Consider belly massage!
3. Consider stress reduction and management. Activities such as yoga, meditation, walking, acupuncture, and reading can help you to manage stress and improve the body's ability to digest.
4. Chew food very well, aiming for 20 chews per bite.

Constipation

Constipation can be caused by a variety of reasons, but magnesium deficiency, hypothyroidism, and low tone in the gut are the ones that most often come to mind.

A great place to start for most people is a magnesium citrate supplement.

If that doesn't help, I would consider dietary changes (as tolerated), taking carnitine and thiamine, and testing for hypothyroidism.

In stubborn cases *H. pylori*, SIBO, parasites, and mold tend to be at the root.

Helpful Dietary Recommendations

- Increase fat intake to 50 to 60 percent of total caloric intake: Fats can be lubricating to the digestive system, and diets too low in fat are associated with constipation. Try increasing your intake of high-quality sources, including olive oil, avocado oil, avocados, coconut oil, and fatty fish (such as wild-caught salmon).
- Eat beets: Due to their fiber content, beets can aid in constipation relief.
- Try pear sauce: Pears contain fiber and because of their high sorbitol (sugar alcohol) content, pears help to draw water into the stool and soften it, making it easier to pass.
- Chew xylitol gum: Natural chewing gum with xylitol can help gently loosen stools, as the act of chewing stimulates digestion and motility.
- Probiotic foods: Fermented foods, which contain probiotics, can help us balance our intestinal flora and improve constipation. Fermented coconut yogurt, fermented coconut water, and fermented cabbage are a few of my favorites. Be sure to choose the kind kept in the fridge to get abundant live cultures. A few words of caution:
  - If your constipation is due to SIBO, you may want to avoid fermented foods, as it can worsen bloat.
  - Fermented foods are high in histamine, so histamine intolerance should be resolved before incorporating probiotic foods.

OTC Medications

OTC laxatives, including lubricants, stool softeners, and suppositories, help trigger movement of the intestinal muscles and elimination. Miralax is a well-known laxative. While these laxatives can provide relief in some cases, I don't recommend them as a long-term solution, as they generally do not target and resolve the root cause of an individual's constipation.

Supplement recommendations

1. Vitamin C: I recommend a total daily intake of 500 to 3,000 mg of vitamin C, as tolerated. Vitamin C can be dosed to bowel tolerance, meaning you can increase your dosage until your bowel movements become regular, better formed, and easy to pass. If you take too much, it may produce a loose stool, and you'll know to decrease the dose. I recommend Rootcology's Electrolyte Blend, Designs for Health's Electrolyte Synergy, or NOW Foods Chewable C-500.

2. Magnesium citrate: Gut motility issues and magnesium deficiency are two of the most common causes of constipation. Supplementing with magnesium citrate promotes gut motility and helps with bowel movements because of its stool-softening properties. Consider Rootcology Magnesium Citrate Powder, Designs for Health's MagCitrate Powder, or Pure Encapsulations Magnesium citrate. The usual starting dose range for magnesium citrate is 400 mg at bedtime but, like vitamin C, magnesium can be dosed to bowel tolerance, meaning you can increase your dosage until your bowel movements become regular, better formed, and easy to pass.

3. Carnitine: Carnitine deficiency can cause smooth muscle dysmotility (changes in speed, strength, or coordination) of the

gastrointestinal tract (similar to what it does to muscle metabolism, causing muscle weakness) leading to constipation. Supplementing with carnitine, alongside more fiber and magnesium, can potentially help alleviate constipation. Rootcology Carnitine Blend, Designs for Health Carnitine Synergy, and Pure Encapsulations L-Carnitine are options to consider.

4. Thiamine: Thiamine may help with motility. Rootcology Benfotiamine, Pure Encapsulations Benfomax, Life Extensions Benfotiamine, or Thiamax Thiamine at 600 mg per day is a good daily starting dosage. I encourage you to work with a practitioner to determine the proper dosage for your needs.

5. Vitamin B_6 (as P5P): Vitamin B_6 promotes the creation of serotonin, which helps with motility. Consider Rootcology P5P, Designs for Health P-5-P, Pure Encapsulations P5P 50, or SFI Health P-5-P.

6. Gallbladder support: Methionine, taurine, ox bile (found in Rootcology's Liver and Gallbladder Support) all support bile flow. Bile helps break down food, and can also help soften stool and speed up gastric motility. This formulation also contains artichoke, which has been shown to promote gastric emptying.

7. Digestive enzymes: A lack of digestive enzymes can lead to constipation. Bitters or supplemental digestive enzymes can be helpful. Bitters stimulate "bitter receptors" which release enzymes throughout the digestive tract, while supplemental enzymes provide the enzymes needed for the digestive process. For bitters, Wellena Digestive Bitters Kit, Quicksilver Scientific Dr. Shade's Bitters No. 9, Nature's Way NatureWorks Swedish

Bitters are high-quality options. For general digestion support consider Rootcology Broad Spectrum Enzymes, SFI Health Ther-Biotic SIBB-Zymes, SFI Health Ther-Biotic Vital-Zymes Complete, Pure Encapsulations Digestive Enzymes Ultra, and Transformation Enzymes Digest.

8. Probiotics: Probiotic supplements can help target common root causes of constipation, such as toxins, inflammation, and infections. I often recommend *Bifidobacterium*-containing probiotics as well as spore-based probiotics to help relieve constipation.

9. SFI Health Ther-Biotic Pro IBS Relief: These clinically supported probiotic strains have been shown to reduce IBS symptoms, including a 79 percent reduction in constipation, in as little as 21 days.

10. Aloe vera: Aloe vera can help alleviate constipation by providing natural enzymes to support digestion, providing prebiotics to feed the microbiome, and reducing inflammation in the small intestine and colon. Consider taking one capsule per day of Rootcology Aloe or Designs for Health Aloe/200x to help relieve constipation.

Some lifestyle strategies I would recommend

1. Incorporate more movement into your life: Moving the body can help to move the bowels. I recommend going for regular walks.

2. Try the Squatty Potty: This popular stool helps you move your stool! It fits at the base of the toilet and elevates the feet,

putting us into a "squat" position, which has been shown to straighten the colorectal canal and decrease the need to strain.

3. Listen to your body's signals: Don't ignore or delay the urge for a bowel movement; rather, go to the bathroom as soon as you feel the need. The more you ignore your body's signals to move the bowels, the weaker they become, leading to constipation.

4. Consider toilet timing: Making time to go to the bathroom at the same time every day (such as first thing in the morning or after meals) trains our migrating motor complex (which moves food through our intestines) to know that now is the time for a bowel movement.

Diarrhea

Diarrhea is a symptom of IBS many of us know all too well! It can be caused by a variety of reasons. A great place to start is dietary triggers, SIBO, stress, and parasitic infections.

I almost always recommend a gluten and dairy free diet as an initial step. If you are still dealing with diarrhea after that, consider getting an IgG food sensitivity test and doing an elimination diet based on the results. Also consider that raw foods, high fiber foods, and food additives may play a role. Coffee and tea can speed up your transit time, so please be mindful there, too.

Next, I would do a parasite test, a comprehensive stool analysis, and a test for SIBO.

If those were inconclusive, I would consider a workup for IBD or a trial of cholestyramine with your doctor to test for bile acid malabsorption.

To find resolution from diarrhea while you heal, consider the following:

Helpful Dietary Recommendations
- Chew: Ensuring that you are chewing your food completely is going to really help your body digest the food.

- Be mindful and don't rush: Enjoy your food! Tasting it, taking your time between bites, and listening to relaxing music, can help get your body into a rest-and-digest state. Stress can cause diarrhea when the body is in fight-or-flight or survival mode.

- Get the right type and amount of fiber: Fiber helps to bulk up the stool, absorbs water, and allows for stools that are more liquid in nature (diarrhea) to firm up and pass more easily. It also acts as a binder to attract pathogens that may be causing the diarrhea, allowing us to eliminate the pathogens through the bowels and stool. However, too much can actually cause diarrhea, so we want to find a happy balance.
    - Soluble fiber: Foods that are rich in this type of fiber are better tolerated by those who have sensitive digestive issues. The soluble fiber creates a gel-like consistency, soothing the digestive tract as you eat it. It's found in oats, peas, beans, apples, carrots, psyllium, and citrus fruits.
    - Limit your intake of insoluble fiber: Foods rich in insoluble fiber can be hard on the digestive system, especially when consumed raw. It's found in nuts, beans, cauliflower, green beans, and potatoes.

- Remove stalks and stems from greens: The leaves are easier to digest.

- Make simple meals: Avoid complex meals with many ingredients, which may be more challenging to digest. This can also help identify any possible food sensitivities, as having minimal ingredients will allow you to more easily identify which foods trigger your symptoms

OTC Medications

Loperamide (Imodium AD) is probably the most effective medication for non-infectious diarrhea. Bismuth Subsalicylate (Pepto-Bismol) would be a better choice if you suspect the diarrhea is infectious.

Helpful supplements may include:

1. Zinc: Take 30-50 mg of zinc picolinate or zinc carnosine. You should see improvement within one to three days of starting (if you're having more than four bowel movements per day, break the capsule apart and add the powder to a cup of water or applesauce, or take it as a liquid). Zinc carnosine options include Integrative Therapeutics Zinc Carnosine, Pure Encapsulations Peptic-Care, and Seeking Health Zinc Carnosine, and for zinc picolinate consider Pure Encapsulations.

2. L-glutamine: L-glutamine may be helpful for diarrhea. Watch for excess constipation, as it is a binder and can work quickly, creating hard stools. Start with ¼ teaspoon per day for two weeks, then increase to ½ teaspoon per day. If diarrhea persists, increase by ¼ teaspoon, with a max of 2 teaspoons per day. Please note, people deficient in B6 may have adverse reactions to L-glutamine and may wish to start P5P first. Consider Pure Encapsulations L-Glutamine or a gut-healing powder that

contains L-glutamine such as Rootcology Gut R&R and Designs for Health GI Revive.

3. Probiotic trial:

    S. boulardii: This yeast based probiotic has been found to help resolve diarrhea of various causes. Start with two capsules per day, and if tolerated, work up to six per day. Consider Rootcology S. Boulardii, Pure Encapsulations Saccharomyces boulardii, Designs for Health FloraMyces, or XYMOGEN Saccharomycin DF.

    SFI Health Ther-Biotic Pro IBS Relief: These clinically supported probiotics have been shown to reduce IBS symptoms, including a 70 percent reduction in diarrhea, in as little as twenty-one days.

    Mutaflor: A therapeutic probiotic product containing the beneficial *E. coli* strain called Nissle 1917, which has been shown to reduce the frequency of acute diarrhea by 2.3 days and chronic diarrhea by 3.3 days.

4. Binders: I have found that taking binders like activated charcoal can help with binding up diarrhea and slowing motility. Please note that binders should be taken away from other supplements and medications, as they can bind to them and reduce their effectiveness. Other binders that may be helpful include:

    Psyllium husk: Take 1 to 2 teaspoons per 8 ounces of water or non-acidic juice (apple, pear, mango); it works well for short bowel syndrome. Additionally, ensure you drink 6-8 glasses of water throughout the day to avoid constipation. Please note psyllium husk can cause anal fissures. Avoid it if you have a history of them.

    Bentonite clay: Add 1 teaspoon of bentonite clay to 4 ounces of water and take once per day. You may increase your intake up to 1 tablespoon, 1-3 times per day as needed.

5. Enzymes: You may find that certain foods trigger your diarrhea, and this could be due to deficiencies in particular enzymes. The following may be helpful:
   a. Broad spectrum enzymes, with high-quality options including Rootcology Broad Spectrum Enzymes, SFI Health Ther-Biotic SIBB-Zymes, SFI Health Ther-Biotic Vital-Zymes Complete, Pure Encapsulations Digestive Enzymes Ultra, and Transformation Enzymes Digest.
   b. Pancreatic enzymes, with high-quality options including Rootcology Pancreatic Enzymes Plus, Designs for Health PaleoZyme, and Pure Encapsulations Pancreatic Enzyme Formula.
   c. Digestive bitters, with high-quality options including Wellena Digestive Bitters Kit, Quicksilver Scientific Dr. Shade's Bitters No. 9, and Nature's Way NatureWorks Swedish Bitters.

6. Thiamine: Diarrhea increases the risk of thiamine deficiency, which may result in ongoing diarrhea. Taking 200–600 mg of thiamine per day may help. Options include: Rootcology Benfotiamine, Pure Encapsulations Benfomax, Life Extensions Benfotiamine, and Thiamax Thiamine.

Some lifestyle strategies I would recommend
1. Wash your hands frequently with soap: This will help reduce the chances of a diarrhea-causing bacteria making its way to your gut.
2. Get plenty of sleep: Lack of sleep is a stressor that contributes to stress hormone imbalance and increases susceptibility to infections, both of which can cause diarrhea. Aim to get at least 7 to 9 hours of sleep per night.

3. **Get a toilet-finder app:** These apps help you to find toilets in your area, which can help you travel and socialize with more confidence.
4. **Make yourself a sh*t kit for peace of mind:** If you have to go somewhere and are worried about an accident, consider bringing a spare set of bottoms, some loperamide, electrolytes, and baby wipes just in case.

Root Causes and Their Associated Symptoms

This table provides a quick reference of the root causes associated with the most common IBS-related symptoms. Use it to help you identify the root causes that may be most helpful for you to consider or identify ones you may have missed. Note ++ and +++ indicate a red flag symptom for me for that root cause.

Root Cause	Diarrhea	Constipation	Acid Reflux	Bloating and Stomach Pain
Dietary Triggers	+	+	+	+
Dysbiosis	+	+		+
Low Stomach Acid and Protein Digestion Issues	+	+	+	+
Pancreatic Enzyme Deficiencies	+	+		+
Low Bile	+			+
Bile Acid Malabsorption	+		+	+
Lactose Intolerance	+			+
Fructose Intolerance	+			+
Sucrose Intolerance	+			+
Fiber Digestion Issues		+		+
Glutamine Deficiency	+			
Zinc Deficiency	+			
Vitamin A Deficiency	+			
Vitamin D Deficiency		+		

Root Cause	Diarrhea	Constipation	Acid Reflux	Bloating and Stomach Pain
Thiamine Deficiency	+	+	+	
Magnesium Deficiency		+		
Omega-3 Fatty Acids Deficiency		+		
Vitamin C Deficiency		+		
Potassium Deficiency		+		
Deficiency of Probiotics	+	+		+
Deficiency of Prebiotics	+	+		+
Intestinal Permeability	++	+		
Intestinal Overgrowths	+	+	+	
Gastrointestinal Hypomotility		+	+	+
Alterations in Stress Hormones	+		+	+
Estrogen Dominance	+		+	+
Alterations in Thyroid Hormones	+	+	+	+
High Toxicity	+	+		
Certain Medications	+	+		
Glyphosate	+	+		
Breast Implant Illness	+			
Mycotoxins (Mold)	+	+		
Viral Infections	+			
Bacterial Infection: Lyme Disease	+			
Bacterial Infection: *H. pylori*	+	+	+++	+
Other Bacterial Infections	+	+		
Protozoan Infections	+++	+		++
Parasitic Worms	+	+		
Inflammation	+	+		
IBD	+++	+		

Chapter Summary
- Dietary adjustments, OTC medications, supplements, and lifestyle strategies can temporarily relieve acid reflux, bloating, cramping, and stomach pain, constipation, and diarrhea while you do your detective work to identify and address the underlying root cause of your symptoms.

Visit https://ibsrootcause.com/bonus for notes on this chapter.

Author's Note

If you've been struggling with digestive symptoms for too long, please know there is hope. There's always a cause, and a path to healing is often a few short steps away, as long as you're heading in the right direction. I hope this book gives you a roadmap to find your way to healing.

I know if you've been on this journey for a while, it may feel overwhelming to learn there may be a lot of causes, but remember little steps help us heal a bit each day. With every step in the right direction, your symptoms will improve.

Making a series of small changes and paying close attention to what your body needs will help you understand what's working best to help you heal. Also remember the journey may look different for everyone.

If you feel frustrated along the way, please don't give up. You'll get there. I know you can do it. And I am here to support you along the way.

Izabella Wentz, PharmD
www.thyroidpharmacist.com
www.facebook.com/thyroidlifestyle
@izabellawentzpharmd

Acknowledgments

I have had many teachers and guides on this journey, and this book would not have been possible without the wisdom, generosity, and kindness of so many individuals.

I'm deeply grateful to the Institute for Functional Medicine and to trailblazers and teachers including Dan Kalish, Liz Lipski, Mark Hyman, Tom O'Bryan, Allison Siebecker, Vincent Pedre, Alessio Fasano, Michael Ruscio, Mark Pimiental, Gerard Mullin, William Walsh, Michael McEvoy, Kiran Krishnan, Donna Gates, and Christa Orecchio, who have inspired my understanding of gut health.

Elena Koles, my first integrative physician, introduced me to the Alletess food sensitivity test, which remains the most accurate test I've encountered and helped me (and now thousands of others) get relief from years of IBS and acid reflux symptoms.

To my dear friends who also happen to be world-class gut experts—Debbie Steinbock, Steve Wright, and Jill Carnahan—thank you for your support and wisdom during one of the most challenging times of our lives. Your generosity in sharing your expertise helped guide us through the maze of inflammatory bowel disease and played a pivotal role in helping Michael find healing. And to Michael, my husband and codetective in decoding IBD—your resilience, curiosity, and trust taught me more than any textbook ever could.

Acknowledgments

To David Tusek, thank you for showing up for our family with such insight and compassion, you helped more than you know.

A heartfelt thank-you to Genevieve Howland (Mama Natural); you may not even know this, but your recommendation for lactation supplements helped me uncover how to reverse dairy sensitivities.

Pejman Katerai, Sheila Kilbane, and Erika Peirson helped me understand carnitine, pancreatic enzymes, bile, histamines, and oxalates in a whole new way, thank you for your brilliance and your care.

To Magdalena Wszelaki, thank you for your beautiful friendship and for nerding out with me about histamines, oxalates, and parasite tests.

To my publishing team at Avery, especially Lucia Watson and Isabel McCarthy, thank you for believing in this project and helping bring it to life with such care and dedication.

Julia Pastore, thank you for taking my ideas and vision and helping to shape them into this manuscript. Your brilliant editorial eye, patience, and professionalism are so appreciated.

To the team at Park & Fine Literary and Media, especially Celeste Fine, John Maas, Sarah Passick, and Melissa Rodman, thank you for your guidance, advocacy, and brilliance every step of the way. Your support has meant the world to me.

To my wonderful team members, thank you for taking the ideas swirling in my head and transforming them into protocols, programs, and healing resources with heart, clarity, and creativity: Tina Chan, Brittany Moore, Stephanie Carson, Emily Penn, Christine Ruggirello, Robin Baker, Mindy Benkert, Tiziana Nenezic, Renee Picard, Sarah Wilson, Diane Blum, and Dave Kinzel. Your brilliance, heart, and passion have not only fueled this work, they've helped bring healing to the world. I'm so grateful to have you on this mission with me.

To my son, Dimitry; my mom, Marta; and my brother, Robert, thank you for being my best guinea pigs, willingly (or at least eventually) trying every odd-smelling supplement, mystery test, and gut-friendly concoction I've thrown your way. Your curiosity, trust, and unshakable support have meant the world to me and made this wild wellness ride a lot more fun.

To my clients and readers, thank you for your trust, your stories, and your unwavering commitment to healing. Your journeys have inspired and shaped every protocol, insight, and word in this book. I'm endlessly grateful to walk this path with you.

Index

acetaldehyde, 205, 283, 291
acetate, 205, 241
acetylcholine, 3–4, 188, 272, 278, 280, 281, 426. *See also* anticholinergics
acid reflux
   author's experience, 6, 8, 36
   causes, 465, 480–482
   as IBS symptom, 24
   medication side effect, 173
   treatment, 333, 355, 384, 461, 465–468
activated charcoal, 165, 291, 293, 439, 470
adaptogens, 355–356
Addison's disease, 349
Additive-Free diet, 407
adrenal issues
   bacteria virulence and, 204, 208, 342
   causes, 189, 208, 342, 346, 348–349
   effects, 292, 367
   support for, 355–357
   testing, 349
Adrenal Transformation Protocol (Wentz), 357
AGES (advanced glycosylation end products), 235
AIP (Autoimmune Paleo) diet, 381–382, 406, 419
airborne toxins, 442
Akkermansia, 227, 442
albendazole, 330, 335

alcohol, 127–128, 137, 235, 236, 284
Alinia. *See* nitazoxanide
aloe vera, 226, 308–309, 310, 384–385, 408, 419, 463, 474
alosetron (Lotronex), 51, 54
Amitiza. *See* lubiprostone
amitriptyline. *See* tricyclic antidepressants
ammonia, 205–206
amphotericin B, 288, 440
amylase, 165–166
Anaspaz. *See* hyoscyamine
andrographolide, 408, 419
angelica, 150, 151
anise seed, 147, 466
antibiotics
   antimicrobial herbs, 332–335, 459
   for bacterial overgrowth, 43, 258, 458
   for diarrhea, 49, 50, 55
   for gut infections, 301, 307, 311, 332–335, 459
   for IBD, 400
   mechanism of action, 49
   resistance to, 306, 310
   side effects, 31, 69, 159–160, 191, 207, 214, 235–236, 284–285, 301, 396, 400, 428
anticholinergic effects, 50, 51–52, 350, 425
anticholinergics, 4, 31, 52, 426. *See also* hyoscyamine

Index

antidepressants (tricyclic antidepressants, SSRIs, mirtazapine)
  indications, 43, 49, 50–51, 55, 276, 350, 410
  mechanism of action, 42, 49, 50–51, 276, 350
  side effects, 31, 276, 425
  types of, 50–51, 410 (*See also* SSRIs)
antifungal drugs (fluconazole, amphotericin B, nystatin, itraconazole), 288, 290, 335, 440–441
anti-*Saccharomyces cerevisiae* antibodies (ASCAs), 398
antispasmodics. *See also* hyoscyamine
  indications, 49, 51–52, 54–55, 426
  mechanism of action, 42, 49
  side effects, 52, 426
  without anticholinergic effects, 52
anxiety, 6, 8, 24, 36, 43, 339–341, 363–364, 410
archaea, 255, 259, 262
artichoke extract, 160, 275
atypical antidepressant, 276
autoimmune conditions, 7–10, 13, 303. *See also* thyroid imbalances and autoimmunity
Autoimmune Paleo (AIP) diet, 381–382, 406, 419

Bacillus-based probiotics, 215, 229
Bacillus cereus, 300
bacterial infections
  causes, 343
  differential diagnosis, 299–302
  effects, 302–312, 396
  overview, 66, 295–296, 337
  post-infectious IBS, 66, 68, 296–300, 369–370
  symptoms and signs, 208, 232, 234, 236, 295–296, 360
  testing, 301
  treatment, 301–302, 334, 458–459
bacterial overgrowth. *See* small intestine bacterial overgrowth
bacteriophages, 219, 228, 268–269, 301–302
Bacteroides, 229, 261, 300
BAM (bile acid malabsorption), 61, 64, 162–165, 168, 170, 475, 480
beneficial bacteria. *See* probiotics
bentonite clay, 478–479
Bentyl. *See* dicyclomine
berberine, 249, 267–268, 289, 293, 307, 310, 332, 334, 416, 440, 459–460
beta-glucan, 115, 205, 222, 224–225
beta-glucuronidase, 207
betaine with pepsin, 154–156, 170, 310, 455
Bifidobacterium, 62, 203–204, 221, 234, 393–394
Bifidobacterium-based probiotics, 213–214, 217, 219, 226, 229, 455
bile acid malabsorption (BAM), 61, 64, 162–165, 168, 170, 475, 480
bile flow (poor), 159–162, 170, 296, 435
binders, 437, 438, 439–440, 478–479
Biocidin Liquid, 228, 302, 460
biologics, 299, 400
birth control pills, 73, 235, 426–427, 428, 431
bismuth subsalicylate (Pepto-Bismol), 4, 47–48, 127, 269, 307, 311, 477
black seed oil, 290, 293, 307, 332–333, 334, 460
black walnut, 290, 293
Blastocystis hominis, 9, 234, 271, 314–317, 325–326, 328–330, 334, 370, 372–373, 394
bloating. *See* gas, bloating, and cramping
blood sugar swings, 346, 352. *See also* metabolic disorders
blueberry extract, 247
Body Ecology Diet, 287–288
bone broth, 147, 243–245, 463, 468
Borellia Burgdoferi, 302–303
boswellia, 408, 418, 419

Index

brain-gut communication, 13, 36, 43, 339–341, 410. *See also* stress and stress hormone imbalances
Breaking the Vicious Cycle (Gottschall), 405
breast implant illness, 443, 481
breathwork, 351
Brown, Benjamin I., 61
Brown, P. W., 26, 384
brush border enzyme deficiency, 165–167, 170
bupropion (Wellbutrin), 350, 410
burdock, 150, 151
Buscopan. *See* scopolamine
butyrate
    food sources and supplements, 241, 409
    function, 66, 204, 205, 212, 232, 409
    indications, 106, 226, 241, 249, 409, 419, 463
    overview, 463
    production, 66, 96, 193, 203–204, 205, 206, 223, 242
B vitamin complex. *See* vitamin B

caffeine, 127, 128–129, 137, 431–432
camel milk, 101, 102
Campylobacter, 203, 269, 299–300, 397
Canasa suppositories, 388, 399, 418
Candida overgrowth, 283–293
    causes, 65, 284, 296, 313
    effects, 397
    overview, 255, 283–284, 294
    relapse prevention, 292–293
    risk factors, 285
    symptoms and signs, 234, 283, 285–286, 481
    testing, 286–287
    treatment, 284, 287–292, 458–459
capsaicin, 130, 235, 236
carbohydrates, 165–166, 265, 284, 381, 404–405, 420
carbonated beverages, 129, 137
carboxymethyl cellulose (CMC), 131, 134
Carnahan, Jill, 389, 394

carnitine, 101–102, 273, 277–278, 383–384, 455, 472–473
carpel tunnel, 6, 8, 366
carrageenan, 132, 134, 416
cat's claw, 251–252, 333, 411, 460
CBT (cognitive behavioral therapy), 351, 355
celiac disease, 92–95, 117, 135, 180, 193, 209–210, 372, 380–381
chamomile, 148, 251–252, 308, 411, 466
Chilomastix, 319–320, 330
Chinese rhubarb, 150, 151
chlorella, 446
cholagogues, 160–161
cholestyramine, 163–164, 439, 475
chronic fatigue, 6, 8, 13, 35, 189–190, 363–364, 418
Chron's disease. *See* inflammatory bowel disease
circadian rhythm, 345–346, 353–354
circulating immune complexes (CICs), 96, 104, 105, 106
citalopram. *See* SSRIs
Citrucel. *See* psyllium husk
citrus, 87, 112, 113, 130, 137, 147, 194
Clostridium difficile infection, 214, 228, 300–301, 334
Clostridium difficile overgrowth, 267
Clostridium spp., 201, 228, 260–261, 300, 397
CMC (carboxymethyl cellulose), 131, 134
cognitive behavioral therapy (CBT), 351, 355
colorectal cancer, 13, 31, 390, 402–403
colostrum, 249–250
constipation
    causes, 183–198, 480–482
    conventional approach, 42, 45–47, 51–55
    medications side effect, 3–4, 425–426
    stress and, 343
    treatment, 470–475
    women-specific issues, 71, 72

491

Index

conventional medicine
  diet and lifestyle changes, 44–45
  one-size-fits-all, 41–42
  over-the-counter medications, 46–49
  overview, 12–13, 39–41, 43–44, 55–56, 60
  prescription medications, 49–55
  root cause comparison, 60
  targets for, 42–43
copper, 177, 180, 384
corticosteroids, 235, 237, 284, 285, 399
cortisol, 254, 341, 349, 356, 430
cramping. *See* gas, bloating, and cramping
Crohn's disease, 391–392. *See also* inflammatory bowel disease
Cryptosporidium, 314, 319, 330, 394
curcumin, 111, 247, 411–412, 418, 419, 447
Cyclospora, 95, 320, 330, 334

dairy-free diet, 175, 454, 468, 475
dairy products, 8, 94, 98–104, 136
dandelion, 150, 151, 161, 438, 448
deglycyrrhizinated licorice (DGL), 251–252, 307, 411, 420, 459, 461, 467
dental health, 285, 292
depletions, 173–198
  causes, 64, 304, 305, 313, 342, 346
  chicken-or-egg problem, 175–177
  constipation and, 183–198
  diarrhea and, 177–185
  overview, 173–175, 198
  testing or guessing, 176–177
depression, 13, 24, 36, 43, 339–341, 410
De Simone, Claudio, 415
desipramine. *See* tricyclic antidepressants
detox pathway support, 438, 445, 446–448
DGL (deglycyrrhizinated licorice), 251–252, 307, 411, 420, 459, 461, 467
diabetes. *See* metabolic disorders
Diantoameoba fragilis, 328

diarrhea
  causes, 177–185, 480–482
  conventional approach, 42, 47–48, 50–51, 53–55
  medication side effect, 427–428
  treatment, 47–48, 475–480
  women-specific issues, 71
dicyclomine (Bentyl), 51–52, 54, 426
Dientoamoeba, 66–67, 234, 320–321, 334
dietary triggers, 83–138
  causes, 62–63, 89–90
  dairy, 8, 94, 98–104, 136
  eggs, 94, 104–106, 136
  elimination diet and, 87–88
  fatty foods, 135
  fructose, 116–118, 136, 165–166, 170, 480
  gluten and wheat, 8, 92–98, 135, 234–235, 236
  high-fiber foods, 112–116, 120, 136, 209, 403–404
  high FODMAP foods, 119–122, 137, 165
  high-protein foods, 135, 175, 480
  histamine, 97, 104–105, 123–124, 137, 262–263, 435
  mechanical triggers, 86, 127–135, 137
  nickel, 73, 96, 109–112, 136
  overview, 83–85, 90–92, 135–138
  oxalate, 124–125, 137, 283, 288
  reintroducing foods, 90
  salicylate, 125–127, 137
  soy, 106–109, 136
  sucrose, 118–119, 136, 165–166, 170–171, 480
  symptoms and signs, 480
  testing, 85, 88–90, 135–138
  types of, 85–87
DIG AT IT, 75
digestion and digestive enzymes, 139–172
  best practices, 141–142, 144–148
  bile acid malabsorption, 61, 64, 162–165, 168, 475, 480

492

brush border enzyme deficiency, 165–167
conventional approach, 45
deficiencies, 234, 473–474
effects, 153, 236, 455
low stomach acid, 153–156 (*See also* low stomach acid)
normal digestive function, 21–23, 38, 142–144
overview, 63, 139–141, 171–172, 340
pancreatic enzyme deficiency, 156–159, 234
poor bile flow, 159–162, 296, 435
supplements, 148–152, 170–171, 455, 469, 473
symptoms and signs, 169, 209
testing, 167–168
digestive bitters, 150–151, 170, 473–474, 479
digestive teas, 147–148, 466
Digestive Wellness (Lipski), 88, 91
DIM (diindolylmethane), 432
D-limonene, 276, 467
dopamine/norepinephrine reuptake inhibitor (bupropion), 350, 410
drotaverine, 52. *See also* antispasmodics
dysbiosis
causes, 96, 199, 207–210, 434
conventional approach, 45
overview, 199–200, 229–230
patterns of, 200–202
symptoms and signs, 210, 480
testing, 210–211, 227–229
treatment (fecal transplant), 219–220, 415
treatment (fiber and prebiotics), 220–226
treatment (probiotics), 211–219, 226–227
treatment plans (tailored), 227–229

E. coli. See Escherichia coli
EFAs (essential fatty acids), 185–188
EGCG (green tea extract), 247
eggs, 94, 104–106, 136
Elavil. *See* tricyclic antidepressants

electrolytes, 352–353
Elemental Diet, 87–88, 108–109, 174–175, 265–266, 269, 295, 404, 419, 454
eluxadoline (Vibrezi), 53–54
EMDR (Eye Movement Desensitization and Reprocessing), 132, 133, 355, 467
Endolimax, 320, 334, 394
Entamoeba, 314, 319, 330, 334, 394
Epsom salts, 192, 270, 447
Epstein-Barr virus, 394, 395
erythritol, 133, 407, 416, 418
Escherichia coli, 228, 259–261, 268–269, 300, 396
Escherichia coli Nissle, 229, 412, 420
essential fatty acids (EFAs), 185–188
estrogen, 292
estrogen dominance, 428–434, 435, 481
exercise, 44, 145–146, 237, 447, 468, 470

Fasano, Alessio, 7, 232
fat digestion problems, 135, 156–157, 159–160, 170, 237
fatigue (chronic), 6, 8, 13, 35, 189–190, 363–364, 413
fecal microbiota transplantation (FMT), 219–220, 415
fennel seed, 148, 150, 161, 466, 468
fermented foods, 146–147, 226, 447, 471
ferritin. *See* iron
fiber
for bile acid malabsorption, 164
for constipation, 46, 48, 224, 471, 473
for detoxification, 439, 447
for diarrhea, 48, 224, 401, 476, 478
digestion of, 144, 152, 171, 203–205, 212, 214, 241–242
digestive/malabsorption issues, 46, 140, 167–169, 171, 480
for estrogen dominance, 431
genetic connections, 214
high-fiber foods as dietary trigger, 112–116, 120, 136, 209, 403–404
IBD precaution, 417

Index

fiber (*cont.*)
  for inflammation, 412–413
  low-fiber diets, 30, 171, 265–266, 403–404
  prebiotics and, 220–226
  short-chain fatty acid production, 203–204, 241–242
  types of, 112–114
FiberCon. *See* psyllium husk
fibromyalgia, 13, 36
"fight or flight," 340, 343–346, 454–455
Finkel, Suzie, 110
Firmicutes, 229
fish oils, 187–188, 408–409, 413–414, 418
5-HTP, 276
5R framework for gut health, 239–240
Flagyl. *See* metronidazole
fluconazole, 288, 290, 291, 440
fluoxetine. *See* SSRIs
FMT (fecal microbiota transplantation), 219–220, 415
food additives, 127, 130–135, 137, 416–417, 454. *See also specific food additives*
food allergies, 62. *See also* food sensitivity/intolerance
food as medicine, 240–247
food poisoning
  bacterial overgrowth risk factor, 257, 259
  causes, 68
  conventional approach, 3–4
  digestive enzyme deficiencies and, 169
  post-infectious IBS, 68–69, 299–300, 369–370
  protozoan infection risk factor, 323
  testing, 28, 74
food reaction types, 85–87. *See also* dietary triggers
food sensitivity/intolerance
  author's experience, 4–6
  causes, 8, 62–63, 305, 306–307, 313, 360
  conventional approach, 45
  symptoms and signs, 236, 237, 314–315
frankincense, 408
fructan, 97, 120
fructooligosaccharides (FOS), 219, 222–223, 225
fructose intolerance, 116–118, 136, 165–166, 170, 480
Fusobacterium, 261

GABA, 151, 350–351, 410
galactooligosaccharides (GOS), 219, 222–223, 225
GAPS (Gut and Psychology Syndrome Diet), 265
garlic, 105–106
garlic oil, 268, 290, 293, 298, 307, 333, 334, 461
gas, bloating, and cramping
  causes, 8, 45, 210, 256, 305, 361, 480–482
  conventional approach, 42, 45, 48, 53
  treatment, 468–470
gastroesophageal reflux disease (GERD), 36. *See also* acid reflux
GasX. *See* simethicone
gentian, 150–151, 161
Giardia, 117, 271, 314, 317–319, 329, 330, 334, 394
ginger, 148, 151, 161, 242, 275, 466, 468
ginseng, 270
gliadin, 92, 93, 234, 236
glucomannan, 439
glucosamine, 244, 251, 252
glucose isomerase, 117–118
glutamine, 73, 177–180, 234, 243–244, 248, 252, 342, 477–478, 480
gluten-free diet, 174, 178, 240–241, 380–381, 446, 454, 468, 475
gluten sensitivity/intolerance, 8, 92–98, 135, 234–235, 236. *See also* celiac disease
glycine-rich foods, 243–244, 445
glyphosate, 97, 207–208, 235, 284, 444–446, 481

GOS (galactooligosaccharides), 219, 222–223, 225
Gottschall, Elaine, 265, 405
grain-free diet, 174, 293, 461
grapefruit seed extract, 289, 293, 461
grape juice recipe, 299
grape seed extract, 247
Graves' disease, 305, 362, 364–365, 373–374, 376–377, 382–383
green tea extract (EGCG), 247
guar gum, 133, 222, 224, 225
Gut and Psychology Syndrome Diet (GAPS), 265
gut-brain communication, 13, 36, 43, 339–341, 410. *See also* stress and stress hormone imbalances
gut infections, 295–338
    bacterial, 296–312 (*See also* bacterial infections)
    conventional approach, 45
    overview, 295–296, 337–338
    parasitic, 312–337 (*See also* protozoal infections; worms)
    viral, 296–299 (*See also* viral infections)
gut microbiome, 199–230
    bacterial by-products, 204–207
    dysbiosis causes, 207–210
    dysbiosis patterns, 200–202
    dysbiosis treatments, 211–229, 415
    overview, 199–200, 229–230
    testing, 210–211, 227–229
    types of bacteria, 202–204
gut motility
    conventional approach, 42
    hypermotility, 272 (*See also* diarrhea)
    hypomotility, 65–66, 271–272, 280, 481 (*See also* constipation)
    support for, 271–272, 274–281, 455, 474, 478
    testing, 273–274

Haas, Sidney, 265, 404–405
Habba, Saad F., 60–61, 162
hair loss, 6, 8, 363

Hashimoto's Food Pharmacology (Wentz), 94, 379, 382
Hashimoto's Protocol (Wentz), 270, 379, 445, 448
Hashimoto's Thyroiditis (Wentz), 9, 369, 379
Hashimoto thyroiditis
    author's experience, 7–10, 359
    causes, 7–10, 313, 315–317, 325–326, 370, 372–374, 380, 446 (*See also* thyroid imbalances and autoimmunity)
    overview, 362
    risk factors, 304, 305
    symptoms and signs, 8, 91, 94, 101, 360, 364
    testing, 367, 369–370
    treatment, 374–375, 380–383, 384–385
    where to start, 457, 458
health plan, 453–464
    overview, 453–454
    Step 1: Fundamental Protocols, 454–455
    Step 2: Testing, 455–457
    Step 3: Advanced Protocols, 457–463
    symptom solutions (acid reflux), 465–468 (*See also* acid reflux)
    symptom solutions (bloating and cramping), 468–470 (*See also* gas, bloating, and cramping)
    symptom solutions (constipation), 470–475 (*See also* constipation)
    symptom solutions (diarrhea), 475–480 (*See also* diarrhea)
Helicobacter pylori infection
    overview, 303–304, 337
    risk factors, 304–305
    sulfate production, 269
    symptoms and signs, 234, 270, 305, 373–374, 481
    testing, 306
    treatment, 48, 306–311, 330, 334
hemorrhoids, 221–222, 392
herbicides and pesticides, 207–208. *See also* glyphosate

Index

high FODMAP foods, 119–122, 137, 165
high-protein diet, 135, 175, 480
histamine, 97, 104–105, 123–124, 137, 206, 262–263, 435
hives (urticaria), 6, 107, 206, 316–317, 372–373
home toxins, 441–442
homocysteine, 156
hormonal contraceptives, 73, 235, 426–427, 428, 431
hormone therapy, 73, 235, 426, 428, 430–431, 433–434
HPA (hypothalamic-pituitary-adrenal) axis, 340–341
H. pylori. See Helicobacter pylori infection
humic acid, 297, 439, 446
hydrogen SIBO, 259–261, 263–264, 268
hydrogen sulfide SIBO (sulfur SIBO), 262, 263–264, 268, 269–270
hydroxocobalamin, 270
hyoscyamine (Levbid, Levsin, Anaspaz, NuLev), 3–4, 51–52, 54, 426
hyperbaric oxygen therapy (HBOT), 414
hypermotility, 272. *See also* diarrhea
hypersensitivity reactions to food, 85–86, 89, 93, 96, 101–109
The Hyperthyroid Healing Diet (Osansky), 379
hyperthyroidism, 361, 363, 364–369, 382–384
hypomotility, 65–66, 271–272, 280, 284, 481. *See also* constipation
hypothalamic-pituitary-adrenal (HPA) axis, 340–341
hypothyroidism, 208–209, 360, 363, 364–369

IBD. *See* inflammatory bowel disease
Iberogast, 275
IBS. *See* irritable bowel syndrome
IBS-C, 25, 28, 30, 201, 218–219. *See also* constipation
IBS-D, 25, 28, 31, 201, 218. *See also* diarrhea
IBS unclassified (IBS-U), 26
IBS with mixed bowel habits (IBS-M), 25, 28
IgE allergies, 107–109
IgG food reactions, 86, 102–104, 105
IgG tests, 89, 96, 101, 103, 106
immunoglobulins, 249–251, 297, 409
IMO (intestinal methanogen overgrowth), 255, 262
Imodium. *See* loperamide
implant illnesses, 443, 481
infections. *See* gut infections
inflammation (intestinal)
  causes, 68
  conventional approach, 43
  degree of, 389–390
  stress and, 346, 354
  symptoms and signs, 482
inflammatory bowel disease (IBD), 387–421
  author's husband's experience, 11, 387–388, 417–419
  causes, 68–69, 393–397
  diagnosis, 34
  differential diagnosis, 29, 31, 32, 75, 389–391, 393, 475
  genetic connections, 62, 214
  misdiagnoses, 69
  overview, 387–389, 420–421
  recurrence prevention, 419–420
  symptoms and signs, 69, 157, 390–392, 482
  testing, 398–399
  treatment, 249, 265, 274, 350, 381–382, 399–415, 417–419
  treatments to avoid and precautions, 215, 415–417
inositol, 161
intestinal methanogen overgrowth (IMO), 255, 262
intestinal overgrowth. *See* small intestine bacterial overgrowth; small intestine yeast overgrowth

intestinal permeability (leaky gut), 231–253
  causes, 64–65, 232–235, 257, 263, 271, 304, 313, 435
  conventional approach, 53, 55
  5R framework for gut health, 239–240
  food as medicine, 240–247
  overview, 231–232, 253
  risk factors, 235–237, 343
  symptoms and signs, 7–8, 238, 481
  treatment, 177, 212, 239, 247–252, 463
  visceral hypersensitivity and, 231–232
intestinal secretagogues, 52–53, 54–55
inulin, 205, 219, 222–223, 225, 258
iodine, 370–371, 376, 377, 446, 448
ION Gut Support, 297, 439, 446
IP. *See* intestinal permeability
iron, 111, 176, 197–198, 396, 426
irritable bowel syndrome (IBS)
  author's experience, 1–12
  conventional approach, 39–56 (*See also* conventional medicine)
  co-occurring conditions, 13, 35–38
  diagnosis, 26–29, 32–34, 37–38
  differential diagnosis, 29–30
  health plan for, 453–464
  misdiagnoses, 30–32
  normal digestive function comparison, 21–23, 38, 142–144
  as real diagnosis, 35
  root causes and associated symptoms (overview), 13, 23–25, 57–79, 480–482 (*See also* depletions; dietary triggers; digestion and digestive enzymes; dysbiosis; gut infections; intestinal permeability; root cause approach; small intestine bacterial overgrowth; small intestine yeast overgrowth; stress and stress hormone imbalances; thyroid imbalances and autoimmunity; toxins and chemical triggers)
  self-education, 37–38
  symptom solutions (*See* acid reflux; constipation; diarrhea; gas, bloating, and cramping)
  types of, 25–26, 28, 30, 31 (*See also* constipation; diarrhea)
  as umbrella term, 70, 84
itraconazole, 288, 440
ivermectin, 335

jello, 245–246

ketogenic diets, 284
Klebsiella, 219, 225, 229, 260–261, 269, 397, 417
Korean Red Ginseng, 270

lactase, 166
Lactobacillus, 203–204, 226, 259–261, 413, 419
Lactobacillus-based probiotics, 212, 215, 217–218, 219, 309
lactose-free diet, 45, 175
lactose intolerance, 45, 94, 98–100, 165–166, 170, 480
L-alanine, 236
larazotide, 250–251
lauric acid, 241
laxatives, 21, 46, 132–133, 472
L-carnitine, 273, 383–384
LDN (low-dose naltrexone), 274, 382, 402–403, 418, 420
leaky gut. *See* intestinal permeability
lecithin, 164
lemon balm, 151, 377, 466
lemon water, 146, 447
Levbid. *See* hyoscyamine
Levsin. *See* hyoscyamine
L-glutamine, 177, 178–179, 252, 463, 477–478
licorice, 356, 466. *See also* deglycyrrhizinated licorice
lifestyle factors, 69, 72–73, 175, 208
linaclotide (Linzess), 53, 54
linoleic acid, 236
lipopolysaccharide (LPS), 206, 218

Index

Lipski, Liz, 88, 91
liver, toxin processing by, 423–424, 445, 448
L-methionine, 161
loperamide (Imodium), 4, 47, 53, 401, 477, 480
Lotronex. *See* alosetron
low-carbohydrate nutrient depletions, 175, 193
low-dose naltrexone (LDN), 274, 382, 402–403, 418, 420
low-fat diet, 175, 186
low FODMAP diet, 44, 55, 121–122, 175, 177, 255–256, 265
low-oxalate diet, 288
low stomach acid
    causes, 153, 181, 304, 310, 337, 361
    overview, 153
    symptoms and signs, 270, 284, 480
    testing, 154
    treatment, 154–156, 170, 310
low-sulfur diet, 405
LPS (lipopolysaccharide), 206, 218
lubiprostone (Amitiza), 53, 54
lycopodium, 469
Lyme disease, 302–303, 394, 395, 481

magnesium, 186, 190–192, 352–353, 356, 384, 428, 433, 438, 448, 455, 470, 472, 481
maltase, 166
maltitol, 133
maltodextrin, 133
Manning criteria, 26–27
mannitol, 133, 238
MAP (*Mycobacterium avium*, subspecies *paratuberculosis*), 397
Marshall, Barry, 311
marshmallow, 148, 251–252, 411, 466
mastic gum, 307, 461, 467
Matula tea, 307
MCTs (medium-chain triglycerides), 134, 241
mebendazole, 330, 335
mechanical triggers, 86, 127–135, 137

medication triggers, 69, 235, 237, 424–428, 481
meditation, 351, 468, 470
Mediterranean diet, 241, 405–406
medium-chain triglycerides (MCTs), 134, 241
mesh implantation illness, 443
metabolic disorders, 37, 65, 200, 280, 346, 352. *See also* thyroid imbalances and autoimmunity
Metamucil. *See* psyllium husk
methane, 206
methane SIBO, 261–262, 263–264, 268
Methanobrevibacter smithii, 255, 262
methionine, 124, 161, 448, 473
methylnaltrexone bromide (Relistor), 54
metronidazole (Flagyl), 329–330, 335
Micrococcus, 261
microscopic colitis, 392. *See also* inflammatory bowel disease
migrating motor complex (MMC), 271
milk thistle, 161, 412, 418, 420
mind-body practices, 351, 468, 470
mirtazapine, 276
mold, 434–441
    causes, 208, 284, 292, 296, 434–435
    effects, 303, 305, 394, 395
    overview, 434
    prevention of mold growth, 441
    symptoms and signs, 435–436
    testing, 436–437
    treatment, 437–439
molybdenum, 106, 270, 283, 291, 293
monoclonal antibodies (biologics), 299, 400
monolaurin, 290, 293, 307, 333, 334, 460
mucilaginous herbs, 148, 251–252, 411, 418, 420. *See also specific herbs*
mucus in stool, 24–25
Mycobacterium avium, subspecies *paratuberculosis* (MAP), 397
mycotoxins. *See* mold
myo-inositol, 383, 384

N-acetyl cysteine (NAC), 105–106, 252, 291, 293, 310, 448
N-acetyl glucosamine (NAG), 251, 252
naldemedine (Symproic), 54, 55
naloxegol (Movantik), 54, 55
Natural Treatment Solutions for Hyperthyroidism and Graves' Disease (Osansky), 379
nickel, 73, 96, 109–112, 136
nitazoxanide (Alinia), 297–298, 330, 335
non-celiac gluten sensitivity (NCGS), 95, 135
non-celiac wheat sensitivity (NCWS), 96, 135
norovirus infections, 296, 298–299, 334
NSAIDs, 235, 237, 396, 425, 427
NuLev. *See* hyoscyamine
Numminen, Lari, 58
nutrient depletions. *See* depletions
nystatin, 288, 440

obesity. *See* metabolic disorders
okra extract, 251–252, 411
olive leaf extract, 247, 289, 293, 462
omega-3 fatty acids, 185–188, 241–242, 251, 408–409, 413–414, 420, 481
omega-6 fatty acids, 236, 241
ondansetron (Zofran), 51, 55, 298–299
onions, 105–106
opiate-induced constipation, 49, 53–54, 69, 425
opiate receptor modulation, 49, 53–55. *See also* loperamide
opioids, 425
Optimizing Thyroid Hormones (Wentz), 378
oral hygiene, 285, 292
oregano, oil of, 267–268, 269, 289, 293, 297, 332, 334, 416, 440, 461–462
Osansky, Eric, 377, 379
oxalate, 124–125, 137, 283, 288
ox bile, 159, 161–162, 448, 473
oxytocin, 354

pain tolerance. *See* visceral hypersensitivity
Paleo diet, 381–382
Pamelor. *See* tricyclic antidepressants
pancreatic enzyme deficiency, 156–159, 170, 234
pancreatic enzymes, 63, 479
parasites. *See* protozoal infections; worms
parasympathetic nervous system, 340, 343–344, 349–355, 454–455
paromomycin, 330
partially hydrolyzed guar gum (PHGG), 222, 224, 225
pau d'arco, 289, 293, 462
Pedre, Vincent, 199
pelvic pain, 13, 36–37
Pentatrichomonas hominis, 320, 334
peppermint, 148, 266, 293, 308, 468
pepsin, 153–156
Pepto-Bismol. *See* bismuth subsalicylate
pesticides and herbicides, 207–208. *See also* glyphosate
P5P (vitamin B_6), 179–180, 186, 245, 276–277, 410, 420, 433, 455, 473, 477
PHGG (partially hydrolyzed guar gum), 222, 224, 225
Pimentel, Mark, 29, 59–60, 255
pinworms, 320–322, 325–328, 334–335, 481
plecanatide (Trulance), 53, 55
polyphenol anti-inflammatory jello, 245–246
polyphenols, 242–247, 329
polysorbate 80, 131, 134
pomegranate extract, 247
post-infectious IBS (PI-IBS), 66, 68, 232, 369–370. *See also* gut infections
potassium, 175, 194–196, 352–353, 481
praziquantel, 335
prebiotics, 220–226, 481
pregnancy, 71, 284, 390–391

Index

probiotics
  best practices for, 215–218
  conventional medicine recommendation, 49
  deficiency, 64, 96, 481
  food sources, 226–227
  genetic connections, 214
  indications (gut motility), 280–281, 455, 474, 478
  indications (infections), 297, 299, 300–302, 307, 309, 330, 334
  indications (intestinal overgrowth), 280–281, 290, 292–293
  indications (intestinal permeability), 248
  indications (overview), 211–219, 227–229, 469–470
  indications (toxin triggers), 439
  precautions, 227, 264
  role of, 203–204
  support for, 462
  types of, 211–217
prokinetics, 66, 274–277, 279, 282
propionate, 205, 241
proteases, 292, 397
protein, 135, 175, 480
proteolytic enzymes (systemic enzymes), 104, 292, 293, 330, 417
protozoal infections
  causes, 66–67, 68, 343, 360, 369–370, 372–373
  celiac disease and, 94–95
  effects, 394
  full moon and, 325
  overview, 295–296, 312–314, 337–338
  pathogenic organisms, 314–322, 326–328
  relapse prevention, 336–337
  risk factors, 323
  symptoms and signs, 117, 208, 234, 236, 271, 284, 323–325, 481
  testing, 325–326
  treatment, 328–335, 458–459
Pseudomonas aeruginosa, 201

psychological distress. *See* anxiety; depression
psyllium husk (Metamucil, Citrucel, FiberCon), 46, 48, 224, 225, 401, 412–413, 420, 478
purple coneflower, 308
Pyrantel, 327–328, 335

quercetin, 246–247, 252

resistant starch, 219, 222–223, 417
"rest and digest," 340, 343–344, 349–355, 454–455
resveratrol, 246, 413
rhubarb, 150, 151
rifaximin (Xifaxan), 50, 55, 60, 267
Rogers, Everett, 40–41
Rome IV Criteria, 27, 29, 33
root cause approach
  conventional approach comparison, 60 (*See also* conventional medicine)
  detective work guidelines, 75–77
  dietary triggers, 62–63 (*See also* dietary triggers)
  digestive enzyme deficiencies, 63–64 (*See also* digestion and digestive enzymes)
  discovering root causes, 59–62
  gut motility, 65–66 (*See also* dysbiosis; gut motility)
  IBD, 68–69 (*See also* inflammatory bowel disease)
  infections, 66–67 (*See also* gut infections)
  intestinal overgrowth, 65 (*See also* small intestine bacterial overgrowth; small intestine yeast overgrowth)
  leaky gut, 65 (*See also* intestinal permeability)
  nutrient depletions, 64 (*See also* depletions)
  overview, 13–17, 57–59, 70, 79

stress hormone alteration, 67 (*See also* stress and stress hormone imbalances)
supplement quality, 77–79
testing (overview), 74–75
thyroid issues, 67 (*See also* thyroid imbalances and autoimmunity)
toxic and chemical triggers, 69 (*See also* toxins and chemical triggers)
Western lifestyle factors, 69, 72–73
women-specific issues, 70–73
rotavirus, 296–299, 334, 461, 462

Saccharomyces boulardii-based probiotics
  indications (infections), 297, 299, 300–302, 307, 309, 330, 334
  indications (intestinal overgrowth), 228, 229, 264, 290, 292–293, 455
  indications (mold), 439
  indications (overview), 462, 469–470, 478
  overview, 214–215, 217–218
salads, 72, 73, 91
salicylate intolerance, 125–127, 137
Salmonella, 300, 397
SCD (Specific Carbohydrate Diet), 265, 381, 404–405, 420
SCFAs (short-chain fatty acids), 144, 185, 193, 202–205, 241. *See also* butyrate
scopolamine (Buscopan), 55
Seacure, 251, 413–414
secretagogues, 52–53, 54–55
seed cycling, 432
selective serotonin reuptake inhibitors. *See* SSRIs
selenium, 111, 136, 174, 382–384, 438
semi-elemental diet, 403, 404, 418
semi-vegetarian diet, 406–407, 420
serotonin
  genetic connections, 62
  gut-brain communication, 36
  medications targeting receptors, 49, 50–51, 54–55, 276, 350, 410
(*See also* antidepressants; opiate receptor modulation)
  production of, 36, 64, 144, 203, 236, 276–277, 325, 410
sertraline. *See* SSRIs
serum-based immunoglobulin, 409
serum-derived bovine immunoglobulin (SBI), 250, 297
sex hormone fluctuations, 71–72, 73, 236, 284
Shabo, Yosef, 102
sh*t kit, 4, 21, 47, 480
Shiga toxin-producing *E. coli*, 300
Shigella, 300
short-chain fatty acids (SCFAs), 204–205, 232, 241. *See also* butyrate
SIBO. *See* small intestine bacterial overgrowth
simethicone (GasX), 48, 469
SIYO. *See* small intestine yeast overgrowth
sleep, 345, 353
slippery elm, 129, 148, 251–252, 411, 466
slowed gut motility. *See* hypomotility
small intestine bacterial overgrowth (SIBO)
  action checklist, 282–283
  causes, 65, 97, 120, 121, 208, 220–221, 295–296, 313
  conventional approach, 43, 45, 50
  diagnosis and tests, 257, 263–264
  IBD trigger, 394
  overview, 255–256, 293–294
  post-treatment motility support, 272–281
  precautions, 212, 219, 220–221, 225, 227
  recurrence prevention, 270–271
  risk factors, 257–258, 262–263, 270–271
  symptoms and signs, 117, 234, 237, 256, 258–262, 360, 372, 481
  treatment, 264–270, 458–459
  types of, 259–262

small intestine fungal overgrowth (SIFO), 283–284. *See also* Candida overgrowth
small intestine yeast overgrowth (SIYO), 283–293. *See also* Candida overgrowth
snacking, 271
SNAS (systemic nickel allergy syndrome), 110
soft and mushy diet, 403, 418, 420
soluble fiber supplements (psyllium husk), 46, 48, 224, 401, 412–413, 478
somatic experiencing, 355
somatization disorder, 36
sorbitol, 133
soy-free diet, 381, 454
soy intolerance, 106–109, 136
soy lecithin, 134
Specific Carbohydrate Diet (SCD), 165–166, 265, 284, 381, 404–405, 420
spore-based probiotics, 215, 217–218, 264, 293, 455
SSRIs (sertraline, fluoxetine, citalopram)
    indications, 49, 50–51, 55, 350, 410
    mechanism of action, 49, 50–51, 276, 350, 410
    side effects, 410
Standard American Diet nutrient depletions, 175
Staphylococcus, 260, 261, 269, 300
Steinbock, Debbie, 266, 269, 389, 403, 415
Steinbock, Roy, 266, 389
steroids, 222, 235, 237, 284, 285, 399
stomach acid. *See* low stomach acid
stomach cancer, 304, 305
"stomach flu" (norovirus), 296, 298–299, 334
stool softeners, 47, 222, 472
Streptococcus, 228, 259–261, 264, 269
stress and stress hormone imbalances, 339–358
    conventional approach, 43
    effects, 208, 235, 237, 305, 341–344, 428–429, 430
    overview, 67, 339–341, 357–358
    stress, defined, 345–346
    symptoms and signs, 292, 339–341, 342–343, 346–348, 468, 481
    testing, 348–349
    treatment, 292, 349–357, 469
sucrase, 118, 119, 166
sucrose intolerance, 118–119, 136, 165–166, 170–171, 480
sugar alcohols, 120, 130–133, 416–417. *See also specific sugar alcohols*
sulfur, 105–106, 405
sulfur SIBO (hydrogen sulfide SIBO), 262, 263–264, 268, 269–270
sunlight exposure, 184, 353
supplement quality, 77–79. *See also specific supplements*
sweet wormwood, 335, 414, 419
sympathetic nervous system, 340, 343–346, 454–455
systemic enzymes (proteolytic enzymes), 104, 292, 293, 330, 417
systemic nickel allergy syndrome (SNAS), 110

taurine, 160, 162, 448, 473
tauroursodeoxycholic acid (TUDCA), 162
TCAs. *See* tricyclic antidepressants
teeth grinding, 324–325
temporomandibular joint syndrome (TMJ), 36
tenapanor, 53, 55
tetracycline, 330
thiamine (vitamin B$_1$), 156, 186, 188–190, 278, 330, 413, 473, 479, 481
thickeners, 133–134
thyme, 308
thyroid imbalances and autoimmunity, 359–386. *See also* Hashimoto thyroiditis
    causes, 67, 305, 315–317, 370–374
    differential diagnosis, 67

effects, 208–209
function of thyroid, 362–363
IBS connection, 360–361
overview, 359, 385–386
symptoms and signs, 363–364, 481
testing, 364–370
treatment, 374–385
tinidazole, 330
titanium dioxide, 131, 133, 417
TMJ (temporomandibular joint syndrome), 36
toxins and chemical triggers, 423–449
airborne toxins, 442
effects, 235, 237, 284
estrogen dominance, 428–434, 435, 481
glyphosate, 97, 207–208, 235, 284, 444–446, 481
in homes, 441–442
implant illnesses, 443, 481
medications targeting receptors, 424–428, 481
mycotoxins, 434–441 (*See also* mold)
overview, 69, 423–424, 449
symptoms and signs, 424, 481
treatment, 438, 445, 446–448
women-specific issues, 73
trauma, 237, 345, 355
traveler's diarrhea, 48
Trichomonas, 330
tricyclic antidepressants (amitriptyline, desipramine), 49, 50, 55, 276, 350, 425
trimethoprim-sulfamethoxazole, 330
Trulance. *See* plecanatide
tryptophan, 236
TUDCA (tauroursodeoxycholic acid), 162
turmeric. *See* curcumin
Tusek, David, 388

ulcerative colitis, 391. *See also* inflammatory bowel disease
ulcers, 311. *See also* Helicobacter pylori infection
undecylenic acid, 290, 293

unsaturated fats, 237
ursodiol, 161
urticaria (hives), 6, 107, 206, 316–317, 372–373

vagus nerve, 65–66, 188, 272, 340–341, 410
vagus nerve stimulation, 279–280
valerian, 151
vegan diet nutrient depletions, 174, 178, 182, 196–197
vegetarian diet nutrient depletions, 174, 178, 182, 196–197
Veillonella, 201, 261
Vibrezi. *See* eluxadoline
Vibrio parahaemolyticus, 300
viral infections
causes, 66
effects, 234, 360
IBD trigger, 394, 395
overview, 295–297, 337
symptoms and signs, 481
treatment, 297–299, 334, 461, 462
visceral hypersensitivity
causes, 65, 223
conventional approach, 42, 50, 53
overview, 231–232
treatment, 42, 50, 53, 65, 212, 350–351
vitamin A, 182–183, 187, 384, 481
vitamin B
for adrenal support, 355–356
B_1, 156, 186, 188–190, 278, 330, 413, 473, 479, 481
B_6, 179–180, 186, 245, 276–277, 410, 420, 433, 455, 473, 477
B_{12}, 176, 196–197
biotin, 291
sources, 384
vitamin C, 111, 192–194, 355–356, 384, 432, 472, 481
vitamin D deficiency, 176, 183–185, 187–188, 411, 420, 481
vitamin E, 111, 187, 384, 433
vitamin K deficiency, 187–188
VSL#3, 415

walking, 146, 468, 470
Warren, Robin, 311
Wellbutrin. *See* bupropion
Western lifestyle factors, 69, 72–73, 175
wheat. *See* gluten sensitivity/intolerance
whey and casein sensitivity, 100–102
whitefish, 251
women-specific issues, 70–73, 284, 390–391
worms, 320–322, 325–328, 330, 334–335, 481
wormwood, 335, 414, 419
Wright, Steven, 389, 394, 411–412

xanthan gum, 133
xenoestrogen exposure, 428, 431
Xifaxan. *See* rifaximin
xylitol, 133, 471
xylose isomerase, 117–118

yeast-based probiotics, 214–215, 217–218, 228, 229. *See also* *Saccharomyces boulardii*-based probiotics
yeast infections, 284, 360, 458–459
yeast overgrowth, 283–293. *See also* *Candida* overgrowth
Yersinia enterocolitica, 300
yoga, 11, 136, 146, 178, 351, 355, 447, 468, 470

zinc
  deficiency, 176–177, 180–182, 186, 234, 248, 432–433, 481
  indications, 111, 252, 309, 477
  sources, 181, 384
Zofran. *See* ondansetron